Larry Bushwick

F5001

JONATHON S. RAKICH, Ph.D.

Associate Professor of Management and Director of Graduate Programs, College of Business Administration, The University of Akron

BEAUFORT B. LONGEST, JR., Ph.D.

Assistant Professor of Health Services Management, Graduate School of Management, Northwestern University

THOMAS R. O'DONOVAN, Ph.D., F.A.C.H.A.

Administrator, Mount Carmel Mercy Hospital and Medical Center

MANAGING HEALTH CARE ORGANIZATIONS

*SAUNDERS SERIES IN
HEALTH CARE ORGANIZATION
AND ADMINISTRATION*

W. B. SAUNDERS COMPANY

PHILADELPHIA • LONDON • TORONTO

W. B. Saunders Company: West Washington Square
Philadelphia, PA 19105

1 St. Anne's Road
Eastbourne, East Sussex BN21 3 UN, England

1 Goldthorne Avenue
Toronto; Ontario, M8Z 5T9, Canada

Library of Congress Cataloging in Publication Data

Rakich, Jonathon S.

Managing health care organizations.

(Saunders series in health care organization and administration)

1. Health facilities—Administration.   I. Longest,
Beaufort, B., Jr., joint author.   II. O'Donovan, Thomas R.,
joint author.   III. Title.   IV. Series.

RA971.R26   658'.91'3621   76–1246

ISBN 0–7216–7451–8

Managing Health Care Organizations   ISBN   0-7216-7451-8

Last digit is the print number: 9   8   7   6   5   4   3

Dedication

To our families, past and present

PREFACE

Health care organizations are among the most complex existing in contemporary society. In the past 20 years the management of these organizations has evolved into an extremely demanding and difficult undertaking. Although their basic missions have remained the same, increased societal demand for more and better health care concurrent with cost containment has placed tremendous pressure on the nation's health care organizations. Other external pressures such as the governmental financing of much of the nation's health care, increasingly organized labor, affirmative action programs, comprehensive planning, and licensure, in addition to health and safety legislation, have collectively placed new burdens of accountability on those who manage health care organizations.

The increasing difficulty of managing these organizations is also evident when one considers the internal structure of modern health care organizations. From our point of view, inputs (in the form of resources) are the basic ingredients that, *properly* transformed through the management process, result in desired output(s). Stated another way, to accomplish organizational objectives, input resources in the form of manpower, material, technology, information, and capital must be planned for, acquired, coordinated, directed, and controlled so that predetermined types and levels of patient care, research, and education can be provided.

In recent years, employees and non-employee members of health care organizations have become increasingly active in seeking larger benefits and more participative influence in organization decision-making. Employee and labor relations now require greater attention than in the past. When this is coupled with the demanding task of coordinating the efforts of an expanding multitude of professional, para-professional, and non-professional employees, the requirement of simply dealing with people alone has added to the complexity and burden of managing these organizations. In addition, increased material requirements and scarcities, technological innovations and requirements, informational needs (both gathering and reporting), and the necessity for the internal allocation of scarce capital resources among competing units of the organization all converge to make the management of health care organizations one of the most demanding tasks in modern society.

***   ***

The basic objective of this book is to provide a framework to help the health care manager function more effectively in today's health care organization. It will provide a frame of reference permitting the manager to cope with the environmental forces that shape the health care delivery system and its organiza-

v

tions, and a set of skills that will enable him to deal more effectively with the internal complexities of the health care organizations.

In writing this book, we have presented management concepts and practices and applied examples to the health care setting. We have specifically taken a *broad process approach* in the presentation of the subject of management rather than one that is narrow and technical in nature. Our intended audience consists of those individuals who presently hold managerial positions in health care organizations and those students who aspire to holding such positions. This book can be used in many settings: at the senior and first year graduate levels in formal health services administration programs, as well as management courses for professionals working in health care organizations. It can also be used in advanced management development seminars and will provide insights for those who have already achieved management level positions in health care organizations.

***   ***

This book follows a structured sequence throughout. Part I begins with a description of the health care system, its scope, and organizations in addition to an examination of the role of management within the system. These serve to establish the *Setting and Framework*. With the development of a *management model* for health care organizations in Chapter 2 from an "Input-Conversion-Output" frame of reference, the reader's attention is turned to the remaining four parts, each of which is linked to that model. They are *Output-Input Determination; Organizational Design and Structure; Organizational Dynamics; and Organizational Control and Change.*

In Part II, *Output-Input Determination*, attention is focused on the decision-making process (Chapter 3), the planning process (Chapter 5), and the formulation of organization objectives and strategies (Chapter 6). Once those objectives (outputs) have been established and decisions on the means to accomplish them made, the prescription of necessary input resources naturally follows.

Because of its link to all of the other management processes, decision-making is presented first. Furthermore, a sequel chapter (4) examining various quantitative decision-making techniques applicable in the health care setting is included. By design, no prior familiarity with quantitative methods, on the part of the reader, is presumed, and this chapter can be omitted without interrupting the flow and basic structure of the book.

In Part III, *Organizational Design and Structure*, the reader becomes acquainted with an overview of classical and contemporary organizational concepts (Chapter 7). Following that, these concepts are applied to and used to characterize health care organizations (Chapter 8) by focusing on the health care delivery system's most prominent and visible organization — the hospital.

Two additional subject areas dealing with the input manpower resource are included in this part, since a substantial portion of organization expenditures concerns employees. From an organizational point of view, these two areas are crucial for promoting efficiency and effectiveness. As a result, manpower acquisition and maintenance (Chapter 9) and labor relations (Chapter 10) are presented.

In *Organizational Dynamics*, Part IV, the activities so important to getting things done through people are examined. Without people, organizations, health care or otherwise, simply would not exist. Because people are different, the interaction among them gives a dynamic aspect to organizations. The specific activities, presented from the manager's point of view, are the motivation of employees (Chapter 11), leadership (Chapter 12), and communication (Chapter 13).

The last part of this book, *Organizational Control and Change*, focuses on three areas. In order to accomplish objectives and ensure appropriate organizational efficiency and effectiveness, activities must be monitored. Through the control process and its techniques this is accomplished (Chapter 14). We then present the subject of change and how it can be facilitated (Chapter 15). Change is a fact of life for those who are involved in managing health care organizations. The external environment imposes it and the internal organization environment generates it. Finally, in the last chapter we conclude with a section concerned with the "Greatest Challenge." Recently there has been a wave of challenges facing those who are part of health care delivery throughout the country, and indeed, the world. As they increase, the need for organizational effectiveness and efficiency becomes even more paramount. Achieving organizational objectives is more likely with sound management behavior. The job can be done. However, it will take teamwork, the coordination of a multiplicity of professionals, sound decision-making, the careful formulation of objectives and strategies, the acquisition of appropriate input resources and their effective utilization, the fine-tuning of organizational dynamics, the control of not only the organization itself but also its output, along with the ability to cope with change. These are the central topics of our text which led to our message — "Managing health care organizations is a complex and difficult endeavor." If this book constructively contributes toward making that task easier, we will have accomplished our objective.

JONATHON S. RAKICH
BEAUFORT B. LONGEST, JR.
THOMAS R. O'DONOVAN

ACKNOWLEDGMENTS

Many people encouraged, reviewed, and supported the writing of this book. We especially thank John C. Neifert, Editor of the Saunders series in Health Care Organization and Administration, for his continuous encouragement, patience, and professionalism, which we have had the opportunity to witness and be a part of. We also thank Elmer Burack, Consulting Editor of the Saunders series in Health Care Organization and Administration and Professor of Management at the Illinois Institute of Technology, whose painstaking reviews of all the drafts of this book greatly improved it; Duncan Neuhauser, Associate Professor of Health Services Administration at Harvard University, for his detailed and most constructive reviews of multiple drafts of this manuscript; Paul Gordon, Professor of Management at Indiana University, for his suggestions which led to the basic structure of this book; Cheedle Millard, Associate Professor of Management at Iowa State University, for his many fine suggestions for improving the book; and James Mitchell, Vice President for Human Resources at Wesley Medical Center, for his assistance in the development of Chapter 9. To each, we give our appreciation. We would also like to thank those individuals who reviewed or commented on portions of this book: Professors Bernard Deitzer, James Inman, Theodore Herbert, Richard Lutz, Gary Meek, Thomas Natiello, and Frank Simonetti.

Our employers, who gave support in numerous ways, also merit our appreciation. They are James W. Dunlap, Dean, College of Business Administration, The University of Akron; Kenneth Black, Dean, College of Business Administration, Georgia State University; Donald P. Jacobs, Dean, Graduate School of Management, Northwestern University; and Sister Mary Leila, R.S.M., Executive Director, Mt. Carmel Mercy Hospital and Medical Center. Without their cooperation and assistance this book would not have been possible.

Special note must be made of those who assisted us in the manuscript preparation during the past three years. In particular, we thank David Hau, David Cox, Susan Lang, Viola Glover, Francine Jordan, Vernell Montgomery, Debora Miller, Irene Astrosky, Mary Malonis, Bea Dagilis, Charlotte Shuff, and Charlene Cook. Those of the W. B. Saunders staff include Lonnie Zienkiewicz, assistant to John Neifert; Patrice Lamb, manuscript editor; and Tom O'Connor and Frank Polizzano of the Production Department, who are responsible for the expeditious production of our book.

Finally, we give our deepest admiration to those we hold dearest — our wives Tana, Carolyn, and Gayle, and our children, Carey, Loren, Brant, Patrick, Lynda, and Julie. The latter have been patient with their fathers. To the former, we recognize that the adage that a wonderful woman stands behind a sometimes not so wonderful and preoccupied man is true in our case. Without our wives' understanding, encouragement, and sacrifices we would not have been able to embark upon or complete this project.

JONATHON S. RAKICH
BEAUFORT B. LONGEST, JR.
THOMAS R. O'DONOVAN

CONTENTS

Part I

THE SETTING AND FRAMEWORK

The two chapters included in Part I establish the setting and framework of this book. Chapter 1, Introduction To Management and the Health Care System, establishes the setting. This chapter also presents our objectives, introduces the reader to the subject of management, and discusses the role of management in health care organizations. In addition, the United States health care system is described by offering a brief orientation of its history, along with its present scope in terms of personnel employed, expenditures, and range of institutions.

Chapter 2, A Management Model for Health Care Organizations, establishes the framework. In this chapter, management is fully defined and described. Furthermore, a model is presented that will serve as the basic framework of this text. Each succeeding part will be devoted to a discussion of its components.

This Chapter Contains:

- Introduction
    - Focus of the Book
    - Objectives

- The Subject of Management
    - Introductory Definition
    - The Role of Management
    - Causes of the Management Revolution

- The Health Care System
    - History of the United States Health Care System
    - Scope of the United States Health Care System (personnel, expenditures, organizations)

- Summary

- Discussion Questions

Chapter 1

INTRODUCTION TO MANAGEMENT AND THE HEALTH CARE SYSTEM

There is ... "a general managerial revolution in the operation of health institutions, a new recognition of the crucial role of efficient management."

(Herman Somers) [1]

INTRODUCTION

A number of significant questions can be inferred from Herman Somers' statement. First, why is a managerial revolution occurring in health care institutions? Second, what is the role of management, and why is it crucial? Third, how does management affect the efficiency and effectiveness of health care organizations? This chapter addresses these questions, introduces the subject of management, and briefly describes the United States health care system. Included is a presentation of (1) the focus and (2) objectives of this book. In addition, this chapter (3) provides an introductory definition of management, (4) discusses the role of management, and (5) addresses the question, "What has caused the management revolution in health care organizations?" Finally, (6) a history and (7) the scope of the United States health care system are described.

FOCUS

This book focuses on managing health care organizations. The subject of management is presented in a way that demonstrates its general applicability to all types of health care organizations, yet offers illustrations pertinent to specific institutions, such as hospitals, ambulatory care facilities, long-term care facilities, clinics, and health departments, among others.

The text has a process orientation providing an *overview* of management, in contrast to a presentation that is detailed and *microscopic*. To make the distinction, a process orientation consists of examining the series of functions, activities, and events that occur to accomplish something, as well as their interrelationship with each other, all within the context of a broad setting. By

---

[1] Herman Somers, "Health services at the crossroads: issues of public policy." *Hospital Progress, 51*:81, October, 1970.

nature the view must be general—encompassing in scope, presenting managerial concepts and techniques applicable at multiple levels of administration and in multiple types of health care organizations.

A detailed microscopic orientation, on the other hand, typically focuses on specifics in a tunneled fashion, without linkage to a broader and, in our opinion, more important foundation. As a rule we will not be concerned with such subjects as the design of a medical record form, the structure and detail of housekeeping services, or the principles of food preparation in the Dietary Department. We will be concerned with some specifics, but only to accomplish our primary purpose, that is, a general presentation of the subject of management as it relates to health care organizations.

OBJECTIVES OF THE BOOK

We address ourselves to two main groups of readers. The first group includes those students interested in health services administration who are being formally exposed to the subject of management for the first time. The second group includes those currently employed by health care organizations who wish to supplement their experiences. A review of the forthcoming material will not make the student an expert, since he lacks an important ingredient—experience. Nor will a review necessarily make those experienced individuals "management experts." However, we hope that both will definitely benefit from this book.

At the minimum, one of our objectives is to present our terminology so that health care organization managers can communicate more effectively with each other. In addition, we offer concepts that may be new to the reader and therefore worthy of constructive consideration. If they are not entirely new but intuitive, we hope to accomplish the objective of reinforcement.

Furthermore, we will attempt to convey a message—namely, that the management of health care organizations is a complex, difficult endeavor; that managers are not born but develop over time, with experience; and that management and those managing must react, change, and adapt themselves and their techniques to suit the specific situation—the time, place, and particular organization in which they find themselves.

Finally, we have as another objective that of helping, perhaps in a small way, health care organizations become more efficient.[2] The term "efficiency" carries many connotations. It is generally used as a synonym for costs; that is, "Is what you are doing more costly than it should be?" If so, it is therefore inefficient. Effectiveness, on the other hand, requires a positive answer to "Are you doing what you do well? Are institutional goals being achieved?" If so, it is therefore effective. We argue that effective management (done well) contributes to organization efficiency (no more costly than it should be).

---

[2]A number of Congressional and Executive Branch studies on health care efficiency have been conducted. Among them see: *Report to the Congress: Study of Health Care Facility Construction Costs,* Comptroller General of the United States, GPO, 1973:725–695/04; and *The High Cost of Hospitalization,* Hearings before the Subcommittee on Antitrust and Monopoly of the Senate Judiciary Committee, GPO, 1971:52–2520.

As we approach the 1980's, the emphasis on cost in health care delivery in the United States has never been greater. This text is intended to provide a vehicle by which present and future managers can become more effective within the health care delivery system and its complex organizations, thereby contributing to organization efficiency.

THE SUBJECT OF MANAGEMENT

Management is not a recent phenomenon. It has been practiced since human beings began organized group activities. The legions of the Roman Empire utilized management concepts dealing with organization structure; specifically, they established line and staff relationships in their military organization. The Catholic Church established a scalar chain of command from priest to Pope; the Egyptians implemented the division-of-labor concept in the construction of the pyramids, and its refinement led to the mass-production systems of this century.

Although management has long been practiced in other fields, the past 100 years have witnessed its ever-increasing application to health care delivery. During this period the delivery of health care has evolved from the direct patient-physician relationship to the patient-physician-health care organization arrangement, which has resulted in the specialization of services, economies of scale, and the ability to care for more people while ensuring higher levels in the quality of care provided. Specifically, the number of hospitals in the United States has grown from several hundred in the 1880's to over 7000 today, and the number of long-term care facilities grew significantly after the enactment of Medicare-Medicaid in 1965, numbering over 30,000 today. Group health insurance organizations began during the 1930's, and in the last 50 years the federal government has assumed a major role in the delivery and financing of health care.

With advances in medical science, specialization of labor has occurred, as exemplified by the rise of the nursing profession from Florence Nightingale's initial efforts in the 1860's to the founding of the first three schools of nursing in the United States in the next decade. Further, the physician board specialization phenomena gathered momentum in the 1930's, and it is now a part of our health care system. Formal organized efforts to set minimum organizational, clinical, equipment, and quality of care standards for care provided in hospitals began initially in 1918 with the "approving" of hospitals by the American College of Surgeons, and this is now implemented by the Joint Commission on Accreditation of Hospitals. Relative to health administration education, graduate degree programs have become commonplace since the first program was begun at the University of Chicago in the early 1930's.

INTRODUCTORY DEFINITION

As a cohesive body of knowledge, management has been developing for centuries. In order to determine what the role of management is and why it is crucial, it is first necessary to answer the question, "What is management?" Simply stated, *management is the set of interactive processes through which the utilization of resources results in the accomplishment of organizational objectives*. It is the catalyst by which organization activity occurs and objectives are fulfilled. It is a complex endeavor practiced in all organizations, and it encompasses various processes, activities, and techniques. When you "practice management" you are getting things done *through people*!

Admittedly, the definition of management provided here is rather general. Our purpose for its inclusion at this point is only to give a brief orientation of the subject to the reader. When coupled with a description of the United States health care system, the *setting* of this book will have been established. In the next chapter we will fully develop a definition of management, describe its characteristics and present the management model that will be used throughout this book.

THE ROLE OF MANAGEMENT

We may now ask the question, "What is the role of management and why is it crucial?" By answering that question we will simultaneously come to realize how effective management affects the efficiency of health care organizations. Management serves the role of a conversion mechanism. It is through management that the objectives of the health care organization are determined. It is the means by which requisite resources are gathered and positioned. It is the means by which things get done.

The role of management is crucial for several simple but important reasons. Without it there would be a lack of purposeful direction, manifested by haphazard activities with no central focus, resulting in inefficiency in terms of the nonoptimal (inappropriate) utilization of resources. Management is a catalytic endeavor, which ensures that the right things occur, when they should and how they should.

Management excellence will contribute greatly toward making any health care organization both effective and efficient. It will contribute to effectiveness by ensuring that the organization is doing what it should be doing. Through management, monitoring means (controls) are instituted in order to make certain that the sum total of organized activity is constantly being carried out as planned, rather than in a random manner. Through effective management, organization resources are acquired, mixed, allocated, used, and coordinated in the most appropriate manner so as to minimize waste. With the establishment of sound objectives and controls and the appropriate utilization of resources, health care organizations can become efficient in what they do, and costs will be minimized relative to the objectives to be achieved.

CAUSES OF THE MANAGEMENT REVOLUTION

"Why are we witnessing a management revolution?" One might answer, on first glance, "costs." However, there is another facet that should be included—"expectations." Since the enactment of the 1965 amendments to the Social Security Act, which created the Medicare-Medicaid programs, the United States health care system has undergone substantial changes. These changes have all, in some degree, contributed to the costs and the expectations of health care. Among these changes are (1) structural changes in the health care delivery system, (2) an increased role of federal assistance programs, and (3) broader third-party health insurance coverage among the population. The latter two, along with an increasing population and a change in consumer expectations (where health care is perceived as a right rather than a privilege), have caused increased demand pressures to be placed upon health care providers. In addition, (4) higher resource costs, particularly for personnel, and (5) advances in technology, which translate into more equipment and the skilled personnel to man that equipment, have contributed to the trend of rising health care costs.[3]

The public's outcry against rising costs has caused the legislative and executive branches of government to direct their attention to the issue. Senator Abraham Ribicoff, former Secretary of the Department of Health, Education, and Welfare, and Senator Edward Kennedy, Chairman of the Senate Subcommittee on Health Care, have been very critical of the current fee-for-service health care delivery system.[4] They, among others, feel that the crisis in the delivery of health care is real, and they are giving attention to the public's dissatisfaction. The basic impact has been the demand for greater accountability by government, consumers, and the community of those who manage health care organizations, along with the exertion of pressure for increased efficiency—that is, quality care at less cost. Since there is no reason to expect that the pressure for accountability and efficiency will decrease, those who manage health care organizations will continue to be held accountable for their organization's performance. As a result, the enormous pressures for managerial excellence in health care administration will continue.

Whether or not one accepts the charge that health care organizations are inefficient, and the resulting implication that those who manage them are at fault (not effective), is not really the important issue. Granted, although managers may have little control over the demand for services, rising resource costs, and technology requirements, they still must function within these constraints. Effective management can play a crucial role in mitigating some of these pressures that have caused renewed attention to be given to management and its role in health care organizations.

THE HEALTH CARE SYSTEM

Up to this point, we have briefly presented the subject of management and its role in health care organizations. In order to complete the setting, the health

---

[3]For an interesting analysis of the increase in hospital costs see: Ronald Anderson and J. Joel May, "Factors associated with the increasing cost of hospital care." *The Annals of the American Academy of Political and Social Science*, 399:62, January, 1972.

[4]For a critical review of the United States health care system see the following: Abraham Ribicoff, *The American Medical Machine*. New York: Harrow Books, Harper and Row, Publishers, 1972. Edward M. Kennedy, *In Critical Condition: The Crisis in America's Health Care*. New York: Simon and Schuster, 1972. Richard Kunnes, *Your Money or Your Life*. New York: Dodd, Mead, and Company, 1971. Alex Gerber, *The Gerber Report: The Shocking State of American Medical Care and What Must Be Done About It*. New York: David McKay Company, 1971. Claire Townsend, *Old Age: The Last Segregation*. New York: Grossman Publishers, 1971. For a positive presentation of the United States health care system see: Harry Schwartz, *The Case for American Medicine*. New York: David McKay Company, 1972.

care system will be described in the remaining two sections of this chapter. We will first direct our attention to a history of the United States health care system and then to its scope.

HISTORY OF THE UNITED STATES HEALTH CARE SYSTEM

In its earlier form, health care delivery was closely associated with the magic and superstition born of ignorance, and medicine was practiced on a one-to-one, healer-patient relationship. Early Greek culture firmly established the delivery of health services as a humanistic responsibility of civilized man, and the medical ethics established by the Greeks still guide the medical profession. Hippocrates developed the oath that still serves as the cornerstone of medical ethics:

> I swear by Apollo the physician, by Aesculapius, Hygeia, and Panacea, and I take to witness all the gods, all the goddesses, to keep according to my ability and my judgment the following Oath:
> To consider dear to me as my parents him who taught me this art; to live in common with him and if necessary to share my goods with him; to look upon his children as my own brothers, to teach them this art if they so desire without fee or written promise; to impart to my sons and the sons of the master who taught me and the disciples who have enrolled themselves and have agreed to the rules of the profession, but to these alone, the precepts and the instructions. I will prescribe regimen for the good of my patients according to my ability and my judgment and never do harm to anyone. To please no one will I prescribe a deadly drug, nor give advice which may cause his death. Nor will I give a woman a pessary to procure abortion. But I will preserve the purity of my life and my art. I will not cut for stone, even for patients in whom the disease is manifest; I will leave this operation to be performed by practitioners (specialists in this art). In every house where I come I will enter only for the good of my patients, keeping myself far from all intentional ill-doing and all seduction, and especially from the pleasures of love with women or with men, be they free or slaves. All that may come to my knowledge in the exercise of my profession or outside of my profession or in daily commerce with men, which ought not to be spread abroad, I will keep secret and will never reveal. If I keep this oath faithfully, may I enjoy my life and practice my art, respected by all men and in all times; but if I swerve from it or violate it, may the reverse be my lot.

The Romans organized the delivery of health care for their armies in much the same way as contemporary public health systems, but their system died with their empire. The Middle Ages saw a renewed interest, mainly on the part of organized religion, in the establishment of places for the care of the poor who were sick. This interest was short-lived, however, because the seventeenth century brought a reversal of the progress that had been made to that date. As described by Hepner and Hepner:

> During the seventeenth century there was a decline in the quality of hospitals; by the eighteenth century, hospital facilities were abysmal and medical practices deplorable. Infection was widespread throughout the institutions; patients were crowded into large rooms and more than one patient often occupied a single bed. Hospitals were considered pesthouses for the poor and places to die. The wealthy did not use hospitals but were treated in their homes.[5]

---

[5]James O. Hepner and Donna M. Hepner, *The Health Strategy Game: A Challenge for Reorganization and Management.* St. Louis: The C. V. Mosby Company, 1973, p. 9.

Modern medicine and health care delivery really began with the scientific discoveries of the late nineteenth century. Among the major discoveries were anesthesia, the germ theory of disease, and the uses of the x-ray, to name a few. Although formal American medical education began in Philadelphia in 1765 with the establishment, by John Morgan, of the first medical school, it was not until after the Flexner report was issued in 1910 that medical education's much needed quality reforms occurred. Thus, in two hundred years, health care in the United States has evolved from its rudimentary infancy to the most complex and most expensive system in the world, particularly within the last seventy years. The evolution has not been smooth, nor is it complete. Anne Somers describes the current state of the system eloquently when she says:

> The proverbial visitor from another planet would surely be baffled by the violently contradictory reports on medical care in the United States that characterize both public and private discussion. So, too, are many Americans — both providers and consumers of medical care.
>
> On the one hand, attention is called to continual evidence of astounding progress: the discovery and application of cures, drugs, diagnostic and surgical techniques that can only be described as "miracles." Imaginative new health care delivery programs, representing billions of dollars, have been inaugurated under both public and private auspices. Some 20 million elderly persons now have protection against at least the most expensive medical care. Several million additional indigent and medically indigent are receiving noncharity medical care for the first time in their lives. Twenty new medical schools have been started in the past decade, as have many additional schools for other health professions. Quality controls and drug testing are more rigorous than ever before.
>
> On the other hand, there are constant allegations of inadequate medical care, unfilled health needs, exorbitant rises in costs, galloping inflation, and apparently widespread discontent with most medical institutions. Every national administration since 1961 has emphasized the "crisis in health care," and prescriptions for dealing with it have become national political issues.[6]

SCOPE OF THE UNITED STATES HEALTH CARE SYSTEM

Personnel.   The American health care system is enormous when one considers the resources used and the people involved. The demand for services is vast. The number of visits to physicians averages approximately 4.6 per person each year — more than 1 billion visits annually. More than 36 million people are admitted to the nation's 7200 hospitals, and another 250 million are treated in hospitals as out-patients. Approximately 990,000 people reside in the 23,000 long-term care and related facilities. At least 1 billion drug prescriptions are filled annually, while a tremendous amount of drugs are purchased over the counter.

Total manpower in the health care system includes approximately 4.5 million people — this represents some 5 per cent of the nation's work force, making health care the third largest industry in terms of employment. Using rounded numbers, there are 375,000 physicians; 110,000 dentists; 950,000 registered nurses; 450,000 practical nurses; 900,000 nursing aides, orderlies, and attendants; and 140,000 pharmacists. About 240,000 other personnel are employed as engineers, scientists, sanitarians, technicians, and aides; the rest are engaged in supportive positions.

---

[6]Anne R. Somers, *Health Care in Transition: Directions for the Future.* Chicago: Hospital Research and Educational Trust, 1971, p. 3.

Expenditures.   Expenditures for health care in the United States are approximately $120 billion annually ($547.00 on a per capita basis), representing roughly 8.3 per cent of the nation's Gross National Product (GNP). In comparison, Great Britain's National Health Service, with its 2700 hospitals, has public health care expenditures in the range of $7 billion, which represents approximately 5 per cent of Britain's GNP and $120.00 on a per capita basis.[7] Canada, with its nearly 1400 hospitals, has health care expenditures in the range of $8.5 billion per year, which represents approximately 7 per cent of its GNP and $375.00 on a per capita basis.[8]

As is evident, health care expenditures in the United States exceed, on both an absolute and a relative (per capita and per cent of GNP) basis, those of Great Britain and Canada. Furthermore, there has been a substantial rise in spending for health care in recent years in the United States, which is attributed to many factors: technical progress and "catch-up" wages, lack of incentives for efficiency, the enormous demand for health services generated by Medicare-Medicaid, and the growth of private health insurance. Figure 1–1 illustrates this growth in health care expenditures in dollars and as a per cent of the GNP since 1950. The implications are obvious; health care expenditures are fast approaching $130 billion per year and are expected to reach $200

---

[7]*Annual Abstract of Statistics, 1974.* No. 111, Central Statistics Office. London: Her Majesty's Stationery Office, 1974, pp. 7, 51, 71, 302.

[8]*National Health Expenditures in Canada, 1906–1973.* Health Programs Branch, Health Economics and Statistics Division. Ottawa, Canada: Ministry of National Health and Welfare, April 1975, pp. 1–2. *Canadian Hospitals, 1975 Statistics.* Health Division. Ottawa, Canada: Authority of the Ministry of Industry, Trade and Commerce, 1975, p. 10.

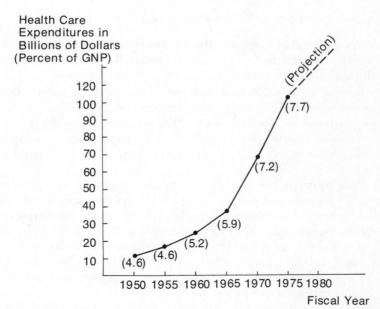

Figure 1–1   United States health care expenditures in billions of dollars and as a percentage of Gross National Product. (Source: National health care expenditures, 1929–1974. *Social Security Bulletin,* 38, February, 1975.)

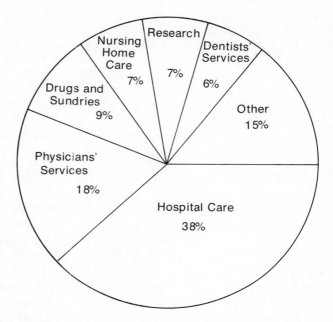

Figure 1–2 Percentage of United States health care expenditures by major classification. (Source: National health care expenditures, 1929–1974. *Social Security Bulletin*, 38, February, 1975.)

billion annually by 1980.[9] In terms of the breakdown of health care dollars, Figure 1–2 presents the percentage of expenditures by major classification, such as hospital and physicians' services.

Organizations.   A large array of organizations makes up the complex set of services and resources needed to deliver health care (Table 1–1). The most important of these organizations are the more than 7200 hospitals in the United States. The American Hospital Association defines the hospital in the following words:

> An establishment that provides—through an organized medical or professional staff, permanent facilities that include inpatient beds, medical services, and continuous nursing services—diagnosis and treatment for patients.[10]

Hospitals may be characterized by their pattern of ownership, such as government (federal, state, local); voluntary (church, community, etc.); or proprietary (individual owner, partnership, investor-owned). They can also be characterized by the type of patients treated, such as general medical-surgical hospitals, geriatric, orthopedic, pediatric, or psychiatric hospitals, to mention a few.

Because of its central importance in the health care system, the hospital will receive extensive treatment in this book. However, the other types of health care organizations outlined in Table 1–1 are also important and have substantial managerial requirements. They also will be treated in this book.

Recognition of the need for management in all types of health care organizations sets this book apart from others on management that deal in a more limited way with only one type or those that focus solely on industrial organiza-

---

[9] Abraham Ribicoff, *The American Medical Machine*. New York: Harrow Books, Harper and Row, Publishers, 1972, p. 71.

[10] Adapted with permission from *Classification of Health Care Institutions, 1974*. Chicago: American Hospital Association, 1974.

Table 1-1   Classification of Health Care Organizations

I. **MEDICAL CARE INSTITUTIONS**
   A. *Inpatient Care Institutions*
       1. *Hospitals*
           a. General
           b. Special
       2. *Nursing Care Institutions*
           a. General
           b. Special
   B. *Ambulatory Care Institutions*
       1. *General*
       2. *Special*
       3. *Day-care Institutions*
           a. General
           b. Special
   C. *Home Health Institutions*
       1. *General*
       2. *Special*
II. **HEALTH-RELATED CARE INSTITUTIONS**
   A. *Intermediate Care Institutions*
   B. *Resident Care Institutions*
   C. *Halfway Houses*

tions. For instance, there are more than 23,000 nursing care facilities in the United States, which can be described as follows:

> An establishment that provides—through an organized medical staff, a medical director or a medical adviser, permanent facilities that include inpatient beds, medical services, continuous nursing services, and health-related services—diagnosis and treatment for patients who are not in an acute phase of illness but who primarily require skilled nursing care on an inpatient basis.[11]

These facilities are similar to hospitals in many ways, as we shall see when they are described in detail in Chapter 8. In addition to in-patient health care organizations, there are out-patient (or ambulatory) organizations. These may be defined as follows:

> An establishment that provides—through an organized medical or professional staff, permanent facilities that do not include inpatient beds, medical services, and health-related services—diagnostic and/or treatment services for patients who usually are ambulatory. The institution may offer a variety of services or a single service.[12]

The patients' homes are often overlooked when thinking about health care delivery, but they compose one of the most heavily-used sites of care. There are formal home health care organizations, defined as:

> Establishments that provide—through permanent facilities, medical services, nursing services, and other health-related services—treatment for individuals at their places of residence.[13]

These must also be considered in the range of health care organizations.

---

[11]*Ibid.*, p. 4.
[12]*Ibid.*, p. 4.
[13]*Ibid.*, p. 5.

Other facilities include laboratories, group-practice clinics, mental health centers, public health agencies, rehabilitation centers, and the like. The full range also includes approximately 140,000 physicians' offices, nearly 85,000 dentists' offices, some 52,000 drug stores, and numerous industrial health departments.

It is clear from this delineation of health care organizations that there is a large array of different organizations involved in the complex health delivery system. They are bound together by two important considerations: (1) the purpose of providing health and/or supportive services, and (2) their need to be more effectively and efficiently managed. This book addresses the latter consideration.

HEALTH MAINTENANCE ORGANIZATIONS (HMO'S)

There are many alternatives to the present organizational patterns for health care delivery. While the possibilities of experimentation are limitless, we will discuss one very important experiment here.

Few subjects have aroused more interest, or generated more discussion in the health care community in the past few years, than the concept of health maintenance organizations or, as they are more commonly known, "HMO's." The term, unfortunately, means different things to different people, and to add to the confusion, some use other terms — "health care corporations" and "comprehensive health service organizations," for example — to mean essentially the same thing.

A number of HMO-type operations have been in existence for many years. The Kaiser-Permanente Plan in California and the Health Insurance Plan of New York are well-known examples. In essence, the major characteristics of an HMO are the grouping of facilities, physicians, and other health personnel into a single organizational entity that provides a full range of medical services to a specifically enrolled population for a fixed fee. The advantages of this organizational arrangement of the delivery of health care, as opposed to the traditional fee-for-service delivery, is that the incentive exists for practicing preventative rather than acute medical care.

It is not clear whether the HMO organizational arrangement of health care delivery will be a more viable alternative to the traditional delivery of care through the patient-physician-health care organization fee-for-service system. However, the federal government has proposed an ambitious program of grants, contracts, loans, and loan guarantees to assist in the planning, initial development, and support of new HMO's, has initiated legislation to provide for an HMO option in public and private health insurance plans, and is attempting to remove or reduce various legal barriers that presently exist to the formation of HMO's.[14] The results in the years ahead will have a significant impact on the health care organizations of the future.[15]

---

[14] Michael Lesparre, "Representative John Heintz speaks out for HMO's." *Hospitals, 49*:55, December 16, 1975.

[15] For the reader who wishes to explore the HMO concept further, the Medical Group Management Association has compiled an excellent bibliography entitled *Comprehensive Bibliography on Health Maintenance Organizations: 1970–1973.* Denver: Medical Group Management Association, 1974.

SUMMARY

In this chapter the basic setting has been established in terms of the subject of management and the health care system. We have identified the focus and objectives of this book. A brief discussion of the role of management was presented, along with recent pressures that have heightened its importance in health care organizations. Furthermore, the history of health care delivery, from the age of magic and superstition to the most complex organizations in modern society, has been briefly traced. The variety of health care organizations in modern society has been described, along with the enormous scope of resources directed at delivering health services.

We have also seen that the health system in the United States consists of a great variety of organizations, ranging from the individual physician's office to the most complex hospital. Each of these organizations shares with the others (to a greater or lesser degree) the need for better management, which will make them more effective and more efficient. In the next chapter the subject of management will be fully developed, and its attributes will be described. Finally, a management model will be presented, which will serve as the foundation and framework for the remainder of this book.

DISCUSSION QUESTIONS

1. Why has attention recently been directed toward the management of health care organizations?

2. What is management's role in health care organizations? What results can be anticipated from managerial excellence?

3. Describe the trend in health care expenditures and its resulting implication for our society?

4. List the various types of health care organizations.

5. What are the characteristics of an HMO, and how does it differ from the traditional health care organization?

6. Read and discuss the following fable:

GOURMAND AND FOOD—A FABLE*

The people of Gourmand loved good food. They ate in good restaurants, donated money for cooking research, and instructed their government to safeguard all matters having to do with food. Long ago, the food industry had been in total chaos. There were many restaurants, some very small. Anyone could call himself a chef or open a restaurant. In choosing a restaurant, one could never be sure that the meal would be good. A commission of distinguished chefs studied the situation and recommended that no one be allowed to touch food except for qualified chefs. "Food is too important to be left to amateurs," they said. Qualified

---

*By Judith R. Lave and Lester B. Lave. (Reprinted with permission from "Health Care: Part I" appearing in *Law and Contemporary Problems*, Vol. 35, No. 2, Spring, 1970. Published by the Duke University School of Law, Durham, North Carolina. Copyright © 1970, 1971 by Duke University.)

chefs were licensed by the state with severe penalties for anyone else who engaged in cooking. Certain exceptions were made for food preparation in the home, but a person could serve only his own family. Furthermore, to become a qualified chef, a man had to complete at least twenty-one years of training (including four years of college, four years of cooking school, and one year of apprenticeship). All cooking schools had to be first class.

These reforms did succeed in raising the quality of cooking. But a restaurant meal became substantially more expensive. A second commission observed that not everyone could afford to eat out. "No one," they said, "should be denied a good meal because of his income." Furthermore, they argued that chefs should work toward the goal of giving everyone "complete physical and psychological satisfaction." For those people who could not afford to eat out, the government declared that they should be allowed to do so as often as they liked and the government would pay. For others, it was recommended that they organize themselves in groups and pay part of their income into a pool that would undertake to pay the costs incurred by members in dining out. To insure the greatest satisfaction, the groups were set up so that a member could eat out anywhere and as often as he liked, could have as elaborate a meal as he desired, and would have to pay nothing or only a small percentage of the cost. The cost of joining such prepaid dining clubs rose sharply.

Long ago, most restaurants would have one chef to prepare the food. A few restaurants were more elaborate, with chefs specializing in roasting, fish, salads, sauces, and many other things. People rarely went to these elaborate restaurants since they were so expensive. With the establishment of prepaid dining clubs, everyone wanted to eat at these fancy restaurants. At the same time, young chefs in school disdained going to cook in a small restaurant where they would have to cook everything. The pay was higher and it was much more prestigious to specialize and cook at a really fancy restaurant. Soon there were not enough chefs to keep the small restaurants open.

With prepaid clubs and free meals for the poor, many people started eating their three-course meals at the elaborate restaurants. Then they began to increase the number of courses, directing the chef to "serve the best with no thought for the bill." (Recently a 317-course meal was served.)

The costs of eating out rose faster and faster. A new government commission reported as follows: (1) Noting that licensed chefs were being used to peel potatoes and wash lettuce, the commission recommended that these tasks be handed over to licensed dishwashers (whose three years of dishwashing training included cooking courses) or to some new category of personnel. (2) Concluding that many licensed chefs were overworked, the commission recommended that cooking schools be expanded, that the length of training be shortened, and that applicants with lesser qualifications be admitted. (3) The commission also observed that chefs were unhappy because people seemed to be more concerned about the decor and service than about the food. (In a recent taste test, not only could one patron not tell the difference between a 1930 and a 1970 vintage but he also could not distinguish between white and red wines. He explained that he always ordered the 1930 vintage because he knew that only a really good restaurant would stock such an expensive wine.)

The commission agreed that weighty problems faced the nation. They recommended that a national prepayment group be established which everyone must join. They recommended that chefs continue to be paid on the basis of the number of dishes they prepared. They recommended that every Gourmandese be given the right to eat anywhere he chose and as elaborately as he chose and pay nothing.

These recommendations were adopted. Large numbers of people spent all of their time ordering incredibly elaborate meals. Kitchens became marvels of new, expensive equipment. All those who were not consuming restaurant food were in the kitchen preparing it. Since no one in Gourmand did anything except prepare or eat meals, the country collapsed.

This Chapter Contains:

- Introduction

- Management Defined
    - Decision-making Process
    - Planning Process
    - Organizing Process
    - Executing Process
    - Controlling Process

- Characteristics of Management
    - Set of Processes
    - Interactive
    - Technical/Social
    - Dynamic

- A Model of Management
    - Inputs
    - Outputs
    - Set of Processes
    - Environmental Interface

- The Model as the Framework

- Summary

- Discussion Questions

Chapter 2

A MANAGEMENT MODEL FOR HEALTH CARE ORGANIZATIONS

"The health care delivery system is undermanaged."

(Gary Filerman)

INTRODUCTION

In an address before the 1975 annual meeting of the Association of University Programs in Health Administration, its president, Dr. Gary Filerman, stated "the health care delivery system is undermanaged." In context his meaning was clear. He did not mean that there were too few people occupying managerial positions. Quite the contrary; his point was that some who have managerial responsibility in health care organizations are not as familiar with the subject as they should be, and they do not manage as effectively as they should. Given that our primary purpose is to present the subject of management as it applies to health care organizations, the remainder of this text will be devoted to management—its processes and activities. This chapter will (1) expand our introductory definition made in the first chapter, (2) describe the characteristics of management, and (3) present a management model which will provide the framework for the following parts of this book.

MANAGEMENT DEFINED

Management has been defined in a number of different ways. Some have regarded it as getting things done through people by providing an organization environment conducive to enabling individuals to accomplish objectives.[1] Others have viewed management as a distinct set of functions such as planning, organizing, and controlling, while other writers include additional functions such as decision-making, staffing, and directing.[2] While there is no precise definition universally accepted,[3] we will define management as follows: *an interac-*

---

[1]Harold Koontz, "The management theory jungle." *Academy of Management Journal, 4*:166, December 1961.

[2]For an excellent classification review of various functions by writers see: Richard M. Hodgetts, *Management: Theory, Process, and Practice.* Philadelphia: W. B. Saunders Company, 1975, pp. 108–109.

[3]For an interesting but not dissimilar definition of management (Health Administration) see: Charles J. Austin, "What is health administration?" *Hospital Administration, 19*:27, Summer, 1974.

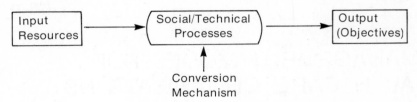

Figure 2-1 Input–Conversion–Output.

tive set of social/technical processes occurring within a formal organizational setting with the purpose of accomplishing predetermined objectives through the utilization of human and physical resources.[4]

Stated another way, management is the totality of interactive processes that (1) are social and technical in nature and (2) that occur within a formal setting. The purpose of these processes is (3) to accomplish organizational objectives, which is done through (4) the utilization of human and physical resources.

In Figure 2-1, an input-conversion-output portrayal of our definition of management is presented. This model demonstrates that input resources, in the form of manpower, material, technology, information, and capital, are utilized by the health care organization in order to generate output. Ideally, that output is desirable in that it corresponds to organization objectives, such as quality patient care. The social/technical processes are the mechanisms (processes of management) by which inputs are converted to outputs.

Figure 2-2 enlarges upon the conversion mechanism and denotes management's role. The five specific processes (often called functions) that constitute management are described as follows: (1) the Decision-Making Process; (2) the Planning Process; (3) the Organizing Process; (4) the Executing Process; and (5) the Controlling Process. These processes are interactive in that each affects the other, they occur simultaneously, they are continuous, and the totality of their interaction results in the conversion of inputs to outputs. Perhaps a few words about each of these important processes are in order.

DECISION-MAKING PROCESS

Decision-making is a technical process that is pervasive in nature, that is, it is inherent in all of the following processes. Specifically, decision-making involves a series of activities that includes, among other things, the definition of problems, the identification of alternatives, and the evaluation of those alternatives. Managerial decision-making in health care is pervasive because it is performed by people throughout all hierarchical levels within any health care organization, ranging from administrator to supervisor. It should be pointed out,

---

[4]For a corresponding view see: Theo Haimann and William G. Scott, *Management in the Modern Organization.* Boston: Houghton-Mifflin Company, 1974, p. 6.

however, that the scope of the decision-making performed and the importance of those decisions will vary, depending on the individual's position in the organization and the responsibilities he has.

PLANNING PROCESS

Planning is a technical process that is concerned with the future. Planning has been described as determining in advance what is to be done. In order for the health care organization to fulfill its purpose, plans must be made. In order for the department head to discharge his responsibilities, he must plan. Characteristic of planning is the formulation of objectives and, of course, the determination of the input resources required. Health care organizations have received a great deal of pressure in recent years to establish sound facility planning in relation to verified community need. Some examples of this include many state laws requiring "certificate of need" by the health care organization for expansion from local health care councils and/or from Comprehensive Health Planning Commissions; Section 1122 of the Federal Social Security Regulation regarding local approvals for certain health care expenditures above $100,000; and the National Health Planning and Resources Development Act of 1974 (PL 93–641), all of which have a considerable impact on planning for health care in America.

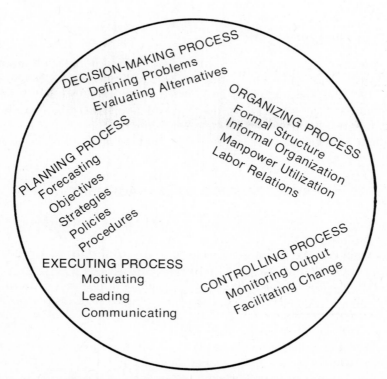

Figure 2–2   Interactive set of social/technical processes.

ORGANIZING PROCESS

The organizing process is technical in nature. It deals with the authority-responsibility relationships within the organization; that is, the formal setting within which group activity is carried out in order to accomplish predetermined objectives. Characteristic activities include the determination of the formal organization structure and the acquisition and positioning of manpower resources in order to ensure that activities can be carried out. The organizing process is also concerned with such activities as departmentation, delegation, and line-staff structures, to name a few. The essence of organizing lies in "dividing up the work" in order to achieve the objectives of organization. No health care facility can maximize the delivery of health care without a proper allocation of resources to achieve such care. This allocation must be organized in such a way that all parts relate to the whole.

EXECUTING PROCESS

The executing process is social in nature and is primarily concerned with initiating action within the organization. It is people-oriented and includes those activities necessary for dealing with the human resources (people) of the organization. The following activities are involved: motivating employees, leading and supervising them, and communicating with them so that planned activities can be initiated and accomplished within the formal setting. This is an extremely important process because of the dominant "people-orientation" of health care delivery.

CONTROLLING PROCESS

The controlling process is technical in nature, and it focuses on monitoring the organization's activity. The gathering and utilization of resources should result in the accomplishment of predetermined objectives. The controlling process entails such activities as determining standards against which the organization's resultant activity is measured, and establishing techniques for measurement and corrective mechanisms, should change be necessary.

CHARACTERISTICS OF MANAGEMENT

Management, as we have defined it, has certain characteristics, among which are the following:

1. Management is a Set of Processes. In order to make this point clearer, we should define the word "process." A process is a series of continuous functions, activities, or actions carried out in the utilization of resources to achieve specific results. Each of the processes in Figure 2–2 represents a series of actions or activities continuously carried out, and the sum of the processes constitutes a full set, which is management.

2. Each of the Processes is Interactive. They are interrelated and affect each other. All are carried out, to some degree, simultaneously with one another, feeding upon the other. For example, *decision-making is interrelated with all* *of the other processes* because each process requires decisions to be made. Decisions are made when formulating objectives, when alterations are made in the existing organization structure, when tasks are delegated to others, when one motivates employees, and when change is indicated and implemented by the control process.

3. The Processes are Technical and Social in Nature. They are technical in that a specific series of activities is involved. They are also social in nature in that they all involve people. People make decisions, establish objectives, and justify their conclusions to others. People make organizational assignments and introduce changes that affect other people. People initiate activity within the organization by causing others to perform certain tasks. People monitor organizational action, and they must deal with others if control actions are warranted. In sum, organizations require human resources in order to function. The people act, interact, and react. Consequently, people in organizations generate a dynamic set of social relationships with which management is concerned.

4. Management is Dynamic. The dynamic attribute of management implies that the set of interactive social/technical processes and their corresponding activities are continuous in an ongoing sense. Furthermore, the word dynamic implies that the formal organization's setting, input resources, outputs, and processes change over time. Thus management is not static and fixed but fluid and adaptive.

A MODEL OF MANAGEMENT

So far we have defined management and briefly described its major characteristics. We have also conceptually presented management (Fig. 2–1) as representing the conversion mechanism by which inputs are transformed into outputs. Figure 2–3 is a more complete model of management, portraying its interrelated elements as follows: (1) inputs, (2) outputs, (3) set of processes, and (4) environmental interface. Each of these elements is described below.

INPUTS

The "inputs" component (1) of the management model presented in Figure 2–3 denotes that certain resources are required by the health care organization in order to generate output (2), that is, to accomplish objectives. Basic inputs are manpower, material technology, information, and capital resources. These are the necessary ingredients that must be acquired and used in order to accomplish the desired output (objectives).

For health care organizations, examples of manpower resources are physicians, nurses, technologists, pharmacists, dentists, dieticians, medical records librarians, and business office and other administrative personnel. The material inputs (resources) range from supplies to food. Technological resources range from sophisticated radiology machines to computers. The information resources range from internal reports, covering such diverse areas as census, supplies, schedules, numbers of personnel, and budgets, to external information relative to governmental legislation covering grants and reporting requirements.

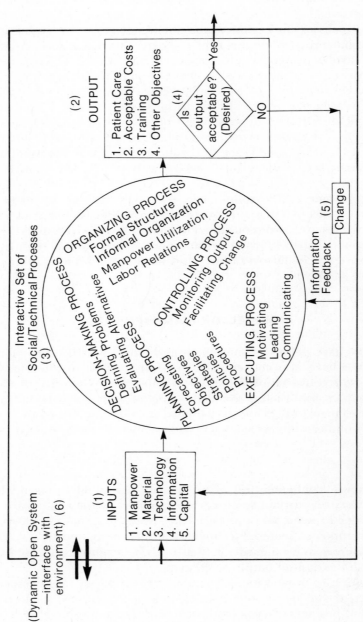

Figure 2-3   Management model.

Finally, capital resources consist of such items as physical plant, equipment, and funds.

All of these input resources are necessary in order for the health care organization to function. Eliminating or restricting any one grouping compromises the effectiveness of the whole organization. For example, the rapid rise in the cost of supplies would certainly affect the total organization. Furthermore, rising interest rates may render capital expansion infeasible because of the shortage of capital funds or its prohibitive cost.

OUTPUTS

The "output" component (2) of the management model presented in Figure 2–3 denotes that organizational output (objectives) results from the conversion of inputs (1) by the set of managerial processes (3). Output for health care organizations can take many different forms. Typically, we call them objectives. Objectives are those ends, missions, goals, and results that are to be accomplished. They are the rationale and purpose for the existence of the health care organization. Desired output consists of those predetermined objectives that the members of the organization wish to achieve, and it can include such things as providing quality patient care to the community, engaging in significant medical research, or the training of health care professionals.

It is the responsibility of the Board of Trustees or an appropriate governing body to establish the purpose(s) of their health care organization. They may wish to fulfill either a multitude of objectives or only one. For example, the skilled nursing facility has the objective of providing quality care to a selected population of patients. On the other hand, the community general hospital may have the purpose of providing various levels of care and serving the whole community. Yet, it may also have the objective of training resident doctors. The Veterans' Administration Hospital may have the purpose of caring for veterans to the exclusion of the general population. The community health center may have the purpose of providing care to the population of the inner-city. In contrast, the university-based hospital may propose to provide not only general patient care but also specialized care, which requires the combination of sophisticated equipment and medical specialists. It may also have the purpose of training health care professionals through resident and nursing programs. Finally it may be heavily research oriented.

Within the delivery system there is a place for organizations that have a multitude of limited objectives. In fact, this is desirable from a resource allocation point of view relative to the whole health care delivery system. Yet, the management of them is essentially the same, and all in some way convert inputs to outputs.

SET OF PROCESSES

The "set of processes" component (3) of the management model was first presented in Figure 2–2. It denotes that through the interactive set of social/technical processes, inputs (1) are converted to organizational output (2). One important consideration is an understanding of the placement and role of the processes relative to the management model under consideration. Through the planning process output-input decisions are made. Through the organizing process organizational design and structure decisions are made. Through the executing process decisions are made to initiate the activity within the organization, thus resulting in organizational dynamics. Finally, through the controlling process decisions are made relative to monitoring activity that is initiated and carried out in the organization.

Viewing the "output" component of the management model presented in Figure 2–3, a decision cell is noted (4). The question asked is "Is output acceptable?" Through control, activity is compared with objectives. If they correspond with each other, desired output is being attained; that is, objectives are being accomplished. If the activity of the organization (patient care, cost levels) does not correspond to its objectives, then the latter are not being accomplished. At this point corrective action in the form of change is necessary. This is denoted by the "change" component (5) of the model.

Flowing from the "change" component (5) is an information feedback loop. It demonstrates that information related to nonattainment of objectives and the change actions required both flow to the "process set" (3) and "inputs" (1) components of the model. Information feedback to the "set of processes" (3), which might indicate that change is necessary, could include rising costs, higher mortality rates, high employee turnover, excess (abusive) utilization of diagnostic tests, and declining daily census, to name a few.

Information feedback to the "inputs" (1) component could indicate, for example, that additional or different types of personnel (manpower) with other skills are needed. Consider the situation of a research hospital that has as one of its objectives the provision of medical care that is on the frontier of the state of the art. Using organ transplants to represent one characteristic of the frontier, the output-measurement-change-information feedback sequence of the model may indicate that personnel (inputs) with specialized skills and sophisticated equipment must be acquired in order to accomplish that objective (output).

Since health care organizations are ever-changing, so is the management of them. The management model represents a circular flow, which is continuous, that is, inputs-processes-output-change (if necessary). It would be very easy to view the model as a closed sequence of events unto itself. However, health care organizations reside within a larger environment; they are not isolated islands. They are affected by the environment, and they in turn affect it. Therefore, when managing those organizations, considerations must be given to the concept of "interfacing with the environment."

ENVIRONMENTAL INTERFACE

Surrounding the health care organization and its managers is the environment. Viewing Figure 2–3, it is noted that the management model is circumscribed by an environmental boundary (6). Health care organizations are affected by, and in turn affect, their external environment. Kast and Rosenzweig make this point when stating that the hospital (and other health care organizations) have "a dynamic interplay with its (their) environment—the community, patients, medical practitioners, governments and many other elements."[5] Simply stated, health care organization managers must interact with the environ-ment.

Environmental influences affecting health care organizations and the management of them are most often represented by constraints within which the manager must act and react. For example, Figure 2–3 demonstrates that input resources are obtained from the environment. Manpower, material, technological, information, and capital resources are typically acquired externally. The manager must compete for those input resources and can be constrained by the source entities existing in the environment. For example, he must compete for capital (financial) resources as well as interact with union representatives who can affect his supply and the cost of manpower resources. Health care's greatest environmental impact is from the government, especially from the federal level.

In addition, the output generated by the health care organization affects the external environment. The quality of patient care provided in the community, the range of services offered, the financial burden placed on patients and on third-party payers, the training of health care professionals, and the breakthroughs in medicine from organized research all affect the external environment.

Furthermore, government programs such as Medicare-Medicaid, regulations such as the necessity of PSRO's, and legislation such as the Taft-Hartley Act can constrain the utilization of inputs, affect the processes, and, therefore, shape the nature of the output.

Health care organizations do not exist in a vacuum, and their management cannot be carried out in isolation. The health administrator, department head, or supervisor must cope with the environmental constraints and must also be responsible to that environment. He must be able to adapt and change in response to external events.

As can be seen from the model just presented, management serves the role of a conversion mechanism. It is through management that the objectives (desired output) of the health care organization are determined. It is the means by which requisite resources (inputs) are gathered and positioned. It is the means by which things get done.

THE MODEL AS THE FRAMEWORK

The management model presented in Figure 2–3 will serve as the structure for the remaining parts of this book. We will present the decision-making and planning processes in Part II (Output-Input Determination). Part III (Organizational Design and Structure) will focus primarily on the organizing process. In Part IV (Organizational Dynamics) the executing process and its characteristic activities will be presented. Finally the controlling process will be discussed in Part V (Organizational Control and Change).

---

[5] Fremont E. Kast and James E. Rosenzweig, "Hospital administration and systems concepts." *Hospital Administration, 11*:18, Fall, 1966.

SUMMARY

In this chapter management was defined as *an interactive set of social/technical processes occurring within a formal organizational setting with the purpose of accomplishing predetermined objectives through the utilization of human and physical resources.* The various characteristics of management were discussed, and a management model applicable to health care organizations was presented and its interrelated elements described. As a result, the framework for the following chapters, which treat the various processes and activities presented in Figure 2–3, has been established.

DISCUSSION QUESTIONS

1. What are the basic elements inherent in the definition of management?

2. Describe the various processes of management.

3. What are some of the characteristics of management?

4. Describe the basic components of the management model and indicate how they are interrelated.

5. Discuss the environmental factors that affect health care organizations and the management of them.

Part II

OUTPUT-INPUT DETERMINATION

In Part I, *THE SETTING AND FRAMEWORK*, the health care system and some of the organizations that are part of that system were described. Furthermore, a management model was presented and it was noted that its component parts will serve as the framework and structure for the subsequent parts of this text. In this Part II, *OUTPUT-INPUT DETERMINATION*, the two processes that are characteristic of output-input determination—the Decision-Making Process and the Planning Process—will be presented. There are four chapters in this part. The first two are devoted to decision-making, and the last two are devoted to planning and its activities.

Basically, output-input determination involves the making of decisions pertaining to the organization's objectives, decisions on how these objectives can be achieved, and decisions concerning what input resources are required in order to achieve those objectives. Viewing the "input-conversion-output" model presented in Figure 2–1, the logical place to start is the formulation of organizational objectives, since they prescribe what inputs are necessary for accomplishing those objectives.

Output-input determination is, in essence, the planning process. Activities characteristic of it are forecasting, objective and strategy formulation, and the development of policies and procedures. In Chapter 5, Planning and Planning Methods, we will describe the planning process along with its characteristic activities. Chapter 6, Objectives, Strategies, and Policies, will serve as a sequel to Chapter 5 and expand upon it.

Chapter 3, Managerial Decision-Making, and Chapter 4, Decision-Making Techniques, precede the two chapters devoted to the Planning Process. The reason for this order is that the decision-making process is pervasive in nature and is an integral part of all of the other managerial processes (planning, organizing, executing, and controlling). In each, decisions are made. As a result of its common nature, an understanding of the decision-making process and familiarity with various managerial decision-making techniques will contribute to a better understanding of those other managerial processes.

In Chapter 3 the decision-making process is presented and its characteristic activities described. In Chapter 4 various managerial decision-making techniques are presented in such a manner that the non-mathematically oriented reader will benefit. Furthermore, Chapter 4 is designed so that it can be omitted, if necessary, by the reader without affecting the flow of the remaining chapters of the book.

This Chapter Contains:

- Introduction

- The Concept of Decision-Making
    Common
    Pervasive
    Dynamic
    Continuous

- Decision-Making Defined

- Classifications of Decisions
    Individual–Group
    Ends–Means
    Administrative–Operational
    Programmed–Nonprogrammed

- Decision-Making Process
    Awareness
    Problem Definition
    Gathering Relevant Information

- Solution Criteria and
    Constraints
        Developing Alternative Solutions
        Evaluating Alternatives
        Choosing An Alternative

- Comprehensive Example

- Factors Influencing Decision-Making
    Decision-Maker's Value System
    Environment And Internal Pressures
    Uncertainty, Timeliness, Experience

- Summary

- Discussion Questions

Chapter 3

MANAGERIAL DECISION-MAKING

". . . if one considers the entire decision-making
process of gathering information and processing it,
making choices from among alternatives, and
effectively communicating decisions made to other
members of the organization, *there is little
managerial activity which could not be considered
within the decision-making framework.*" (Italics
added.)

(Richards and Greenlaw)[1]

INTRODUCTION

Two points are evident from the preceding statement. First, decision-making involves choosing from among alternatives. Second, decision-making is an integral part of all other managerial processes and activities. The first point is important because it states simply the essence of decision-making; the second point is important because it indicates that decision-making is common to all managerial activity throughout health care delivery.

In Chapter 2 we presented a management model (Fig. 2–3), which included the following: (1) decision-making, (2) planning, (3) organizing, (4) executing, and (5) controlling as the set of interactive processes through which the conversion of inputs (resources) to desired output (objective accomplishment) occurs. It was also indicated that in the planning process output-input decisions are made; in the organizing process organizational design and structure decisions are made; in the executing process decisions are made relative to initiating activity; and in the controlling process decisions are made relative to monitoring organization activity.

Decision-making is truly a common process that pervades all health care organizations and that is linked to all of the other processes by reason of the fact that decisions are made in each. This point is displayed in Figure 3–1. Tersine also reinforces this point when contending that decision-making is at the center of management. "The manager," he states, "makes decisions in establishing objectives; he makes planning decisions, organizing decisions, motivating decisions and controlling decisions."[2]

[1]Max D. Richards, and Paul S. Greenlaw, *Management: Decisions and Behavior.* Homewood, Illinois: Richard D. Irwin, Inc., 1972, p. 33.

[2]Richard J. Tersine, "Organization decision theory—a synthesis." *Managerial Planning, 21*:18, July/August, 1972.

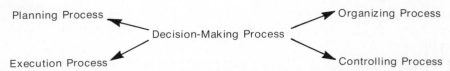

Figure 3-1   Decision-making, common process.

Because of its "common" characteristic, decision-making is a process that eventually affects the effectiveness and efficiency of health care organizations. John McMahon, the President of the American Hospital Association, noted:

> The subject of decision-making—how to make sound decisions in the midst of this changing scene—has not received the attention it deserves. We are beginning to realize that, everything else being equal, the level of effectiveness and efficiency in an organization is directly related to the quality of problem-solving and decision-making.[3]

In the remainder of this chapter we will present (1) the concept of decision-making and (2) define it. We will (3) discuss various classifications of decisions and (4) present the activities characteristic of the decision-making process. Finally, (5) a comprehensive example of a major decision will be given along with (6) a concluding section presenting some of the factors that influence decision-making. The next chapter will present an overview of various quantitative decision-making techniques.

THE CONCEPT OF DECISION-MAKING

Decision-making is a common, pervasive, dynamic, never-ending, and extremely important process. As has already been pointed out, it is common to the other management processes. The pervasive nature of decision-making can be noted when observing that all individuals within health care organizations who have resource responsibilities make decisions. Decision-making is performed not only by the administrator but by all department heads, and supervisors. For example, as Young observes in the following quote, decision-making is carried out by people in the top, middle, and lower levels of management:

> It is not the function of top management to solve all problems or make all decisions. Their fundamental obligation is to supervise the decision-making activities of their immediate subordinates in the middle and lower levels of management in order to assure that their activities are being performed properly.[4]

---

[3]John Alexander McMahon, "Hospital–physician relationships—where do we go from here?" *Michigan Hospitals, 10*:5, December, 1974.
[4]Stanley Young, "Organizational decision-making." *Hospital Administration, 10*:38, Fall, 1965.

For example, members of the board of trustees decide (and modify) the objectives of the organization. The administrator decides to whom to delegate certain authority within the organization, and the supervisor decides to which subordinates tasks will be assigned. Thus decision-making filters through the organization. While all organization members who deal with resources (human or physical) make decisions, it should be pointed out that the scope of their decisions may vary, depending upon the individual's level in the organization hierarchy and the nature of his responsibility.

Decision-making is also dynamic. The fact that a decision needs to be made implies a time frame. The past creates the conditions that give rise to a decision point. The making of decisions occurs in the present, and their implementation occurs in the future. Furthermore, decision-making and its extension — implementation — necessarily involve resources (human and physical) and, generally, change from the present state. Therefore decision-making is dynamic and, as a result, an action-oriented process, as opposed to one that is static. This is particularly true in the health care field because so many of the departments in the skilled nursing facility or hospital *interact* with one another. The delivery of medical care in one department is partly dependent on the quality of performance of members of many other departments. This results in a chain reaction of decision-making effectiveness that is highly unique in the health care field.

Decision-making is also a continuous process. The fact that a decision has been made does not imply that the process stops, because a decision must be implemented in order to be effective. Deciding to do something and then not doing it is not constructive. Therefore additional decisions must be made regarding the implementation of what was decided and control to ensure that it is being carried out as planned. If it is not, the initial decision will need to be re-evaluated. In short, decision-making is not a "one time" event; it is continuous in the "business-related" departments of health care organizations as well as in the "medical departments."

DECISION-MAKING DEFINED

Authorities basically agree that decision-making, in its simplest sense, is the selection of a choice from among alternatives. For example, McDonnell states that "to decide is to choose,"[5] while Ives indicates that decision-making is a rational attempt to consider quantitative and qualitative means in the selection of alternative courses of action.[6]

For our purposes we will define decision-making as the choosing from among alternatives. There are two other elements that are implied in this definition — the recognition that decisions need to be made and the formulation of alternatives. They are preceding but necessary activities that lead to the choice among alternatives. For example, when the head of the Respiratory Therapy Department needs to appoint a midnight shift supervisor, a whole array of decisions is

[5]John F. McDonnell, "The human element in decision-making." *Personnel Journal, 53*:188, March, 1974.

[6]Brian D. Ives, "Decision theory and the practicing manager." *Business Horizons, 16*:38, June, 1973.

amassed. He cannot decide *not* to decide if quality care is to be maintained. He needs to work with the Personnel Department on the job description, selection of the person from applicants brought forth, and the orientation of the selected person.

Our definition of choosing among alternatives has the advantage of being brief and simple; it focuses on the essential activity of decision-making — making a choice. However, to fully grasp the nature of decision-making and how it is performed, we will first examine various classifications of decisions and then the activities characteristic of the decision-making process.

CLASSIFICATIONS OF DECISIONS

Decisions can be grouped into many classification sets, such as major–minor or hard–easy. We will present the following four classifications: (1) individual–group; (2) ends–means; (3) administrative–operational; and (4) programmed–nonprogrammed decisions. These classification sets are presented in order to introduce the terminology. *By no means are they mutually exclusive, each set residing in its own watertight compartment, isolated from the other.* In Figure 3–2 the notion that the classifications overlap is presented. In fact, one might observe that a given decision may encompass one portion of each of these classification sets. For example, a decision to share services with other facilities, or establish a satellite neighborhood health center, could be a decision made by a group or by one person (individual). It would be a "means" decision in that it represents a way of accomplishing the organization's objective(s), such as community service. Furthermore, it would be an "administrative" decision, since it deals with major resource commitment versus one that is primarily operational in terms of carrying out day-to-day activities. Finally, it would be a

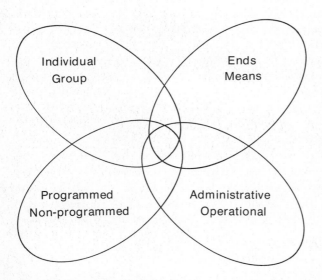

Figure 3–2 Classification of decisions in the health care setting.

Not Mutually Exclusive

"nonprogrammed" decision, since it was not routine but unique in terms of occurring infrequently. With this note of caution against the idea that the following decision classifications are mutually exclusive, a description of each will be made.

INDIVIDUAL–GROUP

There are basically two means by which decisions are made, by an individual or by a group. In some instances group decision-making can be appropriate; however, one hazard is that group consensus can lead to a commonly acceptable decision that may not be the best one. Furthermore, committee or group decisions can blur accountability. Most health organizations are so structured that specific individuals are responsible for various areas of operation and the decisions made relative to those areas. Yet the delivery of health care is strongly characterized by a preponderance of group input to decision-making because the dynamics of patient care involve so many departments and professionals working together.

ENDS–MEANS

"Ends" decisions refer to those dealing with the determination of objectives. That is, what are the ends (objectives) to be accomplished? "Means" decisions are those that deal with the strategies and/or the operational activities that will enable the objectives to be accomplished. Looking at ends–means decision-making in its broadest perspective, we can view the management model "desired output" component (Fig. 2–3) as representing the "ends" to be accomplished by the health care organization.

We may also look at ends–means decisions on a narrower plane. In Chapter 6 we will present the subjects of objectives (ends) and strategy (means) determination as well as the notion that objectives can be arranged in a hierarchy. Specifically, objectives can be nested in a hierarchy with the primary objectives of the organization superseding and embracing the objectives of specific organization units or departments. That is, individual departments may have their own objectives, which when fulfilled, will contribute to accomplishing the organization's *primary or overall* objective(s). Suffice it to say that primary "ends" decisions *for the organization as a whole* are usually made by the board of trustees, with "means" decisions generally made by the chief executive officer of the health care organization. Both have a major impact in terms of the input resources required by and activities that will occur in the organization.[7] By the same token, a department head makes ends–means decisions for his area of responsibility, which hopefully complement the primary ends–means of the organ-

---

[7]For some interesting examples see the following:

Thomas R. O'Donovan, "Contract service: some pros and cons." *Hospital Progress, 48*:70, February, 1967.

Sister Gertrude Bastnagel, Frederick Hyde, Jr., Sister Mary Leila Koeppe, and Julien Priver, "Hospitals consolidate medical services." *Hospitals, 47*:33, July 1, 1973.

Francisco D. Sabichi, and Timothy L. Long, "Association serves 17 hospitals." *Hospitals, 48*: 101, June 1, 1974.

August F. Hoenack, "Outcome is merger." *Hospitals, 47*:55, June 1, 1973.

ization. However, those decisions will not have as great an impact as, nor require the resources of, the latter.

ADMINISTRATIVE–OPERATIONAL

Administrative decisions are those made by individuals who occupy positions at the upper levels of the organization hierarchy. In addition to primary ends–means decisions, other administrative decisions would be those that involve a substantial resource commitment and, therefore, have a major impact throughout the organization. Examples would be the following: (1) the contracting of services such as maintenance, radiology, dietary, laundry; (2) the closing of units such as obstetrics and pediatrics; (3) the sharing or (4) the expanding of services such as emergency, out-patient, intensive care, rehabilitation.

Operational decisions, on the other hand, are those generally made by department heads, heads of services, and supervisors, and which are concerned with the day-to-day operational activities of the particular organizational unit. Operational level decisions may consist of departmental equipment purchases, personnel deployment, and those that deal with specific work assignments.

PROGRAMMED–NONPROGRAMMED

Both programmed and nonprogrammed decisions can occur at the administrative and operational levels. Programmed decisions are those that are repetitive and routine in nature. Since they are repetitive, policies and/or procedures are often formulated to cover those situations and, thereby, provide future guidelines for decision-making. Included would be patient care procedures and wage and salary policies, to name a few. According to Herbert Simon, nonprogrammed decisions are those that are "novel, unstructured, and consequential."[8] In short, they are unique, and they may only be made once.

Perhaps several examples will serve to make the distinction. Decisions to expand facilities, add, close, or share medical services, change employee compensation levels, alter the organization structure, change to a salaried medical staff in the Emergency Department, or add a residency in pediatrics are nonprogrammed types of decisions. They are unique, nonroutine, and may occur once, or at most, very infrequently. Some additional examples of programmed decisions are whether or not to grant maternity leave to employees, reorder supplies, what time of the day to admit patients, and whether to request some prepayment for those patients not having health insurance. In most instances repetitive situations will cause a decision to be programmed; that is, to make a decision once that will continuously be applied and that will be translated into a policy or procedure. Once this occurs, consistency will result, those responsible for discharging the activity will not have to make decisions each time, and their time can be more effectively spent pursuing other tasks.

---

[8] Herbert A. Simon, *The New Science of Management Decision*. New York: Harper and Brothers, Publishers, 1960, p. 6.

THE DECISION-MAKING PROCESS

The decision-making process incorporates a number of activities, ranging from becoming aware that a decision must be made to selecting an alternative and taking the necessary steps for its implementation. The specific activities are as follows:

1. Becoming aware that a decision must be made.
2. Defining the problem.
3. Gathering relevant information.
4. Developing alternative solutions.
5. Evaluating those alternatives.
6. Choosing the most acceptable alternative.[9]

Each activity composing the decision-making process is important. However, we wish to point out that *those activities are not individually isolated events that consume similar time and effort for all people in all decision-making situations. Nor is the stepping through the activities necessarily sequential from "becoming aware of the problem."* Depending upon experience, the value set of the individual decision-maker, the urgency or nature of the problem, and cost implications of a wrong or delayed decision, to name a few, a decision-maker may engage in all or part of the activities representative of the decision-making process, spending little time and effort on some and more on others. Furthermore, there may be recycling through the activities and/or entrance at some point other than the first activity. For example, a situation such as a fire may immediately indicate that there is a problem and also define it. These two activities in the decision-making process consume virtually no time, and the decision-maker basically enters the "gather relevant information" phase (Where is the fire? How intense is it? Has the alarm been sounded?).

Also, depending upon the decision to be made, little or much time and effort might be spent on evaluating alternatives and final selection. That is, some decisions are major and some are minor. Some involve large amounts of resources, some involve little, if any. The major decisions involving large amounts of resources will generally and properly take more time and effort to evaluate. For example, little time would probably be spent on evaluating which of several people a minor task should be delegated to, versus evaluating two alternatives of acquiring or not acquiring a piece of equipment costing, say, $50,000. Recycling can occur when, for example, it is determined that the alternatives available are not appropriate after being evaluated for any number of

---

[9]There are some variations of these activities. For example, see the following:

Mary F. Arnold, L. Vaughn Blankenship, and John M. Hess, *Administering Health Systems.* New York: Aldine, 1971, pp. 337–347.

Paul R. Donnelly. "Corporate decision-making and information flow model." *Hospital Progress,* 55:33, March, 1974.

Richard M. Hodgetts, *Management: Theory, Process and Practice.* Philadelphia: W. B. Saunders Company, 1975, p. 225.

McDonnell, op. cit., p. 189.

Edward J. Spillane, "The anatomy of a decision." *Hospital Progress,* 50:47, April, 1969.

Paul E. Torgersen, and Irwin T. Weinstock, *Management: An Integrated Approach.* Englewood Cliffs, New Jersey: Prentice-Hall, Inc., 1972, pp. 31–34.

Young, op. cit., p. 39.

reasons, such as an incorrectly defined problem or a problem that was not evaluated in sufficient depth. As a result, the decision-maker may recycle to the point of "defining the problem" again. In addition to recycling, the decision-making process is continuous. The fact that a decision has been made will necessarily lead to more decisions, such as how and when to implement what has been decided.

The point that we have made is that the decision-making process is not a fixed sequence of activities that consume the same amount of time and effort. Each activity is important, yet the nature of the situation can effectively permit entrance other than at the first activity. Furthermore, upon reflection, one can observe that cycling can occur, and one decision will often lead to the need to make other decisions.

With this introduction, we will proceed next to a description of the activities characteristic of the decision-making process. They represent events which enable the decision-maker to systematically channel thoughts and efforts in order to focus on the decision that must be made (problem to be solved) and to minimize becoming bogged down in minute details or overwhelmed by irrelevant matters.

AWARENESS

A truly basic activity of the decision-making process is being aware that a decision needs to be made. An effective manager must be sensitive to situations in his area of responsibility that do not meet standards and expectations, as well as be aware of opportunities for improvement. This sensitivity can be termed perceptual skill, often enhanced with experience, and it enables the manager to collect and interpret informational cues from his surroundings, such as abnormally high turnover, rising costs, increased infection rates, higher supply usage, poor morale, low levels of performance, and so on. When no triggering informational cues are picked up by the manager, he will not necessarily become aware that a problem exists. Those with limited perceptual skills, or those who are inattentive, can be oblivious to potential problems until they blossom into full-bloom crises. It is obvious that crisis decision-making does not permit thoughtful and full consideration of events or the evaluation of as much information or range of alternatives as non-crisis decision-making allows. Furthermore, in the crisis setting, the decision-maker is reacting to events, rather than shaping and causing them. Perceptual skills cannot really be taught; they are developed through experience. This is one of the main reasons that managers usually become more effective with experience.

PROBLEM DEFINITION

Problem definition necessitates that a distinction be made between cause and symptom. As in medicine, failure to make this distinction will inevitably lead to unnecessary complications, or worse. Defining the real problem is not always an easy task, because what appears to be the problem might only be a symptom. For example, a supervisor in the clinical laboratory might believe he is confronted with a problem of conflicting personalities when two medical technologists are continually bickering and cannot get along with each other. Upon investigation, the supervisor might find that the real problem is that he has never clearly outlined the functions and duties of each of his subordinates, specifying where their duties begin and end. Therefore, what appeared to be a problem of personality conflict was actually a problem of delegation and responsibility.

Defining a problem can be time-consuming, but it is time well spent. There is no need for a manager to go any further until he is sure the problem has been clearly defined, because nothing is as frustrating as the right solution to the wrong problem. A simple but effective way of getting behind the symptom to the underlying problem is to ask—*why?*

GATHERING RELEVANT INFORMATION

After the problem—and not just the symptom—has been defined, the manager generally acquires information. This means assembling the facts that are *relevant* to the situation. Judgment must be used in deciding what and how much information should be gathered as well as what information should be ignored.

Solution Criteria

In addition to basic information and data, two additional sets of information should be gathered in order to be able to evaluate alternatives. They are (1) the *solution criteria* and (2) the *solution constraints.*

Solution criteria specify the ultimate purpose(s) for which the problem is being solved. It may be to provide better care, foster employee harmony, promote organizational effectiveness and efficiency or any number of criteria that would be appropriate. In other words, before alternatives can be evaluated, the purpose (solution criteria) for solving the problem must be identified.

Solution Constraints

Solution constraints are internal and external parameters within which the solution must reside. There may be authority, resource, cost, humanitarian, ethical, and political constraints, to name a few, that must be considered. It makes little sense to spend time making a decision to increase the pay of one of your better employees who is threatening to leave (the problem) if the organization's wage and salary structure will not permit it. Nor would it be wise to discharge a problem employee when the union contract requires that an oral and written warning be given before discharge can occur, or to refuse to modernize a wing when its present condition is in violation of a code. Expanding the number of beds when financing is not available and/or there is a substantial excess of beds in the area would also be tantamount to ignoring constraints.

Thus, once the problem has been identified, whether its solution requires an administrative or an operational level decision, information must be gathered, including that information related to solution criteria and solution constraints. Only then can the alternatives be evaluated and the "best" of them selected. In other words, intelligent *decisions cannot be made in a vacuum, but they must be considered within the context of the objectives and constraints, both internal and external, that are imposed.* All things being equal, the quality of decisions is obviously related to the number of *relevant* facts that are gathered and analyzed in reaching a decision. Judgment is required in determining when additional facts are needed and in determining whether it is advisable to make a decision even though all necessary facts have not been acquired or analyzed.

DEVELOPING ALTERNATIVE SOLUTIONS

After defining the problem and collecting the relevant information, the decision-maker's next activity is to develop reasonable alternative courses of action. The decision-maker should not always think in terms of "one best solution." More realistically, problems have several reasonable solutions that have both positive and negative characteristics. The task is to develop those alternatives that are satisfactory, then to choose from these the one that seems "best" in light of the solution criteria and constraints along with the costs and benefits and the advantages and disadvantages.

EVALUATING ALTERNATIVES

The effective evaluation of alternatives is a decision-making activity that is often neglected, yet it is extremely important. It is at this point that *the ramifications of each alternative should be fully explored, both in qualitative and quantitative terms.* For each alternative, three considerations should be made. First, will the alternative contribute to the attainment of objectives? In other words, will it satisfy the solution criteria? If a potential alternative does not support stated objectives, perhaps it should not be adopted.

Second, the decision-maker can ask whether the alternative is feasible or capable of execution. This incorporates not only the solution constraints but also, in practical terms, how a particular alternative will be implemented, if selected, in view of the resources that are available.

Third, the decision-maker can ask himself whether the alternative represents an acceptable degree of cost effectiveness or ineffectiveness. In other words, does the proposed solution make the maximum use of available resources relative to other uses of those resources? For example, at the program level, one might ask if society's resources are best utilized by federal support for kidney dialysis treatments or for heart research. The answer will hinge on many social and political factors. That is, what solution criteria are applied, what the solution constraints are, and how the advantages and disadvantages of two alternatives are weighed.

There may be times, of course, when "least" or "lowest" cost *should not* be used as a criterion for decision-making, especially in the area of health care, where quality considerations are so important. However, the costs involved relative to the benefits obtained for any given alternative cannot be totally ignored.

It is strongly emphasized that an *objective* and *subjective* analysis of each alternative be pursued. First, objective evaluation consists of a quantification of cost and benefits. Although some information may be hard to quantify, the attempt is urged. Second, subjective evaluation consists of being aware of those considerations (advantages and disadvantages) that cannot be quantified. The resulting sets of information from both evaluation methods should be considered simultaneously when evaluating each alternative. An intelligent decision cannot be made by considering one without the other. *Both* objective and subjective considerations should be weighed against each other and against the other alternatives. Should an alternative carry large costs, but the decision-maker stipulates that the subjective considerations must outweigh the objective considerations, a rational decision has been made. The reason is that both were considered.

CHOOSING AN ALTERNATIVE

Once the alternatives have been evaluated, one is then chosen. It should be pointed out that, typically, there is no one "best" alternative. There will be advantages and disadvantages to all of them. The example in Table 3–1 pertaining to the closing or not closing of an Obstetrics Department is a case in point. The responsibility of the decision-maker is to judge which alternative has the fewest disadvantages and/or the most advantages, both from a quantitative and nonquantitative point of view.

In addition, it may be found that the results of the objective cost–benefit evaluation should be discounted in light of subjective advantages. It is hard for the administrator to decide not to acquire equipment using a cost rationale, for example, when a subjective benefit is that "it might save a patient's life." What is the price (cost) of one life?

Since one of the constraints of decision-makers is the allocation of scarce resources, choosing among alternatives may involve consideration of where the best utilization of those resources will occur. If a decision is to be made that involves choosing between two pieces of equipment, one costing $100,000 which might save ten lives per year, and the other costing $200,000 which might save eleven lives per year, which should be selected? One might quickly say the latter. However, the answer is not that simple. To extend the situation to governmental policy level decisions, consider the following observation made by Schwartz:

> Hard questions (decisions) arise when the life that is thus painfully and expensively preserved is at or near the vegetable level. Little wonder that there is increasing public discussion of euthanasia, much more of it to date in Britain than in the United States. One reason may be that the economic consequences of unbridled humanitarianism — of the determination to keep people alive as long as possible regardless of cost or of the value of the lives preserved — are more apparent in a socialized than in a private medical system. Certainly British policymakers know that every penny spent on maintaining an eighty-year-old with respirators and the like is a penny that cannot be spent on the health care of the young and of those in productive age groups. And in this country there are hospitals where the doctors and nurses complain about the large proportion of beds occupied by old people who will never recover. In these hospitals it is very difficult to get beds for younger people whose chances of recovery are excellent and who still have energy and talents to contribute to society.[10]

---

[10] Harry Schwartz, *The Case for American Medicine.* New York: David McKay Company, Inc., 1972, p. 53. Copyright © 1972 by Harry Schwartz. Reprinted with permission of the publisher.

The purpose of this quote is to make a point—how does one weigh the objective (cost) and subjective (humanitarian) considerations relative to a decision? This quote is provocative. It indicates that decisions are often not simple or easy, particularly for those responsible for managing health care organizations. The services those organizations provide are unique in that they deal with health and life. The decision-maker must, therefore, be attuned to social, humanitarian, and ethical solution criteria when evaluating alternatives.

Once chosen, specific activities must be implemented in order to carry out the decision. The execution of these activities will consist of (1) communicating the decision to those affected, and (2) a follow-up appraisal in order to determine if the decision is being carried out as intended.

COMPREHENSIVE EXAMPLE

We have pointed out that the decision-making process involves a number of activities that enable the decision-maker to systematically focus attention on the decision to be made. It was also pointed out that each activity does not consume equal time and effort, and that a recycling phenomenon can occur. Furthermore, the nature of the decision affects the time and effort spent in making it. Specifically, some decisions are major, some are minor; some involve large amounts of resources, some little. Some can be made quickly, some take a long time to make. Some can be made relatively easily, some are difficult to make. Finally, decisions can be classified in any number of ways, ranging from administrative to programmed.

In order to present the theme that decision-making is often not an easy task, a comprehensive example displaying the activities in the decision-making process has been presented in Table 3–1. Note that it can be very difficult to attach dollars and cents to some of the alternatives. This fact of life will always be present, and it therefore causes the decision-maker's task to be more difficult. Although not all considerations have been described in the example, a sufficient number are present to enable the reader to visualize the decision-making process and its activities for a major "administrative–means–nonprogrammed" decision.[11]

FACTORS INFLUENCING DECISION-MAKING

Decision-making, whether it be individual–group, ends–means, administrative–operational, and/or programmed–nonprogrammed, does not occur in a vacuum. There are multiple factors that influence and shape the manner in which decisions are made, as well as the final outcome. Although it is not possible to include all of them in our discussion, the following will be presented: (1) the decision-maker's value system; (2) the environment and internal organizational pressures; (3) the degree of uncertainty; (4) timeliness; and (5) ex-

---

[11]For a good evaluation of an administrative decision to close two hospitals, join forces, and build a new facility, see Hoenack, op. cit.

Table 3–1 Example of a Means–Administrative–Nonprogrammed Decision

SETTING:

Lakeview hospital with more than 500 beds is located in a major metropolitan area. It is a member of a loosely organized, four hospital cooperative association that has the objectives of (1) providing high levels of patient care and (2) decreasing costs for its members. The administrators of each of the four hospitals constitute the association's executive committee, which meets monthly. A recent topic of discussion was how the four hospitals could cooperate in the sharing of services in order to reduce costs for all.

PROBLEM DEFINITION:

All four hospitals have experienced a declining occupancy rate in their Obstetrical (OB) Departments. Lakeview's was most pronounced, with an annual 43 per cent OB occupancy for its 70 OB beds. As a result, major losses have occurred, since the costs of maintaining the service were greater than revenues generated by it.

RELEVANT INFORMATION

1. General Information for Lakeview Hospital
(a) The costs of operating Lakeview's Obstetrical Department were $1,100,000 per year, while revenue generated was $750,000 per year.
(b) The State Department of Public Health will require a $1,300,000 remodeling of the OB department if the service is to be maintained.
(c) Deliveries in the area have reached an all-time low, and the birth rate is expected to decline further.
(d) The other three association hospitals are also experiencing low OB occupancy rates.
(e) If the OB service at Lakeview is reduced in terms of bed size or closed, those beds could be converted to medical/surgical (M/S) service use for an expenditure of $300,000.
(f) There is close to 100% occupancy for the medical/surgical (M/S) beds, a lengthy waiting list, and the demand will continue to increase. The cost associated with maintaining those M/S beds will be about the same as for OB beds; however, revenue would more than double because of the higher occupancy rate.

2. Solution Criteria

Lakeview's administrator delineated the following solution criteria:
(a) The decision (alternative chosen) must contribute to the fulfillment of the hospital's primary objectives of ensuring that the community's needs for service are fulfilled, contribute to quality care, and assist in keeping costs reasonable.
(b) The decision (alternative chosen) must contribute to the hospital's secondary objectives of remaining financially viable and fulfilling its responsibilities to employees.

3. Solution Constraints

Lakeview's administrator delineated the following internal and external solution constraints:
(a) It would be extremely difficult to finance the remodernization program required ($1,300,000) if OB is maintained at 70 beds; however, it would be possible to finance the remodernization ($300,000) if the beds were converted to medical/surgical.
(b) The hospital had a contract with a government agency to provide OB services to disadvantaged mothers.
(c) The hospital was unable to increase charges substantially in order to cover OB losses.
(d) It was not possible to increase materially the OB occupancy rate.
(e) If the OB service was closed, there would be a potential risk of losing gynecology surgery.
(f) The physician residency programs would be affected.
(g) The medical staff might vigorously resist any action (decision) other than retaining the OB service.

Table continues on the following page

Table 3-1   Example of a Means–Administrative–Nonprogrammed
Decision (*Continued*)

ALTERNATIVES AVAILABLE

The major alternatives available to Lakeview are:
1. Maintain the OB department at 70 beds.
2. Close the OB department without cooperating with the other association hospitals, and convert to M/S beds.
3. Close the OB department and have the other three association hospitals offer the service, and convert to M/S beds.
4. Reduce the number of OB beds to, for example, 35, which would result in an occupancy rate of approximately 85 per cent.

EVALUATION OF THE ALTERNATIVES

In order to reach an appropriate decision, the administrator of Lakeview evaluated each alternative in light of (1) the solution criteria and (2) solution constraints. In addition, each alternative was (3) evaluated by considering objective (costs–benefits) and the (4) subjective (advantages and disadvantages) factors. Owing to space limitations, only two of the four alternatives will be examined. We leave it to the reader to evaluate systematically the other two alternatives.

Alternative I

"Maintain the OB Department at 70 beds and not convert to Medical/Surgical (M/S) beds."

1. Objective Evaluation (costs)

   a. An annual loss of $350,000.
   b. Remodernization expenditures of $1,300,000, which could be used more effectively elsewhere, if available.
   c. An excess of OB beds in the area with the other association hospitals experiencing low occupancy rates. The effect is a higher total cost of OB service to the community as a whole.
   d. An opportunity loss of over twice as much revenue if the beds were classified as medical/-surgical.

2. Objective Evaluation (benefits)

   None.

3. Subjective Evaluation (advantages)

   a. Service to the community would still be provided.
   b. The hospital would retain its full service image.
   c. There would *not* be an adverse effect on the resident training program nor medical staff.
   d. The probable loss of some of the medical staff to other "full service" hospitals would be avoided.

Table 3–1   Example of a Means–Administrative–Nonprogrammed
Decision *(Continued)*

4. Subjective Evaluation (disadvantages)

    a. The waiting time for M/S would not be reduced.
    b. The present underutilization and light work-load of the OB department personnel might cause employee morale problems in other departments.

Alternative III

"Close the OB department, have the other three association hospitals offer the service and convert to Medical/Surgical (M/S) beds."

1. Objective Evaluation (costs)

    Remodernization expenditures of $300,000.

2. Objective Evaluation (benefits)

    a. Eliminate loss of $350,000/year.
    b. $1,000,000 in remodernization expenditures would not have to be made ($1,300,000 − $300,000).
    c. Other hospitals would increase occupancy rates and thus would be more efficient. Total cost to the community for OB service would decline.
    d. Total revenue generated by the 70 beds would increase from $750,000 to over $1,500,000.

3. Subjective Evaluation (advantages)

    a. Better service for M/S patients.
    b. Potential employee morale problems may be eliminated.
    c. The OB needs of the community are expected to be adequately serviced.

4. Subjective Evaluation (disadvantages)

    a. The hospital would no longer be a full service facility.
    b. The hospital might lose some of the medical staff.
    c. Residency programs will be affected.

CHOOSING THE MOST ACCEPTABLE ALTERNATIVE

The State Department of Public Health has set a deadline of six months from now for the completion of remodeling if OB service is maintained at its present level. Which alternative should be selected? Obviously it is not an easy choice. But a decision (alternative selected) has to be made.

perience. The best way to present these factors is to consider the first two separately, then to consider the last three as a group.

DECISION-MAKER'S VALUE SYSTEM

The value system of the health care decision-maker will influence the manner in which the decision is made and also shape the final outcome.[12] For example, personal characteristics, cultural background, past experiences, aspirations, and the ethics of individuals can influence the speed, willingness to accept unpleasantness, objectivity, and appropriateness of the decisions they make. Some people may make quick decisions with rather superficial evaluation because by nature they are "fast"—always on the move from one thing to another without ever fully finishing anything. Other individuals may be procrastinators who delay making a decision in the hope that the problem will go away. It is also possible to find those who do not like to make unpleasant types of decisions and "bite the bullet" instead of, for example, disciplining an employee or criticizing poor work performance.

Furthermore, the religious, racial, and sexist biases of the individual can influence the manner in which decisions are made and also the final outcome of the decision. Other personal biases, to name a few, could be: "a diploma RN is not as good as a degreed RN"; "all government employees are 'bureaucrats'," including all the negative connotations generally attached to that stereotype; and "all ward assistants are lazy." Certainly these and other biases will influence the objectivity of decisions in such areas as promotion, and possibly in discipline and the delegation of work activities.

Finally, the aspirations of an individual and his ethics may influence him to make certain decisions that may not be appropriate in terms of benefit to the organization. For example, an individual who is very ambitious might make decisions within his area of responsibility that may not be the best ones for the health care facility as a whole, but they may be best from his point of view in terms of enhancing his career—possibly building an empire.

ENVIRONMENT AND INTERNAL PRESSURES

The environment influences decision-making. Specifically, government agencies such as the Department of Health, Education, and Welfare (HEW), associations such as the Joint Commission on Accreditation of Hospitals, resource suppliers, labor unions, state and local health departments, and third-party payers, to name a few, can restrict the various options or alternatives that are available for the decision-maker to select from. They can impose solution constraints. Furthermore, many states have passed Certificate of Need legislation, which has resulted in major restraints, as has the National Health Planning and Resources Development Act of 1974.

In addition, internal pressures can stem from multiple sources in the organization. For example, pressure from one's supervisor to take quick action on a

---

[12]Hodgetts, op. cit., p. 226.

particular activity puts pressure on the individual. Pressure from peers and pressure from subordinates can also affect the manner in which a decision is made.

UNCERTAINTY, TIMELINESS, AND EXPERIENCE

Uncertainty, timeliness, and experience are three additional factors that can influence the outcome of a decision. In a great many decision situations a degree of uncertainty exists, while in other situations there is relative certainty. For example, there may not be much uncertainty pertaining to job perform- ance if a task is delegated to individual A versus individual B. However, there may be greater uncertainty attached to a decision situation that might involve expanding the organization's physical facilities or adding services. Will the demand be there? Can we effectively utilize the space? Will it necessarily enable the organization to accomplish its purpose(s)? Will technological advances make it obsolete?

With uncertainty there is always the chance that the outcome of the decision will not be as expected. Therefore, the decision made, with the occur- rence of other events and hindsight, may have been the wrong one and, therefore, could carry certain negative costs.

Timeliness is the second factor under consideration. Intuitively we are all aware that the timeliness of a decision can be crucial to its outcome. A decision made too quickly and without sufficient consideration could be a wrong decision. Stated another way, a decision made too quickly implies less informa- tion and evaluation, therefore less certainty, and the chances of a wrong decision would be greater. Furthermore, we can usually attach costs to a wrong decision.

By the same token, taking too much time to make a decision may mean that unnecessary costs will result. These costs could be in the form of lost op- portunities or the continuation of costs associated with the existing situation. Applying these concepts to the "saving of patients' lives" serves to bring forth greater awareness of the importance of timeliness. In emergencies, those providing care often cannot afford the luxury of delay. Their training is designed to develop their evaluation and decision-making skills.

Decision Model of Uncertainty, Timeliness, and Experience

The recognition that a decision needs to be made implies that there are costs associated with the present situation that will continue at the present rate or at an accelerated or decelerated rate until a decision is made and imple- mented. For example, the recognition that an ineffective billing system, which results in late bills, and therefore greater "bad debts," implies continued costs. With delay (lack of timeliness) these costs continue. This is presented by curve BB of Diagram I, which appears in Figure 3–3.

As previously mentioned, a decision made too quickly and without appro- priate information and evaluation results in greater uncertainty. Therefore, the chance or likelihood of a wrong decision is greater, and some measure of cost that a wrong decision will be made can be assigned, at least conceptually. This is represented by curve AA of Diagram I in Figure 3–3.

Viewing that diagram, the shaded area under the AA and BB cost curves

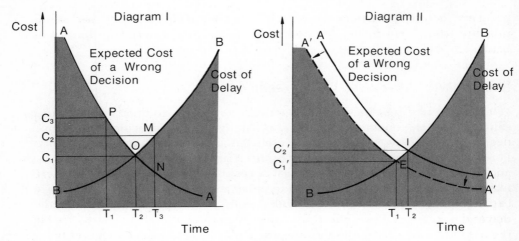

Figure 3–3   Model of uncertainty, timeliness, and experience.

represents cost. A decision made too quickly (greater uncertainty) at time T_1 could result in cost C_3. That is, there is a higher expected cost of a wrong decision (point P on curve AA) than if more time were spent evaluating and making the decision at, say, time T_2 (with cost of C_1).

Furthermore, delaying the decision to time T_3 would enable the decision-maker to collect more information, evaluate it, reduce uncertainty, reduce the likelihood of a wrong decision, and thereby reduce the expected cost of a wrong decision (point N on curve AA). However, by waiting, the cost of not making the decision continues and it would be at point M on curve BB. Thus, even by reducing the expected cost of a wrong decision, the cost of delay (C_2) would increase and be greater.

Point O at the intersection of the cost of a wrong decision curve (AA) and the cost of delay curve (BB) is the minimum cost point with a cost level of C_1. Stated another way, if the decision-maker makes his decision earlier, implying he gathers less information and does not evaluate it as well, there is movement up the AA cost curve from point O; that is, the expected cost of a wrong decision is higher. If he delays, procrastinates, and gathers more information than is necessary, there is movement up the BB cost curve from point O; that is, the cost of delay increases.

How does the decision-maker know when minimal cost will occur (point O)? How does he know if more information will enable him to reduce uncertainty? How does he know if more evaluation will be beneficial?

The answer is—the experience of the decision-maker and of those who advise the decision-maker. Experience has the primary benefit of generally enabling the decision-maker to compress the time factor and thereby benefit from the timeliness of decisions, as conceptually presented in Diagram II of Figure 3–3. He is often able to recognize quickly that he is confronted with a situation that requires a decision to be made. He tends to think very quickly through the decision-making process in terms of defining the problem, gathering the relevant information, deciding how much information he needs, determining how quickly he should make the decision in terms of timeliness, how beneficial further information gathering and evaluation would be, what his range of alternatives is, and making a quick but appropriate evaluation of those alternatives. He is able to weigh the elements without immersing himself in vast quantities of paperwork, unnecessary information collection, and irrelevant evaluations. That is, he can quickly conceptualize the parameters of the situation and the solution criteria and constraints, and assimilate the information.

These skills, gained from experience, have the effect of shifting the expected cost of a wrong decision curve (AA) to the left, as noted by curve AA' in Diagram II of Figure 3–3. The implication of this shift is that the experienced decision-maker can arrive at the *same decision* as an inexperienced decision-maker, but quicker. Thus, there is a lower cost (optimum) point (the difference between C'_2 and C'_1) for the experienced decision-maker (point E) than for the inexperienced individual (point I), since the costs of delay would not be as great.

To the inexperienced individual the skills of the experienced decision-maker may appear to be intuitive. The less-experienced may take a very methodical approach to the decision-making process and can encounter problems when trying to emulate the more experienced decision-maker. (Note the difference between an extern and a head resident.) The point to be made is that knowing when to make the decision, when to delay and gather more information, and when to evaluate alternatives in greater depth is not easy. Also, there is a point when the cost of delaying becomes greater if a decision is not made. There is also a range when a premature decision could be more costly than delay. With experience, the decision-maker is better able to balance uncertainty and timeliness by realizing their influence on the outcome of a decision. Unfortunately experience cannot be taught; however, we can all be made aware of its importance.

It is valuable to note the different approaches to the decision-making processes among health care professionals. When a physician, nurse, medical technologist, or pharmacist makes a patient care decision, he or she is drawing upon the scientific and technological training they have undergone and upon the experience they have had. When these health care professionals become supervisors, department heads, or heads of services, they undoubtedly will be required to make managerial decisions (planning, organizing, executing, controlling) involving resources, which will be quite different from the type of patient care decisions to which they have been accustomed. Furthermore, a different approach, frame of reference, and perspective are required. Instead of being concerned solely with direct patient care, they will have to be concerned with those things necessary to maintain the organizational environment, which will enable the effective and efficient delivery of patient care to occur. As a result, the physician serving in an administrative role will have to shift from an individualistic, unilateral approach used when making patient care decisions to perhaps one that will solicit group input of those who are his administrative peers in the organization hierarchy. By the same token, the registered nurse who becomes a nurse supervisor will have to divert her attention and decision-making from solely patient-care matters to those involving the planning of activities, organizing of work-group effort, executing activities for which she is responsible, and controlling to ensure that her subordinates are doing what they are supposed to be doing.

SUMMARY

This chapter presented the subject of decision-making, which was defined as the *selection from among alternatives.* The nature of decision-making was presented as being common, pervasive, dynamic, and never-ending. In addition, various *non-mutually exclusive* classifications of decisions were made. The activities of the decision-making process were presented, which range from being aware that a decision needs to be made, to the selection from alternatives subsequent to their evaluation.

A comprehensive example of the decision-making process was presented in Table 3–1, with the purpose of demonstrating its wide scope and complexity. Numerous factors that influence decision-making were discussed — among them, uncertainty, timeliness, and experience. Finally, two themes were developed: first, that *decision-making is common to the other processes* of planning, organizing, executing, and controlling. Each of those processes requires that decisions be made and, as a result, decision-making is an integral part of the remainder of this book.

The second theme developed was that the activities characteristic of the decision-making process are not isolated cells consuming the same amount of time and effort. Although sequence may be implied, there is recycling, and the activities are considered differently, in terms of intensity of focus and time, by different decision-makers in different decision-making situations.

DISCUSSION QUESTIONS

1. Explain why "the level of effectiveness and efficiency in a health care organization is directly related to the quality of problem solving and decision-making."

2. List the major characteristics of decision-making, and indicate why each is a major characteristic.

3. Give examples of various decisions, classify them as you think appropriate, and identify the elements that support your classifications.

4. Prepare to discuss the situation portrayed in the quote on page 39 by making a list of the pros and cons of the two alternatives. What solution criteria and constraints are appropriate? If you were in a position to make a decision, what would you do?

5. Presuming you are the administrator, use the information given in Table 3–1 and make a decision by selecting alternative 1 or 3. What steps would you take in order to implement your decision? What would be the likely reactions of other organization members?

6. Presume that you are the administrator of an urban hospital, and because of changing demographic patterns, loss of medical staff, and aging physical facilities, you are considering the alternative of relocating the facility. During the past four months

you have been collecting information, looking at several tracts of land, which do not have hospitals in close proximity, and working on the financial arrangements. So far, you are *not* convinced that the move would be beneficial. For one thing, it would be less costly to remodel your present facility than to build a new one, and for another, you are not sure how you could dispose of your present facility. In addition, if you move you would cause hardship on the population living in the area which you currently serve. Finally, many of your employees will not have transportation to any of the new sites.

Presume that one tract of land is significantly more suitable in terms of location and cost than any of the others, and that your option to buy expires in six months and cannot be renewed. Assume that it will take you three more months to complete your evaluation of all of the ramifications, benefits, and disadvantages of relocating.

Using the model in Figure 3–3, graphically demonstrate and discuss what would happen if you just found out that one of the five zoning commission members in the community where the most preferred tract of land is located will resign in one month and will not be replaced until the next election, 12 months from now. Furthermore, you know that the land is currently zoned for multiple family dwellings and that two of the commissioners would not vote favorably on your petition to rezone the land, while three, including the commission member who will resign, would vote favorably on your petition. (A majority vote is needed to rezone.) Finally, in order for a vote to be held, the land must be purchased.

This Chapter Contains:

- Introduction
- Break-even Analysis
- Capital Budgeting Techniques
- Decision-Making Under Uncertainty
- Statistical Methods
- Simulation
- Summary
- Discussion Questions
- Problems

Chapter 4

QUANTITATIVE DECISION-MAKING TECHNIQUES

INTRODUCTION

There are a number of decision-making techniques which may assist the decision-maker in evaluating alternatives. Emory and Niland state that "decision techniques comprise a body of details or methods" and "they range in scope and sophistication from simple intuitive action to complex mathematical designs."[1] This chapter is a sequel to the preceding chapter, "Managerial Decision-making," which presented an overview of the decision-making process. Its purpose is to describe simply various quantitative techniques which can be of assistance to those having decision-making responsibility.

Since World War II many quantitative techniques, such as mathematical programming, simulation modeling, and systems analysis have been developed.[2] Our purpose is not to present in detail all quantitative techniques, but to describe generally and to present the applicability of selected techniques to health care organizations.[3] The following techniques will be presented: (1) break-even analysis; (2) payback; (3) net present value; (4) decision-making under uncertainty; (5) statistical methods; and (6) simulation.

Before proceeding, it should be pointed out that each technique is presented in its *simplest* form without including the multiple variations each can

---

[1] C. William Emory, and Powell Niland, *Making Management Decisions*. New York: Houghton Mifflin Company, 1968, p. 2.

[2] For a presentation of a number of the methods see the following:

(a) John R. Griffith, *Quantitative Techniques for Hospital Planning and Control*. Lexington, Massachusetts: Lexington Books, 1972.

(b) Russell C. Koza, *Mathematical and Operations Research Techniques in Health Administration*. Boulder, Colorado: Colorado Associated University Press, 1973.

(c) Richard I. Levin, and Charles A. Kirkpatrick, *Quantitative Approaches to Management*. New York: McGraw-Hill Book Company, 1971.

(d) David W. Miller, and Martin K. Starr, *The Structure of Decisions*. Englewood Cliffs, New Jersey: Prentice-Hall, Inc., 1967.

(e) C. M. Paik, *Quantitative Methods for Managerial Decisions*. New York: McGraw-Hill Book Company, 1973.

[3] For an overview of various applications see the following:

(a) Robert L. Gue, "Operations research in health and hospital administration." *Hospital Administration*, *10*:No. 4, Fall, 1965.

(b) Robert B. Fetter, and John D. Thompson, "Patients' waiting time and doctors' idle time in the out-patient setting." *Health Services Research*, Summer, 1966.

(c) Gordon H. Robinson, Paul Wing, and Louis E. Davis, "Computer simulation of hospital patient scheduling systems." *Health Services Research*, *3*:No. 2., Summer, 1968.

(d) David H. Stimson, and Ruth H. Stimson, *Operations Research in Hospitals: Diagnosis and Prognosis*. Chicago: Hospital Research and Educational Trust, 1972.

(e) George R. Wren, *Modern Health Administration*. Athens, Georgia: University of Georgia Press, 1974.

have or the various conditions which would make them more complex. Our purpose is not to make the reader skilled in each application, but only to acquaint him with a general review of selected techniques. To that end, the selected techniques and example problems presented will be relatively un-complicated. For the reader interested in reviewing these techniques in greater detail, it is suggested that he refer to a text specifically written on the subject.

Furthermore, we should indicate that a quantitative evaluation of alterna-tives should not be the only criterion for selection. Health care decisions cannot be based solely on costs, revenues, and profits. While these techniques provide quantitative information, subjective (nonquantitative) considerations should always be given to possible alternatives. Both approaches should be considered before making a decision.

BREAK-EVEN ANALYSIS

Break-even analysis is one of the simplest quantitative decision-making techniques which can be used to evaluate alternatives.[4] The important compo-nents of break-even analysis are as follows: (1) the revenue (R) per unit of ser-vice; (2) the amount of fixed cost (FC) associated with providing the service (those costs which will be incurred regardless of the level of service provided); and (3) the variable costs (VC) associated with providing the service (those costs that would not be incurred if service is not provided or continued). The tech-nique provides a means by which the volume of output needed to "break-even" (i.e., to cover fixed costs and variable costs) can be determined. Any output level above the break-even point would contribute to profit while a volume level below it would result in a loss where costs both fixed and variable exceed reve-nue.

Break-even analysis must be applied carefully in health care settings. Many of the third-party reimbursement mechanisms are based on reimbursing the provider at the level of cost of providing services. For this reason, setting a price for the service based on estimates which later produce a profit (excess revenues over expenditures) may not be possible. Even so, this technique can be useful to the decision-maker who needs to know the volume of a service needed to "break-even" or to cover both fixed and variable costs.

APPLICATIONS

There are many situations in health care organizations where break-even analysis can be applied. Obviously the results derived from break-even analysis should not be the sole criterion for alternative selection; however, it can serve as a useful tool to ascertain the "over-all" feasibility, or "ball park" bene-fits — disadvantages of the alternative under consideration.

Break-even analysis can be used to evaluate any situation which contains volume, cost, and revenue elements; for example, the addition of a new wing to a hospital, the building of a new long-term care facility in the community, or

---

[4]For a clear discussion of break-even analysis see Levin and Kirkpatrick, *Quantitative Approaches to Management*, Chapter 2.

the establishment of a neighborhood health center. Others might be whether or not to add additional services such as rehabilitative, to convert OB to general surgical beds, to subcontract emergency service to a group of physicians, or to have the hospital run the emergency department itself, and whether the usage (volume) of a new x-ray machine would be profitable or unprofitable.

Problem Example

Take, for instance, the consideration by a hospital to add a family practice center. The alternatives are to add or not to add that service. Normally the decision-maker can estimate the fixed and variable costs that would be associated with the alternative to "add the center." If he knows the level of demand, he can then determine, through break-even analysis, what charge (revenue per unit of service) would be necessary for the center to break-even (not incur a loss). Or, if a standard charge is predetermined, he can then determine what volume of service would be necessary to break-even.

Presume that an adjacent building can be purchased for $1,000,000 and will entail a $300,000 remodeling expense. Also presume the following:

1. A service charge of $10 per patient is contemplated. This is the charge made by the organization and does not include the doctor's fee, which is billed separately. Thus, revenue per unit of service to the health care organization will be ten dollars.

2. The *annual* fixed costs are considered to be as follows: (a) depreciation at 5 per cent of the building acquisition and remodeling costs per year (straight line depreciation is over 20 years), or $65,000 per year; (b) heat and electricity are estimated to be $6000 per year; and (c) the depreciation of equipment acquired and periodic replacement of equipment which will average $10,000 per year.

3. The variable costs for employees wages (one R.N.), supplies, etc., are $2 per patient served.

DETERMINATION OF NUMBER OF UNITS OF SERVICE REQUIRED TO BREAK-EVEN: CHARGE GIVEN.

The break-even point is reached when total revenue (RX), which is the charge per unit of service ($10) times the number of people serviced (X), equals total cost (TC). Total cost consists of fixed costs (FC) plus variable costs (VC). Profit or loss (P) is the difference between total cost (TC) and total revenue (RX). When P is set at zero, the break-even point can be determined from the following formula:

$$\text{Break-even point (X)} = \frac{TC + P}{R}$$

or

$$R(X) = TC + P$$

or

$$R(X) = FC + VC + P$$

Using the information given, the equation is:

$$\$10\,(X) = (\$65,000 + \$6000 + \$10,000) + \$2\,(X) + \$0$$

To determine the number of units of service required each year in order to break-even, given the service charge of $10, we must solve for X and set profit at zero. Transferring $2 (X) to the left side of the equation we obtain

$$\$10\ (X) - \$2\ (X) = \$65,000 + \$6000 + \$10,000$$

or

$$\$8\ (X) = \$81,000$$

Dividing both sides of the equation by $8 we obtain

$$(X) = \frac{\$81,000}{\$8}$$

or

$$(X) = 10,125 \text{ units of service}$$

Given the $10 service charge, 10,125 patients per year, or 27.7 per day (10,125 ÷ 365), would have to be serviced in order for the family practice center to break-even, that is, for total revenue to equal fixed and variable costs. This is illustrated in Figure 4–1.

BREAK-EVEN CHART

Figure 4–1 is a graphic portrayal of the information stated in the problem and its solution. The figure demonstrates the following:

1. The fixed cost (FC) line represents the fixed costs ($81,000) associated

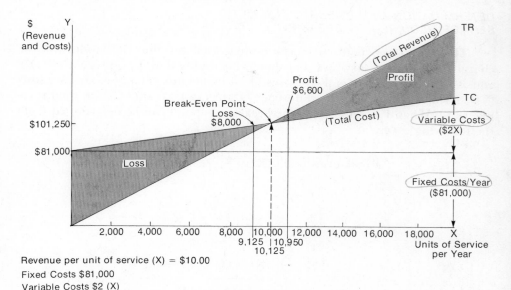

Figure 4–1   Break-even analysis, family practice center.

with the alternative (add the family practice center). Those costs would be incurred whether the center serviced one, 10,000 or 18,000 people each year.

2. The total cost (TC) line starts at $81,000 on the Y axis and slopes upward to the right. The height of the TC curve represents the sum of fixed cost (FC) and variable cost (VC) for a given volume of service which is noted on the X axis (recall that TC = FC + VC). Since variable cost is $2 per person served, variable cost increases as more people are serviced and it is added to the fixed cost. Thus, variable cost is TC − FC for any given number of people serviced. Note that if one person was treated the variable cost would be $2 and total cost would be $81,002. If 10,000 people were serviced each year variable cost would be $20,000, and total cost would be $101,000 ($81,000 + $20,000).

3. The total revenue (TR) line starts at the origin and slopes upward. It is determined simply by multiplying the service charge ($10) by the number of people serviced (X). If one person were serviced, total revenue would be $10. If 10,000 people were serviced, total revenue would be $100,000.

4. The break-even point is determined when TR = TC. The intersection of these lines would be at a volume level of 10,125 people (total revenue = $101,250 and total cost = $101,250).

5. If less than 10,125 people were serviced each year, TC would be greater than TR, and a loss would result. This is noted by the shaded area to the left of the break-even point between the TR and TC curves. The loss is represented by the vertical distance between the TR and TC curves for any given level of service (X), and the dollar amount is read off the Y axis. If, for example, one person were serviced, there would be a loss. Cost would be the sum of the fixed cost of $81,000 and variable cost of $2 or $81,002. The revenue would be $10; therefore, costs would exceed revenues by $80,992. If 8000 people were treated, the loss would be $17,000. It would be determined by TR − TC; at X = 8000 (or $80,000 − $97,000 = loss $17,000).

6. If more than 10,125 people (break-even point) were serviced each year, there would be a profit from the operation because TR would exceed TC. This is noted in the shaded area to the right of the break-even point between the TR and TC curves. The profit is represented by the vertical distance between the TR and TC curves for any given level of service (X). If, for example, 12,000 people were serviced each year, the profit would be $15,000 (TR − TC, at X = 12,000). If 16,000 people were serviced each year, the profit would be $47,000 (TR − TC, at X = 16,000).

The break-even chart can be a useful tool in evaluating alternatives. It represents, in graphic form, the break-even formula and can be used in place of the algebraic computation.

DETERMINATION OF PROFIT OR LOSS: CHARGE AND ANNUAL UNITS OF SERVICE GIVEN.

Continuing our example, if the decision-maker determined that the maximum number of people that could be serviced each day was only 25 (9125 per year) because of space and personnel limitations (capacity) or owing to the limits of demand in the area, given the $10 service charge, there would be a loss of $8000 from the operation (see Fig. 4–1 for a graphic presentation). It would be calculated algebraically as follows:

$$R (X) = TC + P$$

$$R (X) = FC + VC + P$$

$$\$10 (X) = \$81,000 + \$2 (X) + P$$

$$\text{knowing } X = 9125$$

$$\$10 (9125) = \$81,000 + \$2 (9125) + P$$

Transferring:

$$\$10 (9125) - \$2 (9125) = \$81,000 + P$$

Reducing:

$$\$8 (9125) = \$81,000 + P$$

Multiplying:

$$\$73,000 = \$81,000 + P$$

Solving for P:

$$P = \$73,000 - \$81,000$$

$$P \text{ (profit or loss)} = -\$8000 \text{ per year}$$

If the decision-maker determined that the demand would be 30 people per day, or 10,950 per year, given the $10 service charge there would be a profit of $6600 from the family practice center (see Fig. 4–1 for graphic presentation). The algebraic calculation follows:

$$R (X) = TC + P$$

$$R (X) = FC + VC + P$$

$$\$10 (X) = \$81,000 + \$2 (X) + P$$

$$\text{knowing } X = 10,950$$

$$\$10 (10,950) = \$81,000 + \$2 (10,950) + P$$

Transferring:

$$\$10 (10,950) - \$2 (10,950) = \$81,000 + P$$

Reducing:

$$\$8 (10,950) = \$81,000 + P$$

Multiplying:

$$\$87,600 = \$81,000 + P$$

Solving for P:

$$P = \$87,600 - \$81,000$$

$$P \text{ (Profit)} = \$6600 \text{ per year}$$

DETERMINATION OF SERVICE CHARGE TO BREAK-EVEN:
NUMBER OF UNITS OF SERVICE FIXED.

We previously mentioned that if the number of units of service per year (demand) is known (presume 25 per day, or 9125 per year), it is possible to determine the charge needed to break even, when profit (P) is set at zero. Using the same fixed and variable costs, we can solve for the necessary service charge (R) as follows:

The break-even formula is: $R(X) = FC + VC + P$

given demand, $X = 9125$:

$R(9125) = \$81,000 + \$18,250$

dividing both sides of the equation by 9125

$$R = \frac{99,250}{9125}$$

$$R = \$10.88$$

Thus, the service charge required to break-even when a demand of 9125 per year is known is $10.88 per unit of service.

In summary, break-even analysis is a very useful technique for assisting the decision-maker. By knowing the fixed and variable costs associated with an alternative, in our case to add or not to add a family practice center, he can determine the following:

1. Given the service charge and costs, it is possible to determine the volume of service needed to break-even.

2. Given the volume of service (demand), service charge, and costs, it is possible to determine if and how profitable or unprofitable the alternative would be.

3. Given the volume of service and costs, it is possible to determine what the service charge (revenue) must be in order to break-even.

Since it is possible to make these determinations, the information can be helpful to the decision-maker in terms of choosing or not choosing the alternative.

CAPITAL BUDGETING TECHNIQUES

Capital budgeting is the common name given to a group of techniques used for the evaluation of investment alternatives. Those techniques range from payback to internal rate of return to net present value. All but the former require the specification of an interest rate or rate of return.[5] Of the three techniques, payback is the one most commonly used by health care organization decision-makers.[6]

---

[5]For a discussion of the problems inherent in capital budgeting see Roland J. Knobel, and Beaufort B. Longest, Jr., "Cost-benefit assumption in analysis for hospitals. *Financial Management*, 1:64. Spring, 1971.

[6]John Daniel Williams, and Jonathon S. Rakich, "Investment evaluation in hospitals." *Financial Management*, 2:32. Summer, 1973.

PAYBACK TECHNIQUE

Investment alternatives for health care organizations can range from new building programs to the acquisition of equipment, ranging from sophisticated diagnostic and treatment machines to computer systems. Payback essentially determines the length of time required to return the original cost of the investment. Given the fact that the health care decision-maker has limited resources available, he must have some priority system for allocating those resources among various alternatives. When multiple alternatives are evaluated simultaneously, using payback for example, an objective quantitative priority scheme evolves.

The payback technique contains two basic elements. The first is the net investment (NI), which is the cost of the investment (I) less the salvage value (S). The second is the annual net benefit (NB) that would be derived from that investment if it were selected. The net benefit for an alternative is determined by revenues (R) generated plus cost savings (CS) minus the operating expenses (OE) of the alternative under consideration. By dividing the net benefit (NB) into the net cost of the investment (NI), the number of years to return the cost of the investment is determined.[7]

The general formula for the payback period (PBP) would be as follows:

$$PBP = \frac{NI}{NB}$$

or

$$\frac{(\text{Cost of the proposed investment}) - (\text{salvage value})}{\left(\begin{array}{l}\text{revenue generated}\\\text{from the investment}\end{array}\right) + \left(\begin{array}{l}\text{cost saving}\\\text{that would}\\\text{result from}\\\text{the investment}\end{array}\right) - \left(\begin{array}{l}\text{operating}\\\text{expenses}\end{array}\right)}$$

or

$$\frac{NI}{NB} = \frac{I - S}{(R + CS) - OE}$$

It should be pointed out that more than one investment alternative has to be considered; the NB has to be determined relative to another alternative and/or the present situation. Furthermore, adjustments must be made if the investments do not have the same life span. To examine fully the payback method, an example of its use is presented next.

Problem Example

The business office manager of a health care organization is considering the acquisition of one of two pieces of equipment. He has defined his problem to be that his personnel are overworked. As a result, one way of solving the problem is to acquire equipment which would reduce the work load. A second alternative consists of hiring

---

[7]For a discussion of the payback techniques see Paul E. Torgensen, and Irwin J. Weinstock, *Management: An Integrated Approach.* Englewood Cliffs, New Jersey: Prentice-Hall, 1972, Chapter 8.

more personnel; however, a solution constraint consisting of a freeze on net new personnel additions does not make that feasible. Therefore, he has to decide which of the two
pieces of equipment to purchase.

The first piece of equipment being considered is a photocopying machine and the
second is a teletype machine linked to the local Blue Cross office. The former is desirable because it would eliminate the need for using carbon paper. The teletype machine
is desirable because it would eliminate the necessity for the office personnel continually
calling the Blue Cross office for insurance verification.

The department manager has a limited capital equipment budget and can only
purchase one of the machines. Given the information below, and using payback as a
technique to evaluate quantitatively the two equipment alternatives, which should he
buy?

It was found that the photocopying machine would cost $11,800 to purchase, and
it would have a salvage (trade-in or scrap) value of $4000 at the end of its useful life,
which is four years. No revenue would be generated; however, there would be cost
savings in the form of (a) reduced clerical time in using carbons, (b) decreased carbon
paper costs, and (c) a 10 per cent increase in the volume of work performed. Those
savings were estimated to be a total of $4000 per year. However, if the photocopying
machine is acquired, there will be a $1000 per year paper expense (operating expense)
that would not otherwise be incurred if it were not acquired.

When evaluating the teletype machine it was found that its purchase cost would
be $10,000, and it would have a salvage value of $2000 at the end of its useful life,
which is four years. No revenue would be generated, but the cost savings in (a) clerical
time wasted waiting on the telephone, (b) the reduced number of phone lines necessary,
(c) reduction in oral communication errors, and (d) a 5 per cent increase in the volume
of work performed would result in cost savings of $3500 per year. However, if the tele-
type is acquired, a special phone line would have to be leased at a cost of $500 per year
(operating expense).

Table 4–1 displays the calculation of the payback period (the number of years to
return the cost of original investment, less salvage) for both investment alternatives.
The payback period is 2.60 years for the photocopying machine and 2.67 years for the
teletype machine. Thus, the payback evaluation technique would indicate that the photocopying machine should be acquired if no other factors were considered.

PRESENT VALUE TECHNIQUE

One limitation of using the payback technique to evaluate alternatives is
that it does not consider the "time value of money." The present value tech-

Table 4–1   Payback Evaluation of Two Equipment Alternatives

	PHOTOCOPYING MACHINE	TELETYPE MACHINE
I (Investment cost)	$11,800	$10,000
–S (Salvage)	–4,000	–2,000
NI (Net Investment)	$ 7,800	$ 8,000
R (Revenue generated)	$ 0	$ 0
+CS (Cost savings)	4,000	3,500
–OE (Operating expenses)	–1,000	–500
NB	$ 3,000	$ 3,000
PAYBACK PERIOD $= \dfrac{\text{NI}}{\text{NB}}$	$\dfrac{\$7,800}{3,000} = 2.60$ years	$\dfrac{\$8,000}{3,000} = 2.67$ years

nique is a means by which alternatives can be evaluated with the consideration of the time value of money.[8]

Intuitively, we are all aware that a dollar is worth more today than a dollar that is to be received at some future time. In other words, money received a year from now, say $1000, is not worth as much as the $1000 today. The reason is the "time value of money." Specifically, if you had $1000 today and invested it, thereby generating a return of, say, 10 per cent per year, that $1000 would become $1100 a year from now. Consequently, $1000 received a year from now versus today would be worth less by reason of the fact that the potential earnings (return on investment) possible from having it today would be foregone.

Applications.   There are many decisions that are made in health care organizations in which the time value of money may be an important consideration when evaluating alternatives. Let's take an example that would affect most of us. Presume that an organization currently pays its employees at the end of each month, and that the total monthly payroll is $300,000. What effect would there be if the pay period were changed and the employees were paid every two weeks—half of the regular month's pay at the middle of the month ($150,000), and half at the end of the month ($150,000)? The net effect would be that half of the monthly payroll ($150,000) would be paid two weeks earlier than before. Since the total paid out each month would still be $300,000, would it make any difference? Certainly! The organization would be paying out $150,000 two weeks earlier than before. As a result, it would lose or forego the gain (say interest) that it could earn on $150,000 for two weeks. By the same token, the employees would benefit by receiving one-half of their monthly pay two weeks earlier than usual. They could simply place it in a savings account and earn interest.

As demonstrated by this example, the timing of fund flows, both costs (the organization paying part of the payroll earlier) and revenues (the employees getting part of their pay earlier than usual), does have an effect. Whether it is beneficial depends upon whether you are on the receipt or disbursement side. Therefore, any major decision to be made relative to the alternatives of (A) pay earlier or (B) do not pay earlier should consider the time value of money.

In health care organizations, decisions to be made which would affect the flow of funds (revenues and costs) can usefully consider the time value of money. Payroll is one example; billing is another. Is there a benefit to sending out bills promptly to private or third-party payers on the assumption that they would pay sooner than if the bills were mailed out later? Would there be a benefit to installing a computerized billing system versus having a manual system, presuming the former is faster? What happens when the state delays paying Medicaid charges for six months versus three months? Why do doctors dislike submitting Medicare claims?

We can also look at the disbursement side of the funds flow. Would the organization be better off by paying its bills later than usual? Yes, there is a benefit, but what is the "cost" of losing the supplier's goodwill? Is there a

---

[8]For a discussion of present value see Raymond R. Mayer, *Production and Operations Management.* New York: McGraw-Hill, 1975, Chapter 6.

benefit to paying a bill within 10 days if there is a 2 per cent cash discount? To answer these questions we have to consider the time value of money, that is, the potential return derived from retaining funds longer. Another category of decisions where the flow of funds and their timing can be important is investment decisions. This category can include capital expansion and equipment acquisition.

COMPOUND INTEREST

In order to clarify the present value concept, it is first necessary to present the other side of the coin — compound interest which is the return on some principal. If the interest rate (i) were 10 per cent and the principal (p) $1000, the compound interest formula for determining one's return a given number of years (n) from now would be calculated as follows:

$$p(1+i)^n$$ where p = principal
$$i = \text{rate of interest}$$
$$n = \text{number of years}$$

The value received one year from now would be:

$$p(1+i)^1$$

or

$$\$1000(1+.10)^1 = \$1000(1.10)$$

or

$$\$1100$$

The value received two years from now would be:

$$p(1+i)^2$$

or

$$p(1.10)^2$$

or

$$\$1000(1.21) = \$1210$$

Using the concept of interest, we could say that a person would be indifferent if he received $1000 today or $1100 a year from now or $1210 two years from now. The reason is that, if he had the money today, he could invest it at 10 per cent and would have $1100 a year from now. Either way, he is indifferent because he is equally well off. However, he would not be equally well off if he only received $1000 a year from now versus the same amount today.

PRESENT VALUE (DISCOUNTING)

Just as we can determine the compound interest return on a principal invested today over a period of time, we can also determine the compound interest or return on investment *lost* by not having the principal available today. This is known as discounting, and it is central to the understanding of the concept of present value.

The discounting (present value) formula is as follows:[9]

$$P \frac{1}{(1 + i)^n} \text{ where } p = \text{ the principal}$$

$$i = \text{ the interest rate}$$

$$n = \text{ the number of years}$$

The same principal, $1000, to be received a year from now will be used for illustrative purposes. The i is the rate of interest one could receive if the principal were invested, or it can be viewed as opportunity return *lost* by not having the principal today to invest, that is, losing the benefit that could be obtained from using the principal for something else, such as buying new equipment.

The value today of the $1000 that is to be obtained one year from now would be:

$$P \frac{1}{(1 + i)^1}$$

or

$$\$1000 \frac{1}{(1 + i)^1}$$

or

$$\frac{\$1000}{(1 + .10)^1} = \$909.09$$

That is, if $1000 were to be given to you one year from now you would be indifferent to receiving it then or $909.09 today. The reason is that if you received the $909.09 today, you could invest it today at 10 per cent interest and have $999.99 one year from now.

$$p (1 + .10)^1$$

or

$$\$909.09 (1.10) = \$999.99$$

---

[9]Erich A. Helfert, *Techniques of Financial Analysis.* Homewood, Illinois: Richard D. Irwin, Inc., 1967, p. 158.

Similarly, if you were to receive $1000 two years from now it would only be worth $826.45 today. The calculation follows:

$$P \frac{1}{(1 + i)^n}$$

$$P \frac{1}{(1 + i)^2}$$

$$P \frac{1}{(1 + .10)^2}$$

$$\$1000 \times \frac{1}{(1.21)}$$

or

$$\frac{\$1000}{1.21} = \$826.45$$

Thus the *present value* (worth today) of $1000 to be received two years from now is only $826.45 because of the time value of money. The importance of this concept lies in the fact that investment alternatives may have dissimilar revenue (money to be received) and cost (money to be paid out) flows in terms of time. *Therefore, to truly determine the impact of those different flows, all revenues and costs to occur in the future should be discounted to their present value. In this way, they can be appropriately compared with each other, since there is a common basis for comparison.*

Two investments which require the same amount of capital (cost the same) but which generate revenues or costs differently are not equal in terms of merit. We will use a simple example with an i of 10 per cent for two investments which cost the same amount. Alternative A, which generates $2000 in revenue (costs are ignored so as not to complicate the example) two years from now, would not be as beneficial as alternative B, which generates revenue of $1000 at the end of each of the two years. The reason is their different revenue flows in terms of time.

The present value of the revenue ($2000) to be received at the end of year 2 for alternative A would be:

$$\frac{\$2000}{(1 + .1)^2} = \frac{\$2000}{1.21} = \$1652.89$$

The present value of the revenue ($1000) to be received at the end of year 1 for alternative B would be:

$$\frac{\$1000}{(1 + .1)^1} = \frac{\$1000}{1.1} = \$909.09$$

The present value of the revenue ($1000) to be received at the end of year 2 for alternative B would be:

$$\frac{\$1000}{(1+.1)^2} = \frac{\$1000}{1.21} = \$826.45$$

for a total of $1735.54 ($909.09 + $826.45).

Thus alternative B is the preferred of the two because it generates revenue sooner and therefore has a higher present value than does alternative A, even though the nominal amount ($2000) is the same for both.

Present Value Table. In Table 4–2, present value factors for single payments (PVsP) for varying years and rates of interest (opportunity cost) are presented. The factors are the calculated $\frac{1}{(1+i)^n}$ values for the year and interest rate noted. All that is necessary is to multiply PVsP by the revenue or cost flow. For example, the PVsP factor for a sum, say $200, to be received three years from now can be found by moving across the "3 year hence" row to the column with the i to be used. If the interest rate we were using were 8 per cent,

Table 4–2 Present Value Single Payment Factors*

PV_{sp}, Present Value Factors for Future Single Payments

Years Hence	1%	2%	4%	6%	8%	10%	12%	14%	15%	16%	18%	20%
1	0.990	0.980	0.962	0.943	0.926	0.909	0.893	0.877	0.870	0.862	0.847	0.833
2	0.980	0.961	0.925	0.890	0.857	0.826	0.797	0.769	0.756	0.743	0.718	0.694
3	0.971	0.942	0.889	0.840	0.794	0.751	0.712	0.675	0.658	0.641	0.609	0.579
4	0.691	0.924	0.855	0.792	0.735	0.683	0.636	0.592	0.572	0.552	0.516	0.482
5	0.951	0.906	0.822	0.747	0.681	0.621	0.567	0.519	0.497	0.476	0.437	0.402
6	0.942	0.888	0.790	0.705	0.630	0.564	0.507	0.456	0.432	0.410	0.370	0.335
7	0.933	0.871	0.760	0.665	0.583	0.513	0.452	0.400	0.376	0.354	0.314	0.279
8	0.923	0.853	0.731	0.627	0.540	0.467	0.404	0.351	0.327	0.305	0.266	0.233
9	0.914	0.837	0.703	0.592	0.500	0.424	0.361	0.308	0.284	0.263	0.225	0.194
10	0.905	0.820	0.676	0.558	0.463	0.386	0.322	0.270	0.247	0.227	0.191	0.162
11	0.896	0.804	0.650	0.527	0.429	0.350	0.287	0.237	0.215	0.195	0.162	0.135
12	0.887	0.788	0.625	0.497	0.397	0.319	0.257	0.208	0.187	0.168	0.137	0.112
13	0.879	0.773	0.601	0.469	0.368	0.290	0.229	0.182	0.163	0.145	0.116	0.093
14	0.870	0.758	0.577	0.442	0.340	0.263	0.205	0.160	0.141	0.125	0.099	0.078
15	0.861	0.743	0.555	0.417	0.315	0.239	0.183	0.140	0.123	0.108	0.084	0.065
16	0.853	0.728	0.534	0.394	0.292	0.218	0.163	0.123	0.107	0.093	0.071	0.054
17	0.844	0.714	0.513	0.371	0.270	0.198	0.146	0.108	0.093	0.080	0.060	0.045
18	0.836	0.700	0.494	0.350	0.250	0.180	0.130	0.095	0.081	0.069	0.051	0.038
19	0.828	0.686	0.475	0.331	0.232	0.164	0.116	0.083	0.070	0.060	0.043	0.031
20	0.820	0.673	0.456	0.312	0.215	0.149	0.104	0.073	0.061	0.051	0.037	0.026
21	0.811	0.660	0.439	0.294	0.199	0.135	0.093	0.064	0.053	0.044	0.031	0.022
22	0.803	0.647	0.422	0.278	0.184	0.123	0.083	0.056	0.046	0.038	0.026	0.018
23	0.795	0.634	0.406	0.262	0.170	0.112	0.074	0.049	0.040	0.033	0.022	0.015
24	0.788	0.622	0.390	0.247	0.158	0.102	0.066	0.043	0.035	0.028	0.019	0.013
25	0.780	0.610	0.375	0.233	0.146	0.092	0.059	0.038	0.030	0.024	0.016	0.010

*Source: Elwood S. Buffa, *Basic Production Management*. New York: John Wiley & Sons, Inc., 1972, p. 614. Reprinted by permission of John Wiley & Sons, Inc.

the PVsP factor would be .794. The present value of that $200 to be received three years from now could be (.794) times $200, or $158.80.

Present Value Index (PVI).[10] To repeat, the present value technique enables the decision-maker to evaluate the effect of differences in revenue and expenditure flows relative to time among alternatives. A means by which two or more alternatives can be compared with each other is to develop a present value index (PVI). The formula is as follows:

$$\ast \quad PVI = \frac{\text{Present Value (PV) of net operating benefit}}{\text{Present Value (PV) of the net investment}}$$

or

$$\frac{\text{PV (Revenue Generated)} + \text{PV (cost saved)} - \text{PV (operating expenses)}}{\text{PV (total investment cost)} - \text{PV (salvage returned)}}$$

or

$$\frac{\text{PV (R)} + \text{PV (CS)} - \text{PV (OE)}}{\text{PV (I)} - \text{PV (S)}}$$

or

$$\frac{\text{PV (R)} + \text{PV (CS} - \text{OE)}}{\text{PV (I)} - \text{PV (S)}}$$

A present value index can be calculated for multiple alternatives, and the one having the highest PVI is the one which is the best of those examined. Thus the PVI is a means of ranking investment alternatives, much like payback, except that it takes into account the timing of revenue and cost flows, which payback does not.

Problem Example

Using the same data as in the payback example (see Table 4–1), the calculation of the present value indexes for the photocopying machine and the teletype machine are shown in Tables 4–3 and 4–4, respectively. These tables indicate that the PVI for the photocopying machine is 1.05, and 1.10 for the teletype machine. When considering the time value of money, and discounting future funds flows (revenue, cost, and salvage), we find that the teletype machine is the preferred of the two alternatives, whereas, when using the payback technique, the photocopying machine appeared to be the best of the two (2.60 years versus 2.67 years; see Table 4–1). The reason for the difference in attractiveness is the basic assumptions of the payback and present value techniques. The former only considers how many years of net benefit will be required to return the net investment. The present value technique, on the other hand, considers the timing of the fund flows.

The payback method is easy to calculate and use because it is relatively uncompl.cated. However, the present value technique is the preferred of the two.

---

[10]*Ibid.* pp. 158–165.

Table 4–3 Present Value Index Calculation—Photocopying Machine
(i = 10%)

(A) PRESENT VALUE OF NET INVESTMENT =
(PV TOTAL INVESTMENT COST − PV SALVAGE RETURNED)

Time (year)	Formula Component	Value	×	PVsP	=	Net Present Value
present	Initial Total Investment	$11,800	×	1.000	=	$11,800
4	Salvage Value Returned	$ 4,000	×	.683	=	−$ 2,732
	Total PV Net Investment					$ 9,068

(B) PRESENT VALUE OF NET OPERATING BENEFIT = PV FUTURE REVENUES + PV
(COSTS SAVED − OPERATING EXPENSES)

Time (year)	Formula Component	Value	×	PVsP	=	Net Present Value
1	Revenue Generated	0	×	.909	=	0
	Costs Saved − Oper Exp	$4,000 − $1,000	×	.909	=	$ 2,727
2	Revenue Generated	0	×	.826	=	0
	Costs Saved − Oper Exp	$4,000 − $1,000	×	.826	=	$ 2,478
3	Revenue Generated	0	×	.751	=	0
	Costs Saved − Oper Exp	$4,000 − $1,000	×	.751	=	$ 2,253
4	Revenue Generated	0	×	.683	=	0
	Costs Saved − Oper Exp	$4,000 − $1,000	×	.683	=	$ 2,049
	Total PV of Net Operating Benefit				=	$ 9,507

$$\text{Present Value Index} = \frac{\text{PV (Net Operating Benefit)}}{\text{PV (Net Investment)}} = \frac{\$9,507}{\$9,068} = 1.05$$

Table 4–4 Present Value Index Calculation—Teletype Machine
(i = 10%)

(A) PRESENT VALUE NET INVESTMENT =
(PV TOTAL INVESTMENT COST − PV SALVAGE RETURNED)

Time (year)	Formula Component	Value	×	PVsP	=	Net Present Value
present	Initial Total Investment	$10,000	×	1.000	=	$10,000
4	Salvage Value Returned	$ 2,000	×	.683	=	−$ 1,366
	Total PV Net Investment					$ 8,634

(B) PRESENT VALUE OF NET OPERATING BENEFIT = PV FUTURE REVENUES + PV
(COSTS SAVED − OPERATING EXPENSES)

Time (year)	Formula Component	Value	×	PVsP	=	Net Present Value
1	Revenue Generated	0	×	.909	=	0
	Costs Saved − Oper Exp	$3,500 − $500	×	.909	=	$ 2,727
2	Revenue Generated	0	×	.826	=	0
	Costs Saved − Oper Exp	$3,500 − $500	×	.826	=	$ 2,478
3	Revenue Generated	0	×	.751	=	0
	Costs Saved − Oper Exp	$3,500 − $500	×	.751	=	$ 2,253
4	Revenue Generated	0	×	.683	=	0
	Costs Saved − Oper Exp	$3,500 − $500	×	.683	=	$ 2,049
	Total PV of Net Operating Benefit				=	$ 9,507

$$\text{Present Value Index} = \frac{\text{PV (Net Operating Benefit)}}{\text{PV (Net Investment)}} = \frac{\$9,507}{\$8,634} = 1.10$$

DECISION-MAKING UNDER UNCERTAINTY

One method of classifying decisions is by the conditions under which they are made. The "conditions" refer to the degree of uncertainty associated with the alternatives (and their results) which are under consideration.[11] We will present decision-making under conditions of uncertainty. However, before proceeding, its converse, decision-making under certainty, will be discussed.

Decision-making with *complete* certainty as to the outcome of an alternative selected is sometimes possible, but not often. Probably the best examples are "laws of nature." If a person were to make a decision to jump off a high structure, could we be certain of the outcome? Yes, he would fall owing to gravity. However, in medicine, human behavior, or any other areas, could we be completely certain (100 per cent positive) that a specific outcome would occur? Generally not. Decision-making under the condition of certainty implies that the decision-maker has *full* information and can always predict the outcome. Agreed, some things are completely certain, but not many. We will all die—but when?

Decision-making under uncertainty implies that the decision-maker can make *some subjective judgment* about the likely outcome of events.[12] In other words, he can assign some reasonable level of chance (probability) that events will or will not occur. For example, will it rain today? At worst, the likelihood is 50–50. It will or it will not. We could then ask questions and gather information: Are there clouds in the sky? Are they black? Did it rain yesterday? With that information we could provide a better estimate of the likelihood that it will rain, but we can never be certain. Or we could judge, from experience and with fairly good accuracy, the likelihood that a patient would die if an overdose of drug X were given to him. We cannot be certain, but we are far from uncertain. In this situation we can attach some subjective (best estimate) probability, say .99 (with 1.0 representing certainty) that the patient would be harmed.

Thus decision-making under uncertainty is the classification which assumes that we can assign some probability, generally formulated from past experience, to the outcome of an event or events associated with an alternative. Since this is the condition under which we make most of our decisions, it will be presented.

Decision Matrix. One way of evaluating "decision-making under uncertainty" is by using a decision matrix. Its basic components consist of (1) strategies, (2) states of nature, and (3) the determination of expected payoff (benefit or cost). In any decision matrix model the strategies represent the various alternatives available and they can range from two to many. The states of

---

[11] For various discussions of decision-making classifications see the following:

(a) Levin and Kirkpatrick, *Quantitative Approaches to Management*, Chapter 5.

(b) Edward A. McCreary, "How to grow a decision tree." *Harvard Business Review*, 45:13. March-April, 1967.

(c) Max D. Richards, and Paul S. Greenlaw, *Management Decisions and Behavior*. Homewood, Illinois: Richard D. Irwin, Inc., 1972, pp. 80–82.

(d) William A. Spurr, and Charles P. Bonini, *Statistical Analysis for Business Decisions*. Homewood, Illinois: Richard D. Irwin, Inc., 1967, pp. 204–213.

[12] Milton H. Spencer, *Managerial Economics*. Homewood, Illinois: Richard D. Irwin, Inc., 1968, p. 9.

nature consist of the possible outcomes for each strategy (alternative). The determination of expected payoff occurs from identifying the subjective probability associated with each possible state of nature (outcome) for each of the alternatives and multiplying by the presumed cost or gain that would be associated with each outcome, should it occur.[13] Since we are dealing with probabilities, which can range from 0.0 (total uncertainty) to 1.0 (certainty) for each possible outcome, the sum of probabilities assigned for *all* outcomes for each alternative cannot exceed 1.0. Perhaps an example will serve to make these points clear.

Problem Example

In order to demonstrate the evaluation of alternatives under conditions of uncertainty, we will use the following example: it is presumed that the purchasing agent in a health care organization is confronted with two alternatives (strategies). The first is to order and stock 5000 disposable syringes per month. The second is to order and stock 6000 syringes per month. Furthermore, for each alternative two states of nature (outcomes) and the costs associated with each are considered (see Fig. 4–2). The analysis could, of course, be expanded should there be additional alternatives, outcomes, and costs associated with those outcomes; however, for clarity of presentation, only two alternatives, with two outcomes each, will be considered.

From experience, the purchasing agent can determine that the probability (likelihood) of 5000 syringes being used (state of nature or outcome) in any given month is 0.8, while the probability of 6000 being used is 0.2. Stated another way, an average of 5000 syringes will be used in 8 out of 10 months, while only 6000 syringes will be used in 2 out of 10 months. In order not to complicate the presentation, presume that only 5000 or 6000 syringes will be used in any given month, and ignore excess inventory.

The purchasing agent has also assigned various costs to the possible outcomes for each alternative. Specifically, he must allocate storage space, which is expensed at $10 per 1000 syringes. In addition, if he orders and stocks too few syringes, an extra cost of $20 will result for special ordering and messenger pickup. Viewing Figure 4–2, for alternative A (column 1), if 5000 syringes are stocked and the usage during the month is 5000, the storage costs will be $50 (column 3). If 5000 syringes are stocked and 6000 are needed that month, then the costs would be $80 ($60 for storage and $20 for the special order).

For alternative B (column 1), if 6000 syringes are stocked and the usage during the month is 5000, the storage costs will be $60 (column 3). In this instance, the $10 storage cost would be incurred above what was needed ($50 for the 5000 used and $10 for those not used, for a total of $60). If 6000 syringes are stocked and 6000 are used, then the cost would be $60.

The problem is as follows: given the decision-maker's estimated probability of monthly usage, how many syringes should be ordered and stocked in order to minimize costs? The solution lies in determining the lowest expected costs for all possible outcomes associated with each alternative.

If the purchasing agent orders and stocks 5000 syringes (alternative A), then 80 per cent of the time (column 2) he will be correct and only incur a $50 storage cost. However, 20 per cent of the time he will be incorrect and thus incur the $80 storage and reorder cost associated with a usage rate of 6000. By the same token, if he orders 6000 syringes (alternative B), then 20 per cent of the time 6000 will be used and the storage

[13]William Mendenhall, and James E. Reinmuth, *Statistics for Management and Economics.* Belmont, California: Duxbury Press, 1974, Chapter 10.

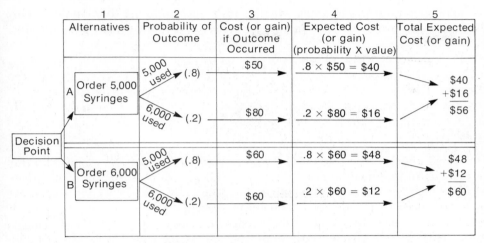

	1 Alternatives	2 Probability of Outcome	3 Cost (or gain) if Outcome Occurred	4 Expected Cost (or gain) (probability X value)	5 Total Expected Cost (or gain)
A	Order 5,000 Syringes	5,000 used (.8)	$50	.8 × $50 = $40	$40 +$16 $56
		6,000 used (.2)	$80	.2 × $80 = $16	
B	Order 6,000 Syringes	5,000 used (.8)	$60	.8 × $60 = $48	$48 +$12 $60
		6,000 used (.2)	$60	.2 × $60 = $12	

Decision Point

Figure 4–2 Disposable syringe decision tree.

cost of $60 will be incurred. However, 80 per cent of the time only 5000 syringes will be used; yet the storage costs would still be $60, with $10 of that storage cost not being necessary.

The decision matrix in Figure 4–2 provides all the needed information necessary to solve the problem—should he order 5000 or 6000 syringes. The alternative to be selected is the one which will result, in this case, in the lowest expected cost.

EXPECTED COST OR GAIN

Expected cost (or gain) is determined by multiplying the probability of occurrence for each possible outcome times the cost or gain associated with it. Let's take a *gain* example to make the point. Which would you rather do: (A) buy a raffle ticket for $1 when you estimate that your chance (probability) of winning a $50 prize is 1 in 1000 (probability = .01), or (B) participating in a baseball pool with 20 other people where you pay $1 for a chance (probability) of winning a $20 prize (probability = .05)?

The expected gain is: (probability) × (value of prize). For alternative A (raffle ticket), the expected gain (EG) would be: EG = .01 × $50 = $0.50. For alternative B (baseball pool), the expected gain (EG) would be: EG = .05 × $20 = $1.00.

If you were attempting to maximize your gain, alternative B (baseball pool) would be selected. You might also note that buying a raffle ticket would never be a wise choice. Each time you bought one, your expected gain would only be $0.50, while the cost of the ticket would be $1.00. Thus, over the long run, you would always lose money.

By the same token, we can use a similar analysis to minimize cost. Specifically, in the syringe problem, two alternatives are available, with each having an estimated probability that given outcomes (the level of demand for syringes) will occur along with the costs associated with each outcome. The decision-maker, through the calculation of expected costs, will seek to select the alternative where expected costs will be minimized.

The general formula which would allow for any number of conditions (our example uses two) is as follows:[14] Expected cost or gain for an alternative =

$$\sum_{\text{all } x} x_i \, p(x_i)$$

where p = the probability of an outcome

x_i = the cost or gain associated with that outcome

Or, stated another way, the expected cost or gain is the sum or addition of the probability of an outcome multiplied by the cost or gain of that outcome *for all possible* outcomes for each alternative. The expected costs associated with each possible outcome are presented in column 4 of Figure 4–2. The total expected cost for each alternative is presented in column 5 of Figure 4–2. If 5000 syringes were ordered the expected cost would be $56, while it would be $60 if 6000 were ordered. Consequently, to minimize costs, alternative A, ordering and stocking 5000 syringes, would be selected.

APPLICATIONS

There are many situations in which the decision-making under uncertainty can be applied. The necessary ingredients are more than one alternative, some estimation of the probability of outcomes occurring, and some measure of cost or gain associated with each of the possible outcomes of each alternative. For example, the physician intuitively thinks through the costs — benefits and probabilities of outcomes occurring when treating patients. For a patient with cancer, he may evaluate the alternatives of whether or not to prescribe chemotherapy. He will consider the probability of the outcomes for each alternative (the patient recovering or not recovering) and the costs or benefits associated with each outcome. The physician's decision can be relatively easy if he considers the cost of "not recovering" to be infinite.

Generally, the administrator will intuitively consider all of the elements (probability of outcomes and costs or benefits of the outcomes) for various alternatives. For example, if, for a multitude of reasons, he wishes to keep his organization union-free, he may consider the alternatives of granting or not granting an across-the-board pay increase to his employees. He can estimate the probability that either action will or will not keep employees from wanting union representation. To translate that information into a decision matrix, the only additional information required is an estimate of the cost of having a union.

One final example should serve to demonstrate the wide applicability of the decision matrix. Recently, health care providers (doctors and facilities) have seen their malpractice insurance premiums increase substantially. Some doctors in high-risk specialties have had their annual insurance premium increase from $5000 to $20,000 in one year. One hospital had an increase in annual premium

---

[14]*Ibid.* p. 257.

from $87,000 to $624,000 in one year.[15] Conceivably, there comes a point where it is more cost effective to self-insure.

Let's presume that a hospital has the alternatives of (A) acquiring malpractice insurance with a 10 per cent deductible per year based on total judgment awards made against it and an annual premium of $87,000, or (B) self-insuring; that is, not buying malpractice insurance and saving the premium money on the assumption that any judgment awards against the facility would be less than the cost of the insurance. For the sake of presentation, consider that the administrator determines that in any one year there are three possible outcomes (ceilings on judgment awards), and he has assigned a probability of 0.7 that the organization will be sued and awards will be given totaling $100,000, a probability of 0.2 that awards will total $500,000, and a probability of 0.1 that awards will total $1,000,000. Obviously, smaller and larger awards (outcomes) are possible, but in order to keep the presentation uncomplicated, only three are considered as being possible.

Figure 4–3 presents the two alternatives, three possible outcomes for each, their likelihood of occurrence, the anticipated cost of each outcome, and the expected cost of each outcome with the total expected costs for the two alternatives.

The expected cost for all possible outcomes if insurance is acquired (alternative A) is $27,000 due to the 10 per cent deductible. The expected cost of self-insuring (alternative B) is $270,000.

In order to complete the evaluation, we have to add the annual premium cost to the expected cost of alternative A. If the premium cost were $87,000, the total annual payout would be the expected cost of $27,000 plus the insurance premium of $87,000, or $114,000. Thus, with a cost of $114,000 if insurance is acquired (alternative A) and an expected cost of $270,000 if insurance is not acquired (alternative B), which alternative would you select? Obviously A. If the annual premium for malpractice insurance were raised to $624,000 per

---

[15]*Akron Beacon Journal,* June 8, 1975, p. H-2.

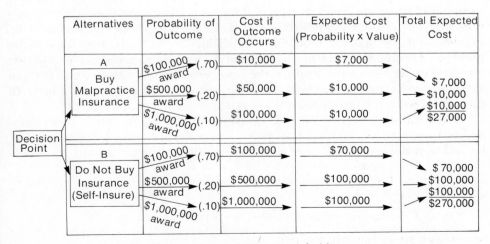

Figure 4–3 Malpractice insurance decision tree.

year with no change in the outcomes or their probability of occurring, which alternative would you select?

STATISTICAL METHODS

Statistics is a very powerful tool which can be useful to the decision-maker in terms of diagnosing and solving problems. For example, it was recently reported that there were 56 cardiac arrests resulting in 16 deaths during a two-month period at a Veterans Administration Hospital.[16] Further, the normal number of arrests for that length of time was 12 to 15. How did the administrator and physicians know that something was wrong? The answer lies in their understanding of statistics. Basically, they knew that on the average there were 6 to 7 arrests each month, on occasion 8; however, there were never 28. As a result, they knew the likelihood (probability) of 28 arrests in one month or 56 in two months happening just owing to chance was so small that there had to be some attributable cause and further investigation was needed.

APPLICATIONS

The subject of statistics encompasses such topics as probability, frequency distributions, testing of hypotheses, sampling methods, and regression analysis, to name a few.[17] The applications of statistical methods in the health care field are many. It is through hypothesis testing that medical research can be conducted. With statistical methods the medical supplier (drugs, surgical kits, etc.) can ensure that the quality of his product meets specifications. It is through sampling that we are able to make an inference (draw a conclusion) about a larger group of things. For example, to determine the incidence of VD in a community do you examine everyone or examine a selected sample and then draw a conclusion about the whole community?

A hospital might ask how we can know if the number of babies delivered in our facility will go up or down next year and by how much. This information can be very important in terms of a decision to reduce or expand OB service. Certainly correlation analysis would help us. Correlation does not indicate causality, but it does demonstrate the degree of association between a dependent and one or more independent variables. What would be related to the number of births per year in a community? How about recession–prosperity, war–peace, the age of the women, the number of women, and so on? If these variables are related to the birth rate, we can make some prediction of birth rates by viewing the trends (directions) of these variables.

With statistics we can provide information which can help the decision-maker to select from among alternatives. In order to demonstrate this point, we will next develop one statistical technique, the z-transformation.

---

[16]"Death Tries 'Repeated' at Hospital." *Akron Beacon Journal,* August 26, 1975, p. 1.
[17]For example, see Donald L. Harnett, *Introduction to Statistical Methods.* Reading, Massachusetts: Addison-Wesley Publishing Company, 1975.

Statistics is basically an attempt to derive information about events, things, and attributes through their description in numerical terms. Many examples come to mind. How many people in the United States are over 65 years of age? How many are under 30? How many of your organization's employees graduated from high school? A professional school? In all of these instances we have asked questions whose answers would describe our population and the education (training) level of the organization's employees in numerical terms.

MEAN

Important to the understanding of statistics are the concepts of mean and standard deviation. The mean is simply the average of a group of observations (measured in numerical terms) which may represent anything such as patient census, number of deliveries, the number of eligible Medicaid recipients in each state, the number of meals served, the number of prescriptions filled, and so on. The formula to calculate the mean is as follows:

$$\text{mean} = \frac{\text{Sum of the numerical values of all observations}}{\text{the number of observations}}$$

The mean of a sample is denoted as $\bar{x}$. Each observation is denoted as x_i where i can range from 1, to 2, to 3, to n where n equals the total number of observations and $\sum$ denotes the sum of all the x_i's. The formula becomes:[18]

$$\bar{x} = \frac{\sum_{i=1}^{n} x_i}{n}$$

Let's take a daily census as an example. Table 4–5 presents the census levels on each day for nineteen days. The mean or average daily census would be the sum of all observations $\left(\sum_{i=1}^{n} x_i\right)$ divided by the number of observations (n).

or

$$\bar{x} = \frac{3857}{19} = 203$$

Thus the mean or average daily census is 203. This can also be viewed in Figure 4–4, which is a frequency distribution of the census data in Table 4–5. Note that 203 is the central value (mean) of the distribution.

STANDARD DEVIATION

The second important concept for understanding statistics is the concept of dispersion or spread that those observations have about the central value

---

[18]Mendenhall and Reinmuth, op. cit. p. 36.

Table 4–5 Daily Census Observations for Nineteen Days

DAY (X_i)	CENSUS LEVEL
1	202
2	205
3	203
4	203
5	204
6	199
7	201
8	206
9	204
10	203
11	200
12	202
13	204
14	203
15	205
16	207
17	201
18	203
19	202

$$\sum_{i=1}^{19} X_i = 3857$$

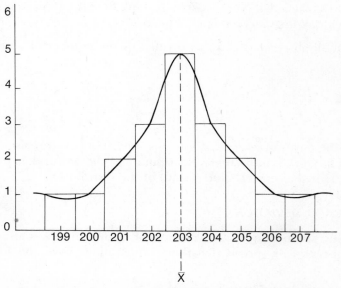

Frequency of
Observations

Figure 4–4   Frequency distribution. Daily census.

(mean). The dispersion of samples can be measured by the standard deviation, which is determined by the following formula.[19]

$$s = \sqrt{\sum_{i=1}^{n} \frac{(x_i - \bar{x})^2}{n-1}}$$

Where s $=$ standard deviation
$x_i =$ the actual observations
$\bar{x} =$ the mean
n $=$ the number of observations

Table 4–6 presents the calculation of the standard deviation for the daily census data in Table 4–5.

NORMAL DISTRIBUTION

Mathematicians can prove that samples which are normally distributed (symmetrical on both sides of the mean) have certain characteristics. Specifically,

[19]*Ibid.* p. 52.

Table 4–6   Standard Deviation for Census Data

	OBSERVATION x_i	MEAN $\bar{x}$	$x_i - \bar{x}$	$(x_i - \bar{x})^2$
1	202	203	−1	1
2	205	203	2	4
3	203	203	0	0
4	203	203	0	0
5	204	203	1	1
6	199	203	−4	16
7	201	203	−2	4
8	206	203	3	9
9	204	203	1	1
10	203	203	0	0
11	200	203	−3	9
12	202	203	−1	1
13	204	203	1	1
14	203	203	0	0
15	205	203	2	4
16	207	203	4	16
17	201	203	−2	4
18	203	203	0	0
19	202	203	−1	1

n $=$ 19

$$\sum_{i=1}^{19} (x_i - \bar{x})^2 = 72$$

$$s = \sqrt{\frac{\sum_{i=1}^{n} (x_i - \bar{x})^2}{n-1}}$$

$$= \sqrt{\frac{72}{18}} = \sqrt{4} = 2.0$$

it can be shown that 68.26 per cent of all observations will fall within ± 1 stand-ard deviation from the mean, that 95.44 per cent of all observations will be with-in ± 2 standard deviations from the mean, and that 99.72 per cent of the observa-tions will fall within ± 3 standard deviations from the mean.[20] This is depicted in Figure 4–5.

In health care organizations many samples drawn can be presumed to be normally distributed. By calculating the mean and standard deviation of a sample and using them to approximate the population mean and standard deviation, we can make probabilistic statements. Specifically, the total area under the normal distribution presented in Figure 4–5 equals 1.0. If we have drawn a large number of sample observations we can calculate the sample $\bar{x}$ and s. We could then make probabilistic statements about the characteristics of an additional observation.

Let's use an example to make the point. Presume we weighed newborn babies over a three-week period and had 200 observations. We could then calculate the mean weight and the standard deviation of the weight for that sample. Presume that from our data we determine the mean ($\bar{x}$) to be 6.5 pounds and the standard deviation (s) to be 1.1 pounds. We can now make probabilistic statements about the weight of children yet to be born. For ex-ample, we know that 99.72 per cent of all babies will have a weight within ± 3 standard deviations (s) of the mean.

$$\bar{x} \pm 3 \ (1.1)$$

or

6.5 pounds ± 3.3 pounds

or

$6.5 - 3.3$ and $6.5 + 3.3$

or

3.2 and 9.8 pounds

---

[20]John E. Freund and Benjamin M. Perles, *Business Statistics.* Englewood Cliffs, New Jersey: Prentice-Hall Inc., 1974, p. 161.

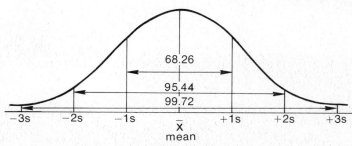

Figure 4–5   Normal distribution.

Therefore, we could answer the question: "What is the likelihood that a newborn will weigh between 3.2 and 9.8 pounds?" The answer is .9972, or almost 100 per cent of those born. Since the area under the normal distribution equals 1.0, we can therefore determine the probability of a specific observation occurring by finding the appropriate area it represents under the curve. In order to do so we must standardize the sample mean $(\bar{x})$ we have determined with respect to the population mean (μ) to conform with the table of "z" values, which are presented in Table 4–7. Specifically, the "z" value table presumes a mean of zero and standard deviation of 1. In order to convert to those tubular constraints, we must subtract the sample mean $(\bar{x})$ from the observation we are seeking information about and divide by the sample standard deviation (s).

z–VALUE

The general formula[21] for the z-transformation is as follows: $\left(z = \dfrac{x - \mu}{\sigma} \right)$ where μ (mu) is the population mean and σ (sigma) is the population standard deviation. However, since μ and σ are not known, we can approximate sufficiently for our needs by using the sample mean $(\bar{x})$ and standard deviation (s). The formula thus becomes: $z = \dfrac{x - \bar{x}}{s}$.

Problem Example

Let's use the daily census example data that were presented in Table 4–5. We know that the sample mean daily census is 203 people, and the standard deviation is 2.0. We wish to know what the likelihood is that we will have a census observation of up to and including 206 people.

$$z = \frac{206 - 203}{2.0} = +1.50$$

What the "+1.50" value means is that a census of up to and including 206 people would be +1.50 standard deviations from the mean. Looking at Table 4–7, we find the z value "+1.50" has an area to the left of "+1.50" of .9332. What this means is that the probability of having a census up to and including 206 people is .9332. This can graphically be displayed as the shaded area under the curve in Figure 4–6 A.

Similarly, we could determine what the probability of having a census greater than 206 people would be. The normal curve represents the distribution of all possible census levels, and the area under the curve equals 1.0. If we know the area associated with having a census of up to and including 206 people (.9332), we can subtract that value from 1.0000 to find the probability of a census greater than 206 people.

$$
\begin{array}{r}
1.0000 \\
-.9332 \\
\hline
.0668
\end{array}
$$

This is represented by the shaded area in Figure 4–6.

---

[21] For a good presentation of z-transformation see Mendenhall and Reinmuth, op. cit., Chapter 7.

Table 4-7   Areas Under the Normal Distribution*

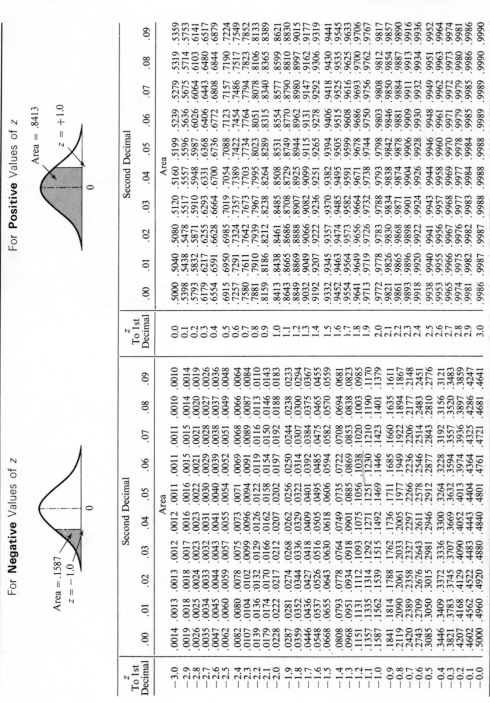

For **Negative** Values of z   For **Positive** Values of z

Area = .1587, z = −1.0   Area = .8413, z = +1.0

For Negative Values of z (Area, Second Decimal)

z To 1st Decimal	.00	.01	.02	.03	.04	.05	.06	.07	.08	.09
−3.0	.0014	.0013	.0013	.0012	.0012	.0011	.0011	.0011	.0010	.0010
−2.9	.0019	.0018	.0018	.0017	.0016	.0016	.0015	.0015	.0014	.0014
−2.8	.0026	.0025	.0024	.0023	.0023	.0022	.0021	.0021	.0020	.0019
−2.7	.0035	.0034	.0033	.0032	.0031	.0030	.0029	.0028	.0027	.0026
−2.6	.0047	.0045	.0044	.0043	.0041	.0040	.0039	.0038	.0037	.0036
−2.5	.0062	.0060	.0059	.0057	.0055	.0054	.0052	.0051	.0049	.0048
−2.4	.0082	.0080	.0078	.0075	.0073	.0071	.0069	.0068	.0066	.0064
−2.3	.0107	.0104	.0102	.0099	.0096	.0094	.0091	.0089	.0087	.0084
−2.2	.0139	.0136	.0132	.0129	.0126	.0122	.0119	.0116	.0113	.0110
−2.1	.0179	.0174	.0170	.0166	.0162	.0158	.0154	.0150	.0146	.0143
−2.0	.0228	.0222	.0217	.0212	.0207	.0202	.0197	.0192	.0188	.0183
−1.9	.0287	.0281	.0274	.0268	.0262	.0256	.0250	.0244	.0238	.0233
−1.8	.0359	.0352	.0344	.0336	.0329	.0322	.0314	.0307	.0300	.0294
−1.7	.0446	.0436	.0427	.0418	.0409	.0401	.0392	.0384	.0375	.0367
−1.6	.0548	.0537	.0526	.0516	.0505	.0495	.0485	.0475	.0465	.0455
−1.5	.0668	.0655	.0643	.0630	.0618	.0606	.0594	.0582	.0570	.0559
−1.4	.0808	.0793	.0778	.0764	.0749	.0735	.0722	.0708	.0694	.0681
−1.3	.0968	.0951	.0934	.0918	.0901	.0885	.0869	.0853	.0838	.0823
−1.2	.1151	.1131	.1112	.1093	.1075	.1056	.1038	.1020	.1003	.0985
−1.1	.1357	.1335	.1314	.1292	.1271	.1251	.1230	.1210	.1190	.1170
−1.0	.1587	.1562	.1539	.1515	.1492	.1469	.1446	.1423	.1401	.1379
−0.9	.1841	.1814	.1788	.1762	.1736	.1711	.1685	.1660	.1635	.1611
−0.8	.2119	.2090	.2061	.2033	.2005	.1977	.1949	.1922	.1894	.1867
−0.7	.2420	.2389	.2358	.2327	.2297	.2266	.2236	.2206	.2177	.2148
−0.6	.2743	.2709	.2676	.2643	.2611	.2578	.2546	.2514	.2483	.2451
−0.5	.3085	.3050	.3015	.2981	.2946	.2912	.2877	.2843	.2810	.2776
−0.4	.3446	.3409	.3372	.3336	.3300	.3264	.3228	.3192	.3156	.3121
−0.3	.3821	.3783	.3745	.3707	.3669	.3632	.3594	.3557	.3520	.3483
−0.2	.4207	.4168	.4129	.4090	.4052	.4013	.3974	.3936	.3897	.3859
−0.1	.4602	.4562	.4522	.4483	.4443	.4404	.4364	.4325	.4286	.4247
−0.0	.5000	.4960	.4920	.4880	.4840	.4801	.4761	.4721	.4681	.4641

For Positive Values of z (Area, Second Decimal)

z To 1st Decimal	.00	.01	.02	.03	.04	.05	.06	.07	.08	.09
0.0	.5000	.5040	.5080	.5120	.5160	.5199	.5239	.5279	.5319	.5359
0.1	.5398	.5438	.5478	.5517	.5557	.5596	.5636	.5675	.5714	.5753
0.2	.5793	.5832	.5871	.5910	.5948	.5987	.6026	.6064	.6103	.6141
0.3	.6179	.6217	.6255	.6293	.6331	.6368	.6406	.6443	.6480	.6517
0.4	.6554	.6591	.6628	.6664	.6700	.6736	.6772	.6808	.6844	.6879
0.5	.6915	.6950	.6985	.7019	.7054	.7088	.7123	.7157	.7190	.7224
0.6	.7257	.7291	.7324	.7357	.7389	.7422	.7454	.7486	.7517	.7549
0.7	.7580	.7611	.7642	.7673	.7703	.7734	.7764	.7794	.7823	.7852
0.8	.7881	.7910	.7939	.7967	.7995	.8023	.8051	.8078	.8106	.8133
0.9	.8159	.8186	.8212	.8238	.8264	.8289	.8315	.8340	.8365	.8389
1.0	.8413	.8438	.8461	.8485	.8508	.8531	.8554	.8577	.8599	.8621
1.1	.8643	.8665	.8686	.8708	.8729	.8749	.8770	.8790	.8810	.8830
1.2	.8849	.8869	.8888	.8907	.8925	.8944	.8962	.8980	.8997	.9015
1.3	.9032	.9049	.9066	.9082	.9099	.9115	.9131	.9147	.9162	.9177
1.4	.9192	.9207	.9222	.9236	.9251	.9265	.9278	.9292	.9306	.9319
1.5	.9332	.9345	.9357	.9370	.9382	.9394	.9406	.9418	.9430	.9441
1.6	.9452	.9463	.9474	.9485	.9495	.9505	.9515	.9525	.9535	.9545
1.7	.9554	.9564	.9573	.9582	.9591	.9599	.9608	.9616	.9625	.9633
1.8	.9641	.9649	.9656	.9664	.9671	.9678	.9686	.9693	.9700	.9706
1.9	.9713	.9719	.9726	.9732	.9738	.9744	.9750	.9756	.9762	.9767
2.0	.9772	.9778	.9783	.9788	.9793	.9798	.9803	.9808	.9812	.9817
2.1	.9821	.9826	.9830	.9834	.9838	.9842	.9846	.9850	.9854	.9857
2.2	.9861	.9865	.9868	.9871	.9874	.9878	.9881	.9884	.9887	.9890
2.3	.9893	.9896	.9898	.9901	.9904	.9906	.9909	.9911	.9913	.9916
2.4	.9918	.9920	.9922	.9924	.9926	.9928	.9930	.9932	.9934	.9936
2.5	.9938	.9940	.9941	.9943	.9944	.9946	.9949	.9949	.9951	.9952
2.6	.9953	.9955	.9956	.9957	.9958	.9960	.9961	.9962	.9963	.9964
2.7	.9965	.9966	.9967	.9968	.9969	.9970	.9971	.9972	.9973	.9974
2.8	.9974	.9975	.9976	.9977	.9978	.9978	.9979	.9979	.9980	.9981
2.9	.9981	.9982	.9982	.9983	.9984	.9984	.9985	.9985	.9986	.9986
3.0	.9986	.9987	.9987	.9988	.9988	.9989	.9989	.9989	.9990	.9990

*Source: From G. W. Summers and W. S. Peters, *Basic Statistics in Business*. Copyright © by Wadsworth Publishing Company, Inc., Belmont, California, 94002. Reprinted by permission of the publisher.

We could also ask: "What is the likelihood of having a census up to and including 202 people. The z-transformation would be as follows:

$$z = \frac{202 - 203}{2.0} = -.50$$

To find the area under the normal curve, we look for $z = -.50$ in Table 4–7 and its corresponding area to the left of the $z = -.50$ point, which is .3085. The meaning is that the probability of a census of up to and including 202 people is only .3085. This is represented by the shaded area in Figure 4–6 C. Furthermore, the probability of a census *greater than* 202 people is

$$\begin{array}{r} 1.0000 \\ -.3085 \\ \hline .6915 \end{array}$$

One final example is required to complete our presentation of z–transformation. We could ask the question: "What is the probability that we would have a daily census between 202 and 206 people, inclusive?" In order to determine the answer we have to find the z value and area under the normal curve to the left of each observation under consideration. The calculation follows:

$$\text{(left of 202) } z = \frac{202 - 203}{2.0} = -.50$$
$$\text{(area} = .3085)$$

$$\text{(left of 206) } z = \frac{206 - 203}{2.0} = +1.50$$
$$\text{(area} = .9332)$$

Viewing Figure 4–6 D, we note that the probability of a census of up to and including 206 people is .9332. The probability of a census up to and including 202 people is .3085. To find the area between 206 and 202, inclusive, we must take the area value for 206 people (.9332) and subtract the area value to the left of 202 people (.3085).

$$\begin{array}{r} .9332 \\ -.3085 \\ \hline .6247 \end{array}$$

Thus the cross hatched area in Figure 4–6 D represents the probability of a census between 202 and 206 people, inclusive. It is .6247.

z–TRANSFORMATION APPLICATIONS

Statistical methods can and should be widely used in health care organizations. We have only presented one (z–transformation), which can be used in many situations. The necessary ingredients are drawing sample observations and determining the mean and standard deviation of that sample. With that information (presuming there is a normal distribution), it is possible to make probabilistic statements about any future observation. To make the point, selected situations follow:

1. If the number of deliveries is expected to decrease from 11 to 8 per day, how many incubators should you keep? The question can be answered by determining the mean and standard deviation of premature births per day. To be on the safe side, figure $\bar{x}$ plus 3 s.

2. If 100 beds are to be added to a facility, how many should be purchased that are eight feet long and how many that are seven feet long (presuming the

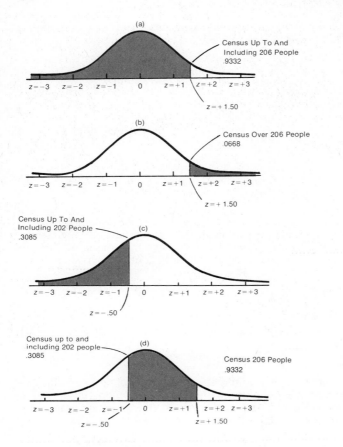

Figure 4–6

cost is appreciably higher for the former)? The answer can be determined by taking a sample of patients over time and measuring their height. Then determine $\bar{x}$ and s. If $\bar{x}$ was 6.0 and s was 0.5, we could use z–transformation to determine the probability of having a patient seven feet or more in height. By multiplying that probability by the 100 beds, we will have our answer.

SIMULATION

Simulation is a powerful technique which can be of great assistance to the health care organization manager when he evaluates alternatives.

Simulation involves the construction of a model representing a set of known phenomena, which permits observation under controlled conditions. The observable phenomena are translated into variables which can then be changed in order to ascertain the impact of those changes without actually tampering with the existing situation.[22]

---

[22]Robert C. Meier, William T. Newell, and Harold L. Pazer, *Simulation in Business and Economics*. Englewood Cliffs, New Jersey: Prentice-Hall, Inc., 1969, p. 1.

In this section we will examine Monte Carlo Simulation. Monte Carlo Simulation has two elements. The first, the simulation model description, consists of translating known phenomena (variables) into some form of mathematical relationship. The second element is random number generating.[23] Random numbers are used to represent the occurrence of events for the model, since any number drawn from a random number table has an equally likely chance of being selected.

APPLICATIONS

Simulation can be used as a training device as well as a planning tool. For example, astronauts and airline pilots train by using cockpit simulators. The controls are linked to computers, which use a mathematical model to simulate speed, altitude, air frame stresses, and so on. It is possible to simulate flying, power dives, and stalls, to name a few conditions, without actually having to fly an airplane or space capsule. Similarly, medical students can train on mechanical manikins, which simulate certain variables, such as heart beat, blood pressure, and other phenomena characteristic of the human body. This is all possible without having to tamper with human patients.[24]

In health care organizations, the applications for simulation are unlimited; if we can identify the variables associated with a situation, we can simulate it. For example, we could determine the impact of the addition of a new surgical complex if the volume of surgery is known. We could answer questions such as what the utilization rate would be and how much support and how many personnel would be required.

We could also simulate the resulting effect from changing the cafeteria food distribution system from, say, one food line for hot and cold meals to two lines, one for each. We could determine if and how many cafeteria personnel would be required and how long employees and visitors would have to wait in line.

Furthermore, we could simulate the results of closing the OB Department, as presented in the previous chapter. Recall that four hospitals in a community were considering consolidating the OB service because of the decline in the community birth rate. One hospital considered closing its OB ward, with the remaining three hospitals providing that service. We could, given demand,

---

[23]Arthur C. Laufer, *Operations Management.* Cincinnati, Ohio: South Western Publishing Co., 1975, p. 147.

[24]For a review of the literature see Stimson and Stimson, *Operations Research in Hospitals: Diagnosis and Prognosis*, Chapter 2.

For an examination of some specific applications see the following:

(a) Robert B. Fetter, and John D. Thompson, "Patients' waiting time and doctors' idle time in the out-patient setting." *Health Services Research*, Summer, 1966.

(b) Paul J. Kuzdrall, N. K. Kwak, and Homer H. Schmitz, "The Monte Carlo Simulation of operating-room and recovery-room usage." *Operations Research, 22*:434, March-April, 1974.

(c) Gordon H. Robinson, Paul Wing, and Louis E. Davis, "Computer simulation of hospital patients scheduling system." *Health Services Research, 3*:No. 2, Summer, 1968.

(d) E. S. Savas, "Simulation and cost-effectiveness: analysis of New York's emergency ambulance service." *Management Science, 15*:No. 12, August, 1969.

(e) C. Swoveland, D. Uyeno, I. Vertinsky, and R. Vickson, "Ambulance location: a probabilistic enumeration." *Management Science, 20*:686, December, Part 2, 1973.

simulate the effect on costs and the possible quality of service in terms of whether the total OB capacity in the community was adequate. However, it should be mentioned that it is not possible to simulate the human reaction (by doctors, patients, and so on) to such a change.

All in all, simulation is a powerful evaluative technique. It provides for the changing of variables which represent the situation from what they presently are without having to make the changes in the actual situation. This is its value, since proposed changes can be evaluated before they are actually implemented. Let us take the admitting office of a hospital as a case in point to present how simulation can be used to evaluate alternatives.

Problem Example

From observation, it has been determined that it takes the admitting clerk an average of four minutes to process patients. We know that new patients wait a minimal amount of time except during the peak busy period from 1:00 P.M. to 1:30 P.M. During that half hour a line forms, patients become angry, and a solution must be found to solve the problem. The reason for the lengthy line is that patients arrive faster than one clerk can service them. One alternative is to assign another individual to the admitting desk during that busy period. However, the department head wishes to determine what effect the addition of another employee would have on patient waiting time and employee idle time before doing so. Monte Carlo Simulation is a technique which will enable that change to be evaluated without actually making it, that is, without tampering with the existing situation.

From the observation of 100 arrivals over a number of weeks between 1:00 P.M. and 1:30 P.M., the time between patient arrivals was determined, as depicted in Figure 4–7. Specifically, it was found that 50 of those 100 sample observations arrived with a "time-between-arrival" of 2 minutes. That is, we observed fifty times that the next person arrived two minutes after the preceding person. Thirty had a time-between-arrival of 4 minutes, and finally, 20 had a time-between-arrival of 6 minutes.

Presuming that these observations actually represent reality (what actually is), we can then assume that if we observe another 100 people, 50 of them would arrive 2 minutes apart, 30 of them would arrive 4 minutes apart, and 20 would arrive 6 minutes apart. We can then transform those actual observations to a scale of 100, as represented in the cumulative frequency distribution presented in Figure 4–7. Using a table of random numbers, it is then possible to assume that a number drawn between 01 and 50 (inclusive) would represent a person with a time-between-arrival of 2 minutes. A drawn number between 51 and 80 (inclusive) would represent a person with a time-between-arrival of 4 minutes. Similarly, a drawn random number between 81 and 100 would represent a person with a time-between-arrival of 6 minutes.

Consequently, it is possible to draw random numbers to represent people arriving at the admitting office, that is, to simulate arrivals. It is now possible to simulate the actual situation in the admitting department. We can determine (1) the number of people waiting in line at any given time; (2) total patient waiting time; and (3) employee idle time with certain variable assumptions. In our case, we wish to determine what will happen to patient waiting time if we change service time from 4 minutes to 2 minutes, presuming that two admitting personnel can process an arrival twice as fast. We can do this by simulation, and we will not tamper with the actual situation. First, let us examine the waiting time when the service time is 4 minutes (one employee).

SERVICE TIME: 4 MINUTES

Table 4–8 presents a series of random numbers which represent for us the arrival of persons. The first random number drawn is 03. Looking at the

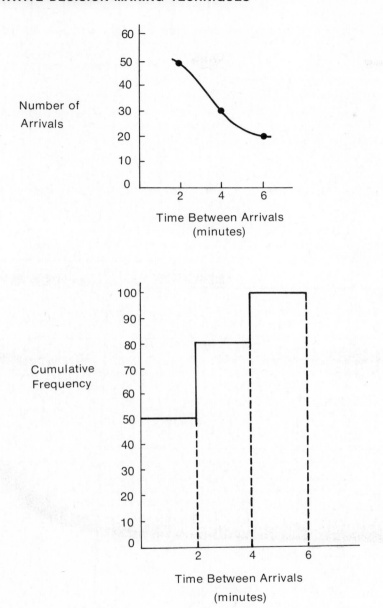

Figure 4–7 Frequency distribution for admitting department arrivals.

cumulative frequency distribution in Figure 4–7, we would note that the random number 03 falls within the 2 minute time-between-arrival classification. Therefore we will say that the first person arrives 2 minutes after the hour of 1 o'clock. To represent the second person arriving, the random number drawn is 72. Looking at the cumulative frequency distribution in Figure 4–7, we find that the value 72 represents an arrival time of 4 minutes after the preceding arrival at 1:06. For the third individual, the random number associated with him is 44. The cumulative frequency distribution in Figure 4–7 shows that the ran-

Table 4-8 Person, Random Number, and Time-Between-Arrival

PERSON	RANDOM NUMBER DRAWN	TIME-BETWEEN-ARRIVAL (MINUTES)
1	03	2
2	72	4
3	44	2
4	25	2
5	37	2
6	12	2
7	86	6
8	58	4
9	02	2
10	48	2
11	35	2

Table 4-9 Simulation of Admitting Department Arrivals, Service, and Waiting Time (Service Time = 4 minutes)

1 Time	2 Time Person Arrives	3 Time Person Serviced	4 Number of People Waiting	Time Each Person Waited
1:00		Employee		
1:02	1	Idle		
1:04		1		
1:06	2		(0)	1 = 0
1:08	3			2 = 0
1:10	4	2	(1)	3 = 2
1:12	5			4 = 4
1:14	6	3	(2)	5 = 6
1:16		4		6 = 8
1:18			(2)	7 = 6
1:20	7	5		8 = 6
1:22			(2)	9 = 8
1:24	8			10 = 10
1:26	9	6	(2)	11 = 12
1:28	10			
1:30	11	7	(3)	Total Patient Waiting Time = 62 Minutes
1:32		8		
1:34			(3)	Employee Idle Time = 2 Minutes
1:36		9		
1:38			(2)	
1:40		10		
1:42			(1)	
1:44		11		
1:46			(0)	

dom number 44 would indicate a time-between-arrival of 2 minutes. Consequently, person number 3 arrives at the admitting office 2 minutes after person number 2. This procedure is followed for all individuals.

Table 4–9 presents the results of the simulation of arrivals at the admitting office with a service time of 4 minutes per person. (Assume no one was being serviced or waiting to be serviced at the start, i.e., 1:00). Column 1 (Time) of Table 4–9 represents the specific time on the clock. Column 2 represents the time between arrivals. That is, the time the person arrives with the time between arrivals determined by the random numbers drawn. Column number 3 represents the time on the clock that the individual is serviced. Column number 4 represents the number of people waiting in line at any given time.

We know from Table 4–8 that individual number 1 arrives 2 minutes after 1:00 P.M. Consequently, between 1:00 and 1:02, the admitting office employee was idle (see column 3, Table 4–9). As soon as individual number 1 arrives at 1:02, service begins. Since all people take (on the average) 4 minutes to service, service ends for the first individual at 1:06 (column 2). The second individual noted in Table 4–8 arrives four minutes after the first individual. Consequently, he arrives at 1:06 on the clock (see Table 4–9). At 1:06 the employee is finished servicing individual number 1 and the service for individual number 2 also begins at 1:06. Therefore, individual number 2 did not have to wait. However, we know that individual number 3 arrived at 1:08, 2 minutes after individual number 2 at 1:06. Since individual number 2 was being serviced until 1:10, individual number 3 had to wait for 2 minutes before being serviced. We know that individual number 4 arrives at 1:10. However, at 1:10 the service begins for individual number 3. As a result, individual number 4's service does not begin until 1:14, and he had to wait in line. The whole process is continued for the full half hour. The values in columns 3 and 4 after 1:30 are only presented in the table in order to indicate the length of time each person had to wait, as well as the waiting line at any given point in time. We have presumed that arrivals stopped at 1:30.

From simulating the arrivals to the admitting desk with a service time of 4 minutes, we found that total patient waiting time was 62 minutes. The employee idle time was 2 minutes (see Table 4–9). The question under consideration is whether the admitting department manager should add an additional employee in order to service more promptly those people who are arriving between the peak period of 1.00 P.M. to 1:30 P.M. The evaluation of that alternative should consider the costs and advantages associated with reducing patient waiting time to something less than 62 minutes.

SERVICE TIME: 2 MINUTES

Let us explore another alternative. The variable that will be changed is service time. By adding another employee, we will assume that service time will be reduced from 4 minutes to 2 minutes. Viewing Table 4–10, we note that the same random numbers were used to simulate arrivals, and the time between arrivals is the same as in Table 4–9. The only thing we have changed is service time. The results from the evaluation in Table 4–10 indicate that total patient waiting time was zero minutes and employee idle time was 10 minutes.

Table 4–10   Simulation of Admitting Department Arrivals, Service, and Waiting Time (Service Time = 2 minutes)

1 Time	2 Time Person Arrives	3 Time Person Serviced	4 Number of People Waiting	Time Each Person Waited
1:00		Employee		
1:02	1	Idle		1 = 0
1:04		1	(0)	2 = 0
1:06	2	Employee Idle		3 = 0
1:08	3	2	(0)	4 = 0 5 = 0
1:10	4	3	(0)	6 = 0
1:12	5	4	(0)	7 = 0
1:14	6	5	(0)	8 = 0 9 = 0
1:16		6	(0)	10 = 0
1:18		Employee		11 = 0
1:20	7	Idle		
1:22		7	(0)	Total Patient Waiting Time = 0 Minutes
1:24	8	Employee Idle		Employee Idle Time = 10 Minutes
1:26	9	8	(0)	
1:28	10	9	(0)	
1:30	11	10	(0)	
1:32		11	(0)	

The question to be asked relative to the alternative of assigning another employee is as follows: Is the reduction in total patient waiting time from 62 minutes to zero worth the cost of assigning another employee for the one-half hour period? Through simulation, the manager has been able to evaluate the effect of a change in service time without tampering with the actual situation. There are many situations in health care organizations where Monte Carlo Simulation can be applied. Examples are: (1) scheduling in the x-ray department; (2) evaluation of waiting time (employee and patient) in the cashier's office; (3) the facility's parking lot; (4) surgical suite scheduling; and (5) the emergency department, to name a few.

The usefulness of simulation should be re-emphasized. It is a technique which can enable a proposed change in a situation to be viewed and evaluated without having to make the personnel and other resource commitments that the change would require. It is therefore possible to see the effect of a change before making it.

SUMMARY

This chapter is a sequel to the preceding one, "Managerial Decision-Making." It specifically focused on various quantitative decision-making techniques which are applicable to health care organizations. Our purpose was not to make the reader an expert nor to present the more complex techniques. It was, however, to make the reader aware that quantitative decision-making techniques have a role in health care decisions—not a singular role in the evaluation of alternatives, but one which can supplement subjective considerations.

The following techniques were reviewed: (1) break-even analysis; (2) pay back; (3) present value; (4) decision-making under uncertainty; (5) the statistical method z–transformation; and (6) Monte Carlo Simulation.

DISCUSSION QUESTIONS

1. Discuss the major features of break-even analysis, areas to which it can be applied in health care organizations, and the kinds of answers it can provide.

2. How does the third party reimbursement system based on total organization cost affect one's use of break-even analysis for a specific component or service?

3. Discuss the advantages of the present value evaluation technique over the payback technique.

4. Discuss the considerations (information that must be used) involved in decision-making under uncertainty. What are some of the deficiencies of the technique?

5. z-transformation has been presented as one statistical method which can assist the decision-maker. Discuss other statistical techniques you have heard about that are used in any area of the health care field.

6. What is simulation and what are its advantages? Give some examples with which you are familiar where simulation could be or has been used.

7. Discuss the range of factors a health care manager might wish to consider in making an important decision. What role should the quantitative techniques presented in this chapter play in the decision?

PROBLEMS

1. A hospital charges $20 for every EKG given. It has been determined that there is an annual fixed cost of $15,000 associated with providing this service (personnel and equipment depreciation). The variable cost is $8 for each EKG. Given this information:
   a. Draw a break-even chart, and visually determine how many EKG's must be performed each year to break-even.
   b. Using the break-even formula, determine how many EKG's will be required to break-even.
   c. Calculate the profit (or loss) if only 1500 EKG's are performed in a year.
   d. If it is estimated that only 1000 EKG's will be performed next year, what should the charge be in order to break-even?

2. The emergency room at Fairview Hospital is run by a corporation of physicians. They estimate that their fixed costs are $60,000 per year. (The doctors are on a profit-sharing system, and the actual emergency room site within the hospital is provided by the hospital, which receives a $15 emergency room fee for each patient above and beyond the doctor's fee. The hospital charge is billed separately.) It is estimated that the supplies and other variable costs for each person treated totals $3.00.
   a. Last year a total of 9000 patients required emergency treatment. Calculate the profit or loss for that year, given that the physician's service charge was a flat fee of $25.00 per person, regardless of the service provided.
   b. It is estimated that 8000 patients will be treated next year. Calculate the profit or loss if the doctor's fee is $25 per patient.
   c. Given the doctor's fee of $25 per patient treated, calculate the break-even point in terms of the number of people that would have to be treated.

3. An investor is considering building a skilled nursing facility in a certain area. He estimates the total annual fixed expenses for the building, property and equipment will be $240,000 (this includes the annual depreciation on the building and property). The total monthly variable expenses for personnel, heat, electricity, etc. will be $350 per patient. The maximum capacity of beds is 120.

    a. How much should he charge per patient each month in order to break-even, presuming that every bed is occupied throughout the year?

    b. If an average of 100 beds are always filled, what would be the annual profit (loss) if the charge is $650 per patient per month?

    c. What do you recommend that the investor charge per month if the average occupancy rate will be 75 per cent and a total gross profit of $120,000 per year is desired.

4. A hospital administrator is considering purchasing a piece of equipment (A) which would cost $15,000 and have a salvage value of $4000 after 5 years. The piece of equipment will reduce present costs by $5500 per year, but the expenses that will be incurred in maintaining the equipment will be $1500 per year. An alternate piece of equipment (B) is also being considered. It would only cost $10,000 and have no salvage value at the end of 5 years. Cost savings for the second piece of equipment are estimated to be $5000 per year, and it would have operating expenses of $1500 per year. Determine the payback period for both pieces of equipment.

5. Two pieces of diagnostic equipment are being considered for purchase. Because of budget limitations, only one can be bought. The first piece of equipment (A) would cost $20,000, have a life of eight years and a trade-in value of $4000. The second piece of equipment (B), which performs the same function as A, would cost $15,000 and would have a salvage value of $2000 after eight years of useful life. Both pieces of equipment can generate revenue amounting to $12,000 a year and result in cost savings of $2500 per year. However, the annual operating expenses for A are $6000 and $7000 for B. By using the payback technique, which piece of equipment should be chosen?

6. Two investment alternatives are being considered. The first (A) has an initial investment cost of $200,000 and a salvage value of $50,000 after eight years. The second (B) has an initial cost of $300,000 and a salvage value of $70,000 after eight years. A will generate revenues of $40,000 per year, while B will generate revenues of $70,000 per year. However, B's annual operating expenses will be $15,000, while the annual operating expenses for A will be $10,000. What is the payback period for each alternative?

7. Using the data in Problem 4, and assuming that the interest rate is 8 per cent, compute the present value index for each alternative and determine which piece of equipment is preferred.

8. Using the figures in Problem 5 and assuming that 10 per cent is the interest rate, compute the present value index for each alternative and determine which piece of equipment is preferred.

9. The number of patients serviced each day in the emergency room of Fairview Hospital (250 beds) was recorded over a 17-day period. The following is a record of the observations for the 17-day period: 35, 36, 33, 32, 34, 35, 37, 36, 38, 35, 33, 37, 35, 36, 34, 35, 34.

    a. What is the mean number of patients serviced over this period?

    b. What is the standard deviation of the observations?

    c. Determine the probability that the number of people serviced in the emergency room will be 33 or greater on any given day.

    d. Determine the probability that the number of people serviced on any given day will fall between 33 and 36, inclusive.

10. The daily census at Freeland Hospital was compiled in the office of admissions for the past 30 days. It was found that the mean census was 450 and the standard deviation was 15. Given this information:

a. What is the probability that the number of patients will be 470 or more in a single day?

b. Find the probability that the number of patients will be 436 or less.

c. Find the probability that the number of patients in any given day will be between 436 and 470 inclusive.

11. The Smith General Hospital has a $1 million endowment, half of which is invested in real estate and the other half in liquid assets. The comptroller has been asked to prepare a report for the administrator which would indicate how the liquid portion of the endowment might be invested in stocks in order to maximize the hospital's gain.

Two alternative stock investment plans were explored. The first plan calls for buying growth stocks which would have an estimated probability based on past stock market performance of .80 for a 10 per cent market value appreciation; a probability of .10 for a 10 per cent loss in stock value; and a probability of .10 for zero appreciation in the course of a year. No dividends would be paid.

The second stock investment plan would consist of buying "blue chip" stocks. For these stocks there would be no appreciation in market value; however, dividends would be paid in the amount of $30,000 per year. The comptroller estimated that there is a probability of .40 that there would be a 20 per cent dividend yield increase above the base amount (due to higher dividends being paid) during the year; a probability of .10 that there would be a 10 per cent decline in dividends; and a probability of .50 that dividends from the blue chips would remain at their present level. Which of these alternatives would maximize the hospital's return and by how much?

12. A long-term care facility has a total of 125 nonprofessional employees, such as nurse's aides, ward assistants, and dietary department workers. At present each is being paid an average of $10,000 per year. Recently many facilities in the area have been unionized. The administrator is considering granting an 8 per cent increase in pay for all 125 employees, estimating that if the pay increase were given, the probability of their unionizing would be .30. However, if the pay increase is not granted, the administrator places a probability of .90 that they will vote for a union. Based on area agreements the administrator feels that if he did not grant an 8 per cent pay increase and if the employees unionized, they would bargain for and receive a 12 per cent wage increase. Further, if he were to grant the 8 per cent wage increase he is considering and the employees still unionized, they would obtain an additional 8 per cent (Total = 16 per cent) wage increase on top of what he awarded previously. By examining the costs on an annual basis, recommend one of the two alternatives (grant or not grant the 8 per cent wage increase) to the administrator by means of decision matrix analysis.

13. In the hospital cafeteria, hot and cold lunches are presently served from one line. During the period between 12:00 and 12:30 it was found that time-between-arrival for customers was one minute and that every other arrival wanted cold food. The average service time of a cold food customer (they served themselves) was one minute, and it takes twice as long to serve a hot food customer. As a result, a waiting line would build rapidly during the half-hour period. Since it is extremely costly to have the professional staff wait in line, the food service manager was considering changing the service system.

a. What is the total waiting time for the present food distribution system (determine for only 30 arrivals, with the first arrival being a cold food customer)?

b. What would the total waiting time be if a cold service line and a hot service line were established?

This Chapter Contains:

- Introduction

- Planning Defined

- Necessity of Planning
      Imposed Requirements
      Effectiveness and Efficiency

- The Planning Process Related to the Management Model
  (Output–Input Determination)

- Planning Process Activities
      Premises (Planning Assumptions)
      Forecasting
      Objective Formulation (Reformulation)
      Developing Plans of Action

- Planning Process Model

- Benefits of Planning

- Who Plans?

- Approaches to Planning

- Planning Methods
      PPBS
      Budgets
      Network Programming

- Summary

- Discussion Questions

- Incidents

Chapter 5

PLANNING AND PLANNING METHODS

"The planning process . . . entails setting objectives
and formulating the steps necessary to reach these
goals."

(Richard M. Hodgetts)[1]

INTRODUCTION

How have the present objectives of a health care organization been determined? How is the determination of what they should be at some point in the
future made? How can the health care organization anticipate the future
demands that will be placed on it? How does it prepare itself in terms of the
kinds of input resources, manpower and otherwise, that will be required, and
what are the organizational structural changes and decisions that will be needed
in order to meet those future demands? How does the health care organization
go about determining the means — the specific steps that need to be taken — by
which those objectives can be accomplished and expected demands satisfied?

The opening statement to this chapter sheds light on these questions.
Specifically, Hodgetts implies that through the planning process the health care
manager can determine in advance the framework necessary to guide the organization's future actions. Basically, that framework includes the determination
of the objectives of the organization, the means that will be used to accomplish
them, and the input resources that will be required — that is, the what, when,
how, and why things *will* be done.

PLANNING DEFINED

Planning has been defined in a number of different ways. One view considers planning to be an orderly manner by which the health care organization
can deal with the future.[2] Another definition views planning as "deciding what
to do and how to do it before action is required"[3] while yet another definition
considers planning as anticipating the future.[4]

---

[1] Richard M. Hodgetts, *Management: Theory, Process and Practice.* Philadelphia: W. B. Saunders
Co., 1975, p. 130.

[2] Charles M. Ewell, Jr., "Setting objectives: first step in planning." *Hospital Progress, 53*:68, September, 1972.

[3] Russell L. Ackoff, *A Concept of Corporate Planning.* New York: John Wiley, 1970, p. 2.

[4] Phillip H. Goodwin, and James D. Harvey, "The intra-institutional planning processes." *Hospital Administration, 14*:114, Fall, 1969.

Each of these definitions incorporates at least one of the distinct attributes of planning. First, planning can be considered as futuristic, since it deals with anticipating future events and determining what activity will be required of the organization in the future. Second, it involves decision-making because the determination of what is to be done by the organization, when, how, and for what purposes, requires that alternatives be evaluated and that decisions be made. Third, an implied attribute of planning is that it is dynamic, meaning that planned activities are affected by future events as they occur and may necessitate that those planned activities be changed. Finally, the essence of planning is to enable the health care organization manager to anticipate the future and to decide what organization action is necessary to cope with it—all for the purpose of accomplishing objectives which have been formulated.

Thus, incorporating the above attributes, we will define planning as *anticipating and making decisions about the future*. The manner in which this occurs is through the planning process. It consists of a series of activities which include the collection and analysis of relevant information from the past and present and the assessment of probable future events so that specific plans can be determined (decided) that will enable the organization to accomplish the objectives that have been formulated.

At first glance, it might appear that planning is a relatively uncomplicated subject. However, upon reflection, it is possible to state that, quite the contrary, it is an involved and important process. In fact, one writer, Charles Ewell, has stated that "no management concept is more misunderstood and bothersome to trustees, physicians and administrators than planning. . . ."[5]

In order to substantiate this point, the remaining sections of this chapter will (1) examine the necessity of planning; (2) show its important relationship to the management process model in terms of output-input determination; (3) present the activities characteristic of the planning process; and (4) demonstrate the inter-relationship among those activities by means of a model. Furthermore, (5) the benefits of planning will be pointed out; (6) a discussion of "who plans" will be made; and (7) various approaches to planning will be described along with (8) various planning methods.

NECESSITY OF PLANNING

One might ask, why is planning necessary? There are two major reasons. First, the need to plan has been imposed on health care organizations by others. Specifically, governmental, association, and other organizations have made planning mandatory. Second, planning is necessary in order for the health care organization to function rationally, effectively, and efficiently.

IMPOSED REQUIREMENTS

In recent years, federal and state governments have imposed regulations which require health care organizations, such as hospitals and skilled nursing

---

[5] Ewell, op. cit.

facilities, to plan. As a prerequisite for participation in the federal Medicare program, for example, health facilities must involve themselves in a significant level of institutional planning. To abide by these regulations, health care organizations must have the following: (1) an annual operating budget that includes all anticipated income and expenses; (2) a three-year capital expenditure plan that identifies projected expenditures for all capital projects in excess of $100,000; and (3) participation by the institution's governing body, medical staff, and administrative staff in the preparation and annual review of the budget and the health care plan.

In addition, Public Law 93–641, The National Health Planning and Resources Development Act of 1974, emphasizes the role of health planning. It calls for the establishment of Health Systems Agencies (HSA's) which will be responsible for health planning at the local level. Included are forecasting, developing area-wide plans in terms of services and facilities, and providing planning assistance to individual health care organizations. The Act also calls for the establishment of State Health Planning and Development Agencies (SHPDA) and induces those states (approximately one-half) without "certificate of need" legislation to enact it.[6]

This federal initiative, along with state licensure requirements, has had the effect of forcing health care organizations to plan carefully. They must not only plan relative to their own organization, but that planning must embrace the needs of the community and other providers within it.

Another source of pressure for planning for quality health care delivery has come from the Joint Commission on Accreditation of Hospitals, which inspects hospitals and examines virtually every facet of quality patient care. The primary purpose of the Joint Commission is to encourage organizations which comprise the voluntary health care system to work together in order to maximize quality patient care for the community.

EFFECTIVENESS AND EFFICIENCY

The second necessity for planning is that it enables the health care organization to cope with the environment and to function more effectively and efficiently. If the health care organization does not plan, then it must passively accept whatever role the environment thrusts upon it.[7] Its destiny will more likely be shaped by others through default. If the organization does not have well-thought-out objectives, haphazard activity will likely result, there will be no sense of direction, and inefficiency will probably occur. If the demand for service is not anticipated, the patient and/or community may suffer because the organization will not be prepared to meet those service requirements; thus, ineffectiveness will result. Finally, if resource requirements are not anticipated and

---

[6]Donald F. Phillips, "Health planning; new hope for a fresh start." *Hospitals, 49*:35, May 16, 1975. For a good discussion on the status of Certificate-of-Need see William J. Curran, Richard J. Steele, and Ellen W. Ober, "Government intervention on increase." *Hospitals, 49*:57, May 16, 1975. For a discussion of the implications of PL 93–641, see Arnold J. Rosoff, "Health planning and certification of need under the new health planning act." *Hospital Administration, 20*:60, Summer, 1975.

[7]Germain B. Boer, "Extending the hospital planning horizon." *Hospital Administration, 17*:51, Winter, 1972.

planned for, maldistribution of resources will probably occur, possibly including shortages of funds, skilled personnel, and so on. To reinforce the point that planning is necessary and important, relative to organization effectiveness and efficiency, we will next demonstrate how the planning process relates to the management model.

THE PLANNING PROCESS RELATED TO THE MANAGEMENT MODEL
(Output-Input Determination)

In Chapter 2, a management process model was presented (Fig. 2–3) which used an "input-conversion-output" frame of reference. Planning, as one of the managerial processes, can be viewed as the basic means by which output-input determination is made. More specifically, one of the primary activities of the planning process is the formulation and reformulation of the organization's objectives. It can be stated that planning should begin with the consideration of the objectives that the organization is attempting to achieve. Reviewing our discussion of the model in Chapter 2, objectives for our purpose are considered as being synonymous to "Desired Output;" that is, what the organization is trying to achieve. Linked to output determination is input determination—the identification of the specific resources, manpower and otherwise, that will be needed in order to accomplish those objectives. Furthermore, planning is interrelated with the other processes. First, output-input determination requires that decisions be made. Consequently, it is intertwined with the decision-making process. Second, through the executing process planned activity is carried out. Finally, the planning process is materially related to the controlling process, since objectives, or desired output, become the criteria against which actual performance is measured.

PLANNING PROCESS ACTIVITIES

There are a number of activities characteristic of the planning process. They are as follows: (1) making premises; (2) forecasting; (3) objective formulation and reformulation; and (4) the development of specific action plans. Although these activities have been enumerated in a serial fashion, it is not meant to imply that they occur in exact numerical order. This will be demonstrated in the following section; however, for the purpose of presentation, each will be discussed separately, then linked together by means of a planning process model.

Premises (Planning Assumptions)

When planning, it is necessary to make certain assumptions about the future. Premises are planning assumptions that are made relative to the external or internal (organization) environment.[8] In order to decide what the organization's objectives should be, whether they should be changed, what plans of action will best enable those objectives to be accomplished, and what input resources and organizational design changes will be necessary to accomplish them, the health care manager will have to make assumptions about the future.

EXTERNAL PREMISES

Basically, when making premises about the external environment, assumptions in several general categories will be made. Those categories and representative examples which are of concern to the planner follow:

1. The State of the Economy:
Will inflation continue, or will there be a recession?
Will the federal government reimpose wage and price controls?
Will there be high unemployment, with people losing health care insurance coverage provided by their former employer?

2. Governmental Action:
Will basic medical research funds be increased, decreased, or will they remain at the same level?
Will there be significant reimbursement method or eligibility changes made in the Medicare or Medicaid programs?
Will National Health Insurance be enacted? If so, when and in what form?
Will governmental action restrain facility expansion, reshape the delivery system, or regulate facilities much like utilities are regulated?

3. Resource Supply and Technology:
Will there be an acute shortage of health professionals such as physicians, registered nurses, or technicians?
Will material supplies substantially increase in price, or will there be shortages of materials?
Will physicians withhold services because of the inability to obtain malpractice insurance?
Will the trend of unionization in health care organizations increase or decrease in intensity?
Will technology breakthroughs occur, requiring new types of equipment and the personnel to man them?
Will medical procedures advance to the point where new and unique means of diagnosis and treatment will be available, such as wider application of laser surgery?

4. Demand:
Will the demand for health care increase or decrease? If so, in what areas and in what form?
Will demographic patterns result in a lower or higher birth rate or a shift in population centers?
Will the incidence of specific diseases change, and will cures occur (cancer or heart disease)?

---

[8] For an excellent review of premises, see George A. Steiner, *Top Management Planning.* New York: The Macmillan Company, 1969, pp. 199–202.

Will a larger portion of the population be covered by health care insurance in the future? If so, how will the demand for health care change?

Although we have only mentioned four general categories and some examples of each which relate to the environment external to health care organizations, there are others. Furthermore, depending upon the assumptions made relative to some of the examples in each category, the objectives, resource requirements, and action plans of a health care organization will be affected and will differ.

For example, if the health care organization has as its objective the provision of a wider range of services to the community, and if it plans to accomplish this by expanding the facility, what will happen if events indicate, and it is assumed, that the economy will deteriorate, capital funds will not be available at reasonable cost, and philanthropic contributions will decline? The planned expansion and increase in services probably will have to be delayed. In other words, plans will have to be changed. Or, for another example, presume that a national health insurance act will be passed within two years and will greatly increase the demand for service placed upon the nation's health care organizations. Should this be the case, it will be necessary to formulate plans today in order to be able to satisfy that future demand. Or, as one further example, presume that the health care organization includes basic research as one of its objectives. How would that change if there were an indication that federal grants would be terminated or substantially reduced?

We might even consider whether the supply of health manpower will meet future needs. If not, what should the hospital, for example, do if a shortage of RN's is anticipated? Perhaps it would modify its set of objectives to include teaching and start an RN diploma program. Furthermore, consider that data indicate that demographic changes will result in population and medical staff shifts from urban areas, and that the number of births will decline. What effect would this have on an urban hospital? Or consider that the number of elderly people will substantially increase in absolute numbers. What effect would this have on long-term care facilities? Should they expand? When? Where?

As can be noted, it is necessary to establish premises. That is, reasonable assumptions must be made about the future in order to formulate and modify objectives along with the long-term plans that are necessary in order to accomplish those objectives. In addition, one's planning assumptions will certainly have an impact on and affect the input resources required by the organization. Although it is not always possible to assume with certainty, making premises will help to reduce future uncertainty by making the planner more aware of the world around him. This will reduce the likelihood of making wrong decisions and also reveal opportunities that might not otherwise be considered. For example, how many long-term care facilities anticipated (planned for) the explosive growth in demand that occurred after the enactment of the Medicare and Medicaid programs? Probably not many.

INTERNAL PREMISES

In addition to making assumptions about the external environment, planning assumptions (premises) should also be made relative to matters internal to the organization. Those assumptions can be classified into many categories. Some of those categories, along with examples, follow:

1. Internal Resources:
Will the personnel turnover rate increase or decrease?
Will RN's leave to work for other facilities?
Will the cash flow cycle for third-party reimbursement shorten or lengthen?
Will supply costs increase or decrease?

2. Specific Demand:
Will the occupancy rate increase or decrease?
Will there be a shift in demand by services such as Medical/Surgical, OB, Pediatrics?
Will ancillary services require additional equipment due to technology or demand changes? If so, which service?

3. Physical Facilities:
Will changes have to be made in the physical plant, perhaps remodernization?
Will security be a problem?
Will defensive medicine require increased medical records storage space and/or overburden other services such as x-ray and lab?

Forecasting

Admittedly, it is difficult to project into the future and assume; nevertheless, assume we must. Depending upon one's expectations of the future, different plans to deal with it will be developed. Unfortunately there are many variables affecting plans over which the health care manager has no control. However, forecasting is a planning activity by which much uncertainty can be minimized, resulting in more accurate planning.[9] Basically, forecasting entails collecting information about the past and present, analyzing it, and making projections into the future. As one would expect, it is much more difficult to forecast political, economic, and human events (that is, the external environment), than it is to forecast the internal environment. However, when information can be quantified, such as birth rates, the incidence of disease, life expectancy, and so on, it is possible to use the data about the past to shed some light on what is likely to happen in the future.

For health care organizations, anticipation of future demand is extremely important in order that adequate facilities, personnel, equipment, supplies, and other input resources will be available to provide services. As a whole, the facility must estimate or forecast the number and type of in-patients who will require service in the next month, year, or years. Forecasts can also be made for separate services. For example, the expected number of out-patient visits, the anticipated number of laboratory tests and types that will be needed, the amount of drugs that will be used, and the number of x-rays that will be taken, to name a few, can usually be forecasted.

There are a number of ways of forecasting. One way is to ask consumers

---

[9] Ernest C. Miller, *Advanced Techniques for Strategic Planning.* American Management Association, 1971.

what their intentions are. This is called the "User's Expectation Method."[10] However, it is not truly applicable to health care organizations. It is generally impossible for the "user" (patient) to know if he will be sick tomorrow, next week, or next year; nevertheless, some areas, such as elective surgery, would be predictable. Another method of forecasting is the Delphi technique. In this method, health care managers, outside experts, and others are asked independently to give their predictions for the future. These predictions can range from forecasting the demand for specific services to predictions regarding changes in technology, scientific breakthroughs, political events (e.g., the enactment of national health insurance), and the like. After each participant has given his opinion, each is informed of the predictions of the other participants and, with that information, they each predict again.[11] Such a consensus without rigorous data analysis is necessarily subjective and based in part on experience, hunch, or possibly luck.

Perhaps one of the best methods of forecasting that is available to planners is time-series analysis. Basically, it involves the statistical identification of trends, cycles, and seasonal patterns based on historical data. For example, examining the monthly data on tonsillectomies covering many years may reveal the following: (1) a decline in the total number of tonsillectomies performed from 1940 to the present; (2) a seasonal variation, with the tendency of more occurring during the summer months; and (3) a cycle which follows the birth rate cycle by five to ten years, with an observable peak after major wars. Given this information, the planner can more accurately predict demand for tonsillectomies, make assumptions about it, and thereby allocate resources to or from that service as demand warrants.

Regression analysis is also another statistical method that uses historical data and which enables planners to draw inferences about the future. For example, statistically, there is a high correlation (degree of relationship) between the number of heroin addicts and the number of cases of hepatitis. Thus, if the number of heroin addicts is increasing in a specific geographic area, the administrator can expect more demand upon his facility to treat more cases of hepatitis.

Although time-series and regression analyses are helpful forecasting methods, model building is also a powerful tool.[12] The most familiar models are those that predict economic activity. The development of sophisticated Gross National Product models was made possible by the growing use of computers during the late 1950's. A requirement of models is that phenomena must be translated into mathematical equations. For example, economists have translated the economy, in its simplest sense, into the following equation: Gross National Product equals Consumption plus Investment, plus Governmental Expenditures plus Net Exports. This is expressed mathematically as

$$GNP = C + I + G + E_n.$$

[10] Hodgetts, op. cit. p. 137.

[11] *Ibid.* pp. 429–430.

[12] For a discussion of models relative to physician supply and demand see: Judith R. Lave, Lester B. Lave, and Samuel Leinhardt, "Medical manpower models: need, demand and supply." *Inquiry*, *12*:97, June, 1975.

In the health care area it is possible to construct models. For example, observation of historical data may indicate that the number of children born each year is a function of the following: (1) the number of married women of child-bearing age; (2) the average level of disposable income; (3) the percentage of the family units having third-party hospitalization insurance; and (4) inversely related to the number of children currently within the family unit. A truly sophisticated model would incorporate other variables to represent (5) war-time-peacetime conditions; (6) cultural background; (7) religious values; and (8) the availability of family planning services, to name a few.

As a matter of practicality, there are several reaons why model building is generally not feasible for individual health care organizations. First, models are expensive to develop, validate, operate, and maintain. Second, it is extremely difficult to refine the equations to the point where the model can forecast for a specific facility. Thus, models of this type are primarily of use to state public health agencies, the U.S. Public Health Service and to associations like the American Hospital Association (AHA) and the American Medical Association (AMA). However, the individual health care organization administrator may be able to take national predictions of births, for example, and then extrapolate on the basis of the population density of his community in order to estimate births.

Objective Formulation (Reformulation)

A primary activity of the planning process is objective formulation (and reformulation). As previously indicated, objectives represent the "desired output" of the health care organization. They become the targets toward which all organizational effort can be directed. One might ask what the typical objectives of health organizations are. Examples for nonprofit hospitals can range from providing an increased scope of health care services to the community, providing quality care at reasonable costs, having educational programs, to a combination of these. A profit-making hospital may have the objective of providing only a limited range of services to the exclusion of others in order to minimize costs. Long-term care facilities may have such objectives as providing services for those who need skilled nursing care, resident care, or both. Health System Agencies may have the objective of providing forecasting, planning, and coordinative services to community facilities which offer direct patient care. A neighborhood health center may have the objective of serving those in the immediate area and functioning as a screening mechanism for referring those acutely ill to other provider organizations. The HMO may have the objective of exclusively serving enrolled members, and it may have a greater orientation toward preventive medicine.

Thus, one of the most important activities of the planning process involves the determination of the organization's objectives. This subject will be presented in greater depth in the following chapter; however, at this point it should be indicated that the overall objectives of the health care organization are generally formulated by the governing body while individual units within may have their own objectives which should be supportive of those for the organization as a whole. Furthermore, objectives will on occasion have to be changed. If events occur which force the modification of initial planning assumptions (premises) or if, through forecasting, data indicate that trends in demand, utilization, and so forth will differ from what was expected, it may be necessary to reformulate objectives. For example, as we saw in Chapter 3, the phenomenon of declining birth rates caused a group of hospitals in a community to consider consolidating various services, with one giving up its Obstetrics Department, thus modifying its objectives of a "full range of services" in order to fulfill the other objective of minimizing overall community health care costs through cooperation.

Developing Plans of Action

Depending upon the assumptions made relative to the nature of the external-internal environment, the information obtained through such means as forecasting, and the specific objectives that have been established (or modified), various plans of action are then developed in order to guide, channel, and direct organizational activity. In other words, given the determination of *what* the organization seeks to accomplish, the *how, when* and *by whom* it is to be accomplished completes the cycle of activities of the planning process.

Of necessity, means to accomplish organization objectives must be evaluated, selected, and implemented. Thus, the *how* translates into the formulation of strategies, Furthermore, the *when* must address itself to the time-frame of planned activities. Long-range planning will focus on the *when* over a considerable number of years, while short-term planning will focus on those requisite activities that must be planned and executed within a short period of time.

PLANNING PROCESS MODEL

In linking the planning process activities together we will refer to the Planning Process Model presented in Figure 5–1, and we will refer to the code numbers above each cell. In almost every instance the manager, whether it is the administrator, department head, or supervisor, functions within a health care organization which currently has specifically stated or at least implied objectives. When the manager plans, those objectives (cell 2) become his point of origin. In order to direct the organization activity for which he is responsible, the manager will of necessity make assumptions about the future (internal and external premising) (cell 1a) and judge whether the objectives for his department or the organization as a whole are reasonable in light of those assumptions. As those assumptions are modified by external events, such as new legislation or by information derived through forecasting (cell 1b), the existing objectives of the organization or the individual department may have to be modified (cell 2) or new ones established. This is denoted by the dual arrow flow between cells 1 and 2.

Given an awareness of the future and a clear formulation (or reformulation) of objectives, it is possible to construct and develop plans of action, both long-range and short-term (which will guide the organization) in order to meet and fulfill those objectives. Depending upon whether assumptions have changed and/or objectives have been modified, previously formulated plans

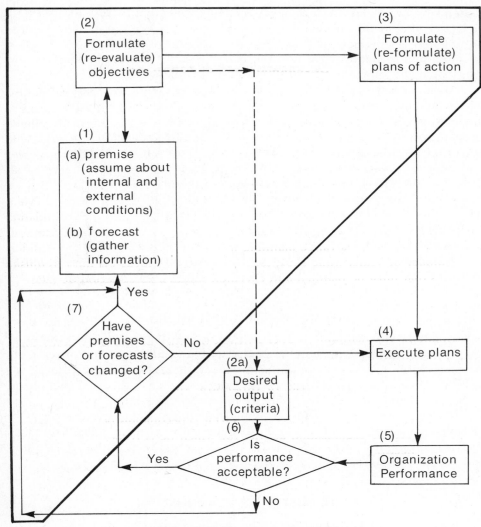

Figure 5–1 Planning process model.

may be left as they are, or they may be reformulated and modified (cell 3). These plans then represent the anticipated activities which must be done, indicate how they should be done, and by whom. For example, plans (cell 3) to add a new wing, expand the range of service, or acquire sophisticated equipment may already be in existence, with their purpose being that of providing a means to increase the scope of quality patient care services at reasonable cost to the community (objective-cell 2). However, subsequent to the formulation of those plans, events may have changed which indicate that there is an excess of beds, lack of demand for planned services, and so on. As a result, the organization's objectives of increased services at reasonable costs (cell 2) would not be accomplished through expansion, for example, and the reformulation of the long-range and short-term plans (cell 3) would be necessary.

As can be noted, the planning process activities do not necessarily flow in a fixed sequential order. Furthermore, the lower right-hand portion of the model presents the relationship that the Planning Process has to the other managerial processes. Note that once plans have been formulated and/or reformulated they must be carried out. The Executing Process is concerned with initiation of action; that is, carrying out or executing (cell 4) planned activities (cell 3) within the organization, which results in organization performance (cell 5). In addition, the objectives delineate the desired output (objectives to be fulfilled) (cell 2a) and become the Controlling Process criteria against which actual performance (cell 5) is compared (cell 6).

Should the actual performance (cell 5) of the health care organization compare favorably (cell 6) to the criteria (cell 2a), then it can be assumed that objectives are being met (cell 2), provided that internal or external events have not occurred which require that premises or forecasts be modified (cell 7). Should premise or forecast changes not be indicated (cell 7), then previously formulated plans can continue to be executed (cell 4). However, should organization performance not correspond to desired output (cell 6), the indication would be that the external/internal environmental planning assumptions and/or forecasts are inaccurate or have changed, thus requiring that they need to be modified (cell 1) and/or that the objectives are unrealistic relative to the capability of the organization and should be re-evaluated and reformulated (cell 2), or both.

In conclusion, one specific fact this model attempts to convey is that the planning process activities are not discrete and mutually exclusive. They never end and are continuous, meaning that the whole process of planning is on-going and has no end point.

BENEFITS OF PLANNING

If one synthesizes the activities represented in the planning process model and looks at it as a whole, a number of benefits of systematic planning can be observed. First, the very act of planning requires that attention be focused on the objectives of the organization; specifically, what is it trying to achieve? Once attention has been focused on objectives, planning identifies the input resources and activities that are necessary to attain them. It therefore provides a means for unifying the action of all the organization members toward common ends and for making sound decisions in regard to staffing, building, equipment, and financing needs.[13] A second benefit of planning is that it reduces role ambiguity within the organization.[14] By determining what the objectives are and the translation of future activities which are required into plans of action, areas of responsibility can be assigned. Each manager becomes aware of his responsibilities and the future performance required of him and his subordinates. When the personnel of health care organizations know the direction in which they are headed and the steps that are planned to get there, all activity can be more effectively coordinated.

A third benefit of planning is that it enhances the capability of the organization to cope with the external environment and reduce uncertainty.[15] The very act of trying to anticipate and make premises about future events obviously enhances the capability of the organization to effectively react. Another benefit of planning is that it enhances the quality of decision-making. Miner observes, "The very process of planning tends to lead to decision-making that deals with more factors and takes more considerations into account."[16] By making premises, and by forecasting and evaluating alternatives in a systematic manner, better decisions will be made and costs can be managed and contained.[17] Finally, systematic planning facilitates control. Control implies comparing actual results with some predetermined standards. Planning involves the establishment of these standards; this is known as desired output. The more clearly they are articulated, the easier it is to monitor the present and future activity of the organization.

WHO PLANS?

In answering this question, our response is—*everyone*. It is evident that those with managerial responsibilities involving resources, whether manpower, financial, material, and so on, must plan. Furthermore, those individuals who simply have a specific job to perform plan their activities to some degree.

INDIVIDUAL

The time devoted to planning, the scope and importance of planning, and the nature of the planning that an individual engages in are typically dependent upon the following: (1) his level in the organization hierarchy; (2) the job responsibilities of the individual; and (3) the amount and type of resources within his jurisdiction. For example, the administrator of a health care organization is responsible for the total organization. Thus, he has a wide planning scope which may include participation in objective formulation for the organization as a whole, making internal and external planning assumptions about the future, forecasting, and the development of the means (i.e., strategies) to

---

[13] Ewell, op. cit. pp. 71, 74.
[14] John B. Miner, *The Management Process: Theory, Research, and Practice.* New York: The Macmillan Company, 1973, p. 126.
[15] *Ibid.* p. 126.
[16] *Ibid.* p. 127.
[17] Harold E. Green, "Developing a master plan." *Hospitals,* 49:75, February 1, 1975.

accomplish those organizational objectives. Since he is responsible for all of the resources used by the organization, he will therefore spend a great deal of time planning. The department head will also plan but will have a narrower planning scope than the administrator. He will be concerned with his department's objectives, which should complement those of the organization as a whole. He will also forecast and make plans relative to the resource needs and service demands for which he is responsible.

The supervisor also plans. The scope of his plans will be fairly narrow, dealing primarily with the operational requirements of his job. These encompass the day-to-day things required to supervise the work of others, such as scheduling, perhaps training, coordination of activities, and so on. Little time will be spent in forecasting, long-range planning, or making external premises. The supervisor's planning will thus require much less time than the administrator's or department head's, and tend to focus on the work group.

The individual employee will also plan, but to a more limited extent. Of concern will be those matters related to the completion of his job. The time frame may consist of what to do and when to do it, such as today or tomorrow, along with how he will complete his job tasks. However, the employee will rarely involve himself in planning activities other than those specifically related to performing his job.

INSTITUTIONAL

Having indicated that all managers and individual employees plan, at least to some degree, it should be pointed out that the degree and scope of planning performed by different health care organizations will vary. Certainly, most, if not all, of the planning process activities will be activated—meaning that objectives will be formulated, some assumptions will be made about the future, forecasts may or may not be made, and specific plans will be developed. However, the degree and focus may vary depending upon the character of the organization. For example, a health system agency will devote most of its effort to planning, formulating premises, forecasting, and developing long-range community plans, since that is its primary function. Of concern will be the future health care needs of the community, the evaluation of existing provider organizations in its area of jurisdiction, and plans to elicit cooperation among them.

Governmental organizations, such as the Department of Health, Education, and Welfare, will be concerned with planning as related to the total health care delivery system, the demand expected in the future, the resource requirements in terms of aggregate numbers of physicians, dentists, nurses, technicians, number of hospitals, long-term care facilities, population center shifts, and so on. In short, its focus will be very broad. Of concern will be how to effect changes in the delivery system through such means as legislation and funding, in order to change the system to meet the nation's health care needs.

The individual hospital or long-term care facility will plan, but its focus will be relatively narrow. Specifically, concern will be directed to itself and to its future resource needs, with some attention given to other institutions in its geographic area.

APPROACHES TO PLANNING

Regardless of who plans, various approaches to planning can be taken. Among them are the following; (1) overt-reaction planning; (2) developmental-adaptive planning; and (3) optimizing-satisficing planning.

OVERT-REACTION PLANNING

Overt planning is planning that is systematic and formalized[18] so that future events can be anticipated and means can be devised in order to cope with them. Reaction planning is basically default planning. It is planning done on the rebound, planning that is *ad hoc* and done in reaction to external or internal events rather than in anticipation of them. For example, the manager who is overworked owing to a lack of organizational support will of necessity become a reaction type of planner through no fault of his own simply because there is not enough time to reflect about and anticipate future events. Whether the overt or reaction planning approach is followed is often a function of the administration's philosophy, its recognition of the importance of planning, and its resource commitment to planning in terms of money and manpower, along with the personal attitudes of the planner.

DEVELOPMENTAL AND ADAPTIVE PLANNING

Another approach to planning can be labeled as developmental-adaptive.[19] Developmental planning implies a high degree of autonomy, few constraints in setting objectives, and the means to accomplish them. Often new governmental programs represent developmental planning where minimal constraints exist. One example is the development and implementation of Medicare-Medicaid programs.

Adaptive planning implies the converse: that autonomy in setting objectives and the long-range and short-term plans to reach them are heavily contingent upon and constrained by environmental factors, both internal and external. Planning in individual health care organizations can generally be considered as adaptive. It would be extremely difficult for a hospital, for example, to change its basic purpose or to function on a "cash-only" basis for services rendered and not in cooperation with third-party insurers. The individual facility must adapt to and operate within the context and constraints of the delivery system and its other providers. However, viewing health care delivery as a whole, agencies responsible for area-wide planning would tend to engage in developmental planning, since they contribute to the identification of the overall health care requirements of a geographic area (desired output) and the role of individual health care organizations in fulfilling those area needs.

A fact of life for the health care administrator is that he must manage his organization within the broad context of the entire delivery system. That means that certain constraints are placed upon him. Often the means by which adaptive planners (individual facilities) influence developmental planners is

---

[18] Goodwin and Harvey, op cit., p. 116.

[19] John Friedmann, "A conceptual model for the analysis of planning behavior." *Administrative Science Quarterly, 12*:229, September, 1967.

through political manipulation. In making this point between developmental and adaptive planning, Friedmann states:

> In adaptive planning, there will be a tendency to push decisions upward to centers of developmental planning where the parameters for choice at lower levels may be changed. In attempting this, lower-level planning systems will generally rely on political manipulation to achieve their ends.[20]

That is, political pressure by representatives of individual health care system constituents (such as hospitals, long-term care facilities, physicians, and dentists, to name a few) is used to influence the initial planning done by developmental planners, which will eventually affect the individual provider. A case in point would be the attempts by the American Hospital Association and the American Medical Association to shape the nature of proposed national health insurance legislation. Another example was the attempt by the AMA to block the establishment of Professional Standards Review Organizations (PSROs).

OPTIMIZING AND SATISFICING

Planning can also be classified relative to administrative philosophy. The two standard classifications are "optimizing" and "satisficing" planning. In describing these two classifications, Ackoff indicates that optimizing planning seeks to translate objectives and the means (plans) to accomplish them into quantifiable measures. Furthermore, optimizing implies attempts to (1) minimize resource inputs and their costs in order to obtain a specific level of performance (quality care); or (2) maximize performance (quality care) given the resources available.[21]

Satisficing planning, on the other hand, is characterized as planning design to "do well enough, but not necessarily as well as possible." This type of planning attempts to achieve an "acceptable" balance between performance (quality care) and the costs of providing it (resources used). Satisficing planning usually occurs when desired output, such as quality patient care, cannot be precisely measured in quantitative terms or when solution criteria and/or constraints are such that maximizing minimizing are not part of the decision choice (alternative) set (see Chapter 3), and plans must therefore be satisficing in nature. Obviously, quality patient care cannot easily be evaluated in quantifiable terms. In fact, from an optimizing point of view, there are instances in which quality patient care is inefficient. For example, organ transplant teams may cost more to assemble and equip than the revenue derived from the operations they perform. Similarly, stand-by sophisticated equipment that "may save a patient's life" may not be justified on an optimizing philosophical basis in terms of minimizing resource (input) costs because of self- or externally imposed solution criteria and constraints. The point is that by necessity the health care organization must satisfice plan because of the nature of its services. Since much of quality patient care cannot be quantified, there is no way

---

[20] *Ibid.* p. 230.
[21] Ackoff, op. cit. pp. 12–13.

to employ optimizing planning truly — nor should it always be employed. While cost benefit planning cannot be totally ignored, decision-making and planning solely on the basis of costs, revenues, and profits are not appropriate in the health care setting.

Since overt rather than reaction planning is good management in and of itself, its merits are readily recognizable. Since adaptive planning is generally imposed on the health care organization administrator, there is little he can do about it. Since satisficing planning is a necessity by reason of the service and humanitarian nature of the health care organization, the administrator must follow that philosophy.

PLANNING METHODS

Planning consists of anticipating the future and making decisions about it. We have presented forecasting as one activity which assists the manager in developing plans of action. At this point we will conclude this chapter with a presentation of several procedural methods which can assist the health care manager in planning. They will include the following: (1) the Planning, Programming and Budgeting System (PPBS); (2) Resource Budgets; and (3) Network Planning, comprised of the Program Evaluation Review Technique (PERT) and the Critical Path Method (CPM).

PPBS

The Planning, Programming and Budgeting System (PPBS) is a planning procedural tool that was first developed for and widely implemented in governmental agencies, in particular, the Department of Defense (DOD). PPBS was formally implemented as a required procedure for federal agencies in 1965.[22] Specifically, it is a procedure by which the planning and development of programs and the budgeting of required resources are integrated into a whole and considered simultaneously rather than each of the activities being carried out in a disjointed fashion. Inherent are (1) the specification of objectives, (2) the identification and evaluation of alternatives to accomplish those objectives, and (3) the minimization of costs or maximization of benefits; all are accomplished through systematic analysis.[23] This constitutes the PPBS procedure.

The planning portion of PPBS involves objective formulation and identification of alternatives and means to accomplish those objectives. The programming portion consists of delineating those resources (manpower, material, financial, facilities) required of each alternative. The budgeting portion includes assigning dollar costs to the resources required by the program.[24]

---

[22]David J. Ott, and Attiat F. Ott, "The budget process." *In*: Fremont J. Lyden and Ernst G. Miller, eds, *Planning, Programming, Budgeting: A Systems Approach.* Chicago: Markham Publishing Company, 1972, pp. 43–44.

[23]*Ibid.* p. 44.

[24]David Novick, "The Department of Defense." *In*: David Novick, ed., *Program Budgeting.* New York: Holt, Rinehart and Winston, Inc., 1969, p. 91.

In commenting on the application of PPBS in the Department of Defense, Seidman observes:

> When the program structure was developed in the Department of Defense, there were two reasons that it was regarded—and rightly so—as a significant advance. First, expenditures had previously been grouped by types of activities or inputs, such as motor pool, quartermaster, equipment repair, and the like. It was impossible to relate these activities to any specific objectives, and it was equally impossible to relate costs to outputs since they were not defined. Therefore, grouping costs by missions (objectives) was a major advance in understanding the cost of achieving specific objectives. Second, these individually defined missions were then placed in a "hierarchy of objectives" with the highest levels having the most generalized goals. This was the first time that high-level DOD officials could see what proportions of their expenditures were being allocated to various broad goals.[25]

Examples of DOD programs or missions include (1) strategic retaliatory forces, (2) continental air and missile defense forces, and (3) reserve and National Guard forces. In the Department of Health, Education, and Welfare, three representative Health Services programs are Health Services for the Aged, Health Services for the Poor, and Health Services for the Indians.[26]

PPBS is widely used in governmental agencies, and it tends to be "macro," meaning "broad in scope." As a procedure, it can be applied to individual health care facilities. A given facility, for example, could have (1) quality patient care, (2) research, and (3) professional training as its three distinct objectives. Through PPBS the administration could translate those objectives into programs, budget the costs of each, evaluate each in terms of benefits, pay off, and output, and then select any or all of them within the constraint of the total resources available.

Budgets

Resource budgets are considered to be operational plans translated into numerical form.[27] As a procedural planning method, budgets are necessary in order to manage a health care organization effectively. There are long-term and short-term budgets, comprehensive and partial budgets, and flexible and fixed budgets.

Generally, budgets are drawn up by functional areas such as administration, business office, pharmacy, medical records, surgery, and the like. They translate the manpower, material, equipment, and anything else required by each unit into dollar terms.[28] As an operational plan, budgets indicate the inputs in terms of dollars that are required of the organization or unit within the organization in order to fulfill its obligations. Of the many benefits result-

---

[25] David R. Seidman, "PPB in HEW—Some management issues." *In:* Ott and Ott, op. cit., p. 319.
[26] *Ibid.* p. 318.
[27] Leon E. Hay, *Budgeting and Cost Analysis for Hospital Management.* Bloomington, Indiana: Pressler, 1963, p. 126.
[28] Richard L. Durbin and W. Herbert Springall, *Organization and Administration of Health Care.* St. Louis: C. V. Mosby Company, 1969, p. 155.

ing from the act of preparing budgets, the American Hospital Association succinctly observed:

> A complete budget program, coordinating planning and control, benefits management, including the governing board:
> (1) it provides assistance in establishing goals and setting policies that will influence the attainment of the goals;
> (2) it aids in coordinating activities and responsibilities of employees at all levels;
> (3) it provides a standard for comparison of actual results with estimates, which will assist in intelligent evaluation of the cost of activities and provide a means to evaluate performance;
> (4) it stimulates cost consciousness throughout the organization; and
> (5) it assists management in anticipating working capital needs so that financial arrangements with lending agencies may be made in advance and at favorable rates. Budgeting is an essential part of the management process.[29]

Network Programming

There are two network programming planning methods that can be used by health care organizations, the Performance Evaluation Review Technique (PERT) and the Critical Path Method (CPM).[30] Both are procedural methods typically used for large-scale, complex, one-time types of projects which require the project manager to plan, schedule, and control a great number of activities. It is particularly suited for implementation through the project management organizational arrangement described in Chapter 7.

Characteristic of any large-scale project is the fact that many of its activities are interrelated and independent of each other and must occur in a specific sequence. For example, in a building project, the architectural design would occur before construction would begin. It would be necessary for the plumbing and electrical work to be completed before the finished carpentry and painting are done and installation of equipment can occur.

In this very simplified example it can be noted that a multitude of activities have to be planned and sequenced in a specific order. With PERT, which was initially developed by the United States Navy in the late 1950's to plan, schedule, and control the Polaris missile submarine construction project, it is possible to plan, schedule, and control large projects.[31]

PERT involves the sequence of activities, and estimates of three times of completion are made for each activity (optimistic, pessimistic, and a probabilistic expected time for completion). By diagramming (sequencing) the activities on a time axis, and taking the optimistic, pessimistic, and expected times for completion, it is possible to ascertain three different time requirements for the

---

[29]American Hospital Association, *Budgeting Procedures for Hospitals.* Chicago: American Hospital Association, 1971, p. 4.

[30]A basic presentation of PERT and CPM can be found in (a) Paul Barentson, *Critical Path Planning: Present and Future Techniques.* Princeton, New Jersey: Brandon Systems Press, 1970. (b) John R. Griffith, *Quantitative Techniques for Hospital Planning and Control.* Lexington, Mass: Lexington Books, 1972; (c) Jerome D. Wiest, and Ferdinand K. Levy, *A Management guide to PERT/CPM.* Englewood Cliffs, New Jersey: Prentice-Hall, 1969.

[31]Wiest and Levy, op. cit., p. 3.

Table 5–1   Nursing Station Remodeling Project

(1) JOB NAME	(2) DESCRIPTION	(3) IMMEDIATE PREDECESSOR	(4) TIME (DAYS)
A	Construct temporary nursing station (N.S.) work area in a vacant room	–	1
B	Move N.S. records, phones, etc. to temporary facility	A	1
C	Remove original N.S. counter, desks, etc.	B	1
D	Construct new N.S. shell	C	3
E	Install electrical wiring	D	2
F	Install heating and air-conditioning	D	4
G	Install dry-wall	E, F	2
H	Install floor	G	2
I	Paint	H	1
J	Replace equipment from temporary N.S. work area	I	1

total project. It is also possible to know which activities must be completed before other activities can be started.

To develop the network requires planning. Specific activities that will have to be done must be identified. How those activities are going to be completed in terms of the equipment needed and the manpower required must be determined. Finally, it is necessary to plan the sequencing of activities so that the whole project can be completed. Gue for instance, indicates the usefulness of PERT and CPM in health care organization planning by stating the following:

> They may be used by architects, engineers, and administrators to plan construction and finance large scale hospital projects in such a way that costs are minimized, time schedules are maintained and potential bottlenecks are located.[32]

The Critical Path Method (CPM) is very similar to PERT in that it focuses on project activities and the sequencing of those particular activities, but it does not incorporate the probabilistic determination of "expected time" for activity completion. It uses one estimated time.

With CPM, the planner establishes the sequence of activities. He estimates the time of completion for each activity. He can also identify those activities which could delay the whole project if not completed on time if others cannot be started until they are completed. This is known as the Critical Path. He can then determine whether (1) to assign more resources, such as manpower, to an activity behind schedule, or (2) to work overtime to speed up the completion time of a given activity so that the project could be completed faster.

CPM EXAMPLE

Table 5–1 and Figure 5–2 present a simplified example of how CPM can be utilized in the remodeling of a nursing station. Table 5–1 presents the required activities "A" through "J" and their description (column 2). In addition, the immediate predecessor activity (column 3) is recorded. This indicates the required sequencing of activities; in other words, the electrical wiring (activity E) cannot be installed until after the shell is constructed (activity D). Finally, column 4 indicates the estimated time required to complete each activity of the project.

---

[32] Ronald L. Gue, "Operations research in health and hospital administration." *Hospital Administration, 10:*13, Fall, 1965.

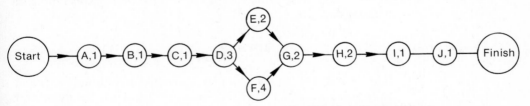

Total Project Time: 16 Days
Critical Path: A, B, C, D,
F, G, H, I, J
Slack Time: Activity E, 2 Days

Figure 5–2   Nursing station remodeling network diagram of activities.

Figure 5–2 presents the information appearing in Table 5–1 in diagram form. Each activity is labeled with its required days (A, 2). The arrows denote the required sequencing of activities. For example, activity B must be completed before activity C can be started.

The minimum project completion time is 16 days. The critical path is A,B,C,D,F,G,H,I, and J. A delay in any one of those activities would delay the entire project. The only slack time in the total network is activity E. Activities E and F cannot begin until activity D has been completed. Similarly, activity G cannot begin until activities E and F have both been completed. F takes four days and E takes two days. Thus, E could take two additional days and still not delay the project.

The planner has several options. First, if any of the critical path activities are delayed, the whole project will be delayed. If, upon reexamination, it is found that activity H, for example, will take three additional days (five instead of two) then the total project time will increase from 16 to 19 days. If assigning an extra work crew to the activity of installing the floor (H) for one day will keep it within the original estimate of two days, at a cost of 200 dollars, it may be advantageous. In deciding whether to add another crew, the project officer would consider a number of factors. One might be a cost-benefit analysis. Assume that the scheduling of another crew to help lay the floor would cost 200 dollars. If the revenue foregone by having the temporary nursing station in a semi-private room for three additional days was greater than 200 dollars, a decision would probably be made to add the crew.

A second option, for example, would be to decrease the total completion time of the project from 16 days to 14 days. Note that activity F requires four days while activity E requires two days. If F could be reduced two days by assigning more workers, it will enable the project to be completed two days earlier. The planner must evaluate his alternatives. If, for example, the cost of assigning an additional crew of workers to activity F (air-conditioning) was 800 dollars and the revenue lost from the semi-private room was 500 dollars, what should the planner do?

The benefits of network programming are that it is extremely useful as a planning and control device. For our purpose now we are interested in network programming as a planning device. PERT and CPM require advanced planning. All the activities of the total complex operation have to be identified, estimates of time for completion of the activities must be made, and the required manpower and resources needed in order to carry them out must be acquired. In other words, it is anticipation of the future, it is expectation of events, and it is making decisions.

SUMMARY

This chapter presented the subject of planning. It was defined as *anticipating and making decisions about the future.* The planning process was described as consisting of the activities of (1) making premises, (2) forecasting, (3) objective formulation, and (4) the development of plans of action, both long-range and short-term. Reviewing the management process model presented in Chapter 2 (Fig. 2–3), it was pointed out that planning entails output-input determination; that is, the determination of the desired output (objectives) of the organization and the input resources that are required by it.

Furthermore, the planning process activities were described, linked to each other, and linked to the decision-making, executing, and controlling processes by means of the model presented in Figure 5–1 of this chapter. Some of the benefits of planning were described. In addition, a discussion of who plans and approaches to planning was given. Finally, this chapter concluded with a presentation of various procedural planning methods.

Brief attention was given to objective formulation and the development of means (plans) to accomplish these objectives. In the following chapter these subjects will be presented in greater depth, along with a discussion of policies, procedures, and rules.

DISCUSSION QUESTIONS

1. Discuss the various reasons why you feel planning is important in order to manage effectively.

2. It has been stated that "Planning is the most important of the managerial processes." Do you agree? Why?

3. A number of benefits resulting from planning were presented in this chapter. Identify others and discuss why you think they are beneficial.

4. Regardless of your current status (administrator, department head, employee, or student), reflect for a moment about the organization with which you are identified (health care or educational organization). Turn to the Planning Process Model (Figure 5–1), and note what you perceive to be the official position of the organization relative to each activity. What assumptions about the future have been made? What are its objectives? What plans of action, both long-range and short-term, can you identify?

5. Viewing the Planning Process Model in Figure 5–1, make notes about each activity with regard to your personal life. In particular, answer the following questions: What assumptions about the future have you made? What are your objectives? Have they recently changed because events forced the alteration of your assumptions? What long-range and short-term plans do you have to accomplish those objectives? Have you been accomplishing the activities that will presently or eventually result in the accomplishment of those objectives?

6. It was mentioned that optimization as a planning approach was not suitable for health care organizations. Do you agree or disagree? Discuss your answer.

7. How do decision criteria and constraints (see Chapter 3) which are internally or externally imposed force health care organizations to satisfice plan? What are some examples of those constraints?

8. Presume that you are a health care organization administrator, that national health insurance was recently enacted to be implemented in one year, and that demand for all services provided by your organization would increase by 15 per cent. What things would you have to consider and do to meet that demand?

INCIDENTS

1. SHARING SERVICES—CONSIDERATIONS

A certain community has a population of 400,000, with six general acute hospitals. At none of these hospitals is there a formal program of ambulatory surgery. These hospitals have banded together to discuss the implications of establishing programs of ambulatory surgery, since this concept has begun to sweep the United States. One of the ways that they could do this would be to erect a freestanding center owned and operated by the six hospitals. Another idea they are considering is for some or all of the hospitals to establish a program of ambulatory surgery within their individual hospitals in such a way that the out-patients would be merged with the in-patients.

A. What major factors should be taken into consideration as to how these hospitals should proceed to develop the proper level of ambulatory surgery for their community?

B. What are the advantages and disadvantages of some of the alternate approaches that they may consider?

C. What committees might be formed that would be valuable to help resolve these issues?

2. SHARING SERVICES – PROBLEMS

Five hospitals in your area have been working together to share services in order to reduce cost and improve patient care while avoiding the duplication of community facilities. One of these hospitals has agreed to provide psychiatric employees in your Emergency Department. As administrator you have examined the overall concept and feel that it is very important to have psychiatric help available for some of the patients that come through a busy Emergency Department. You have the most active Emergency Department in the city, but you do not have a Department of Psychiatry in your hospital. The hospital nearby has an active department, and they have trained both psychiatric nurses and psychiatric social workers who could be assigned to your hospital. The employees from the other hospital work regular shifts and receive their pay and fringe benefits from the other hospital, and you are billed for their services for their direct payroll cost plus 25 per cent in fringe benefits. Occasionally, in the past few weeks, conflicts have arisen between some of the employees in your Emergency Department and these "outsiders" from the neighboring hospital. As far as you can determine, all the patient care implications are excellent, but the interpersonal behavior problems are creating quite a problem.

A. As administrator of this hospital, what steps would you take to help resolve this situation?

B. Is such an arrangement automatically destined for failure?

C. How would the proposal help fulfill your organization's objectives?

D. What plans would you make before implementing the arrangement to ensure its success?

Activity Job Name	Description	Immediate Predecessor	Time (weeks)
A	Look for and select location	—	4
B	Arrange for and obtain financing	—	6
C	Design of building	A	6
D	Requests for bids and select	A,B,C	2
E	Building construction	D	24
F	Order equipment and have delivered	C	20
G	Install equipment	E,F	2
H	Recruit, hire, and train key personnel	C	16
I	Obtain Medicare-Medicaid and state certification	G,H	2
J	Facility inspection by fire and health officials	G	2
K	Inform public and other acute care providers and seek patients	I	1
L	Open doors	J,K	—

3. BUILDING A LONG-TERM-CARE FACILITY

A proprietary group of investors has decided to build a 50-bed long-term-care facility. Having planned the project, they determine that the following activities would be necessary, and they have estimated the times of completion (in weeks) for each:

A. Draw a CPM chart using the data presented above.

B. How long will it be before the long term-care facility's doors can be opened for the admission of patients?

C. Which activities represent the critical path?

D. Which activities can be delayed, and for how long can they be delayed without affecting the completion of the total project?

E. What would happen to the project if the equipment supplier was struck by its employees (as soon as the equipment was ordered) for 12 weeks? (It takes 20 weeks to manufacture and deliver the equipment once the order has been placed.)

This Chapter Contains:

- Introduction
- Objectives
    Multitude of Objectives (Primary-Secondary)
    Hierarchy of Objectives
- Strategies
    Hierarchy of Strategies
- Policies
    Hierarchy of Policies
- Formulation and Linkage
- Policies Revisited
    Characteristics of Good Policies
- Procedures
- Rules
- Summary
- Discussion Questions
- Incidents

Chapter 6

OBJECTIVES, STRATEGIES, AND POLICIES

"Organizational objectives may be described as 'hoped for results, goals or targets.'

... strategies may be viewed as specific *major* actions or patterns of action for attainment of objectives.

Policies may be described as broad guides for managers, supervisors and other employees for the achievement of objectives."

(Paine and Naumes)[1]

INTRODUCTION

We are often confronted with the words "objectives," "strategies," and "policies." We are told, for example, that one objective of the federal government is full employment. From observation, it can be determined that the strategy (means or plans of action) used to accomplish that objective includes deficit spending and direct or indirect support of various economic sectors such as transportation and construction. Policies that guide behavior as the strategy is carried out may range from the unshelving of public works projects when unemployment rises to a given level, to the taking of specific steps for lowering the rate of interest.

In the health care area, the objective of the federal government (or society) is to ensure that quality health care is available to all at an affordable price. The strategy used to accomplish this objective may include sponsoring federal health care programs, either for specific segments of the population (Medicare-Medicaid) or for the whole population (National Health Insurance), supporting the construction of new facilities (Hill-Burton Act), and sponsoring basic research and the training of health professionals. Policies to guide behavior and decision-making during the execution of this strategy might be to determine eligibility for service or funds, the manner of disbursement of funds (for example, whether copayments are required), the manner in which priorities for construction of facilities are established, and which types of educational programs will receive support and attention.

In dealing with the objective of quality care at an affordable price, a strategy might consist of cost containment possibly including specific actions such as

---

[1]Frank T. Paine and William Naumes, *Organizational Strategy and Policy*. Philadelphia: W. B. Saunders Company, 1975, pp. 6–7.

demonstration grants for the investigation of incentive reimbursement systems, funding for various forms of delivery, such as the HMOs, and the need for comprehensive health care manpower and facility planning. Complementary policies might include establishing an admission review procedure and requiring that generic rather than brand name prescriptions be issued.

How are objectives, strategies, and policies formulated? How are they interrelated? How do they relate to individual health care organizations, and what is the link between them and the management of those organizations?

In this chapter we will endeavor to answer these questions. As the introductory quotes indicate, objectives, strategies, and policies are defined differently, and yet, as we will demonstrate, they are linked together.

In the preceding chapter, "Planning and Planning Methods," the planning process and its characteristic activities of (1) making premises, (2) forecasting, (3) formulating objectives, and (4) developing plans of action were presented. Also discussed was the fact that the planning process entails output-input determination and that it is, therefore, linked to the other management processes of (1) decision-making, (2) organizing, (3) executing, and (4) controlling. This chapter will expand further upon the subjects of objectives, strategies, and policies.

WHAT ARE OBJECTIVES, STRATEGIES, AND POLICIES?

OBJECTIVES

Objectives were previously described as the goals, missions, or targets of the health care organization. In terms of the management model presented in Chapter 2 (Fig. 2–3), *we have used the term "desired-output" to denote objectives—what the organization wishes to accomplish*. It was further indicated that without clear-cut objectives, haphazard activity, misdirected behavior, and inefficiency would be likely to occur. This lays the foundation for the statement that "only when objectives have been thought out and articulated can the resources required by the organization, its plans of action, and the execution of organization activity logically occur." Having given examples of objectives for various types of health care organizations in the previous chapter, we will now follow up with a discussion of the multitude and hierarchy of objectives.

Multitude of Objectives (Primary-Secondary). Most health care organizations have a multitude of objectives, which can be classified as primary and secondary. For most of these organizations, the primary objective will be quality patient care. Many organizations will have additional objectives which might be classified as secondary, since they do not carry as high a priority as the primary objective. Some of these objectives may relate to employees; for example, providing stability of employment. Another objective might be that of maintaining an innovative institution in terms of medical care. Other objectives may be growth and survival. In the case of hospitals, Georgopoulos and Mann observe

The chief objective of the hospital is, of course, to provide adequate care and treatment to its patients (within the limits of present day technical-medical knowledge, and knowledge of organizing human activity effectively, as well as within limits that may be imposed by the relative scarcity of appropriate organizational resources or by extraorganizational forces). Its principal product is medical, surgical, and nursing service to the patient, and its central concern is the life and health of the patient. A hospital may, of course, have additional objectives, including its own maintenance and survival, organizational stability, and growth.[2]

Any or all of these secondary objectives may be adopted, survival typically being one of them. The set or sum total of primary and secondary objectives becomes the "desired output" of the organization. The implication is that many objectives—not just one—will be adopted by health care organizations.

Hierarchy of Objectives.   Within any organization a hierarchy of objectives will exist. The health care organization will have primary and secondary objectives. In addition, the operating departments or units within that particular organization will have specific objectives of their own. These departmental or unit objectives will be subsidiary to the overall primary and secondary objectives, and should be consistent with and complement them. They are established in order to give direction to the activities of the various departments; their fulfillment will contribute to the fulfillment of the organization's overall objectives. In order to make the distinction, Table 6–1 provides examples of the primary and secondary objectives of a health care organization along with sample objectives of specific departments within it.

STRATEGIES

Basically, strategies are defined as broad sets of action plans designed to accomplish the organization's objectives. Paine and Naumes state that "strategies may be viewed as specific *major* actions or patterns of action for attainment of objectives."[3] In the previous chapter, we discussed the need for the organization to develop long-range and short-term plans. *The broad set of present and planned activities of the organization constitutes the strategy or means by which the organization seeks to accomplish its objectives.* Strategy, then, is the *means* by which objectives are to be accomplished.

The long-term care facility may have a primary objective of delivering quality patient care and a secondary objective of remaining financially solvent. Its broad strategy, the means to accomplish its primary objective, may include having the most modern facilities and employing qualified personnel. Relative to the secondary objective, it may have the strategy of containing costs and promoting mutual cooperation with the state nursing home association to explain the need for adequate state per diem payments for Medicaid patients.

Hierarchy of Strategies.   As in the case of objectives, there will exist in each organization a hierarchy of strategies. This means that the organization will have an identifiable strategy (means by which it seeks to accomplish objectives) and that each department or unit will develop a strategy to fulfill its own objectives. In order to present the concept of strategy hierarchy, Table 6–2

---

[2]Basil S. Georgopoulos and Floyd C. Mann, *The Community General Hospital.* New York: The Macmillan Company, 1962, p. 5.

[3]Paine and Naumes, op. cit. p. 7.

Table 6–1 Examples of Primary, Secondary, and Departmental Objectives

PRIMARY OBJECTIVES:	*A hospital may have primary objectives of:* Maximizing the level of patient care using the resources available and providing a wide range of services to meet the needs of the whole community.
SECONDARY OBJECTIVES:	*Secondary objectives could consist of:* Providing a sound medical education program, being a responsible employer and a cost efficient organization, and conducting medical research.
DEPARTMENTAL OBJECTIVES:	*(A) Objectives of the dietary department, for example, which would be subsidiary to the primary and secondary objectives of the organization, might be:* To serve food to patients, personnel, and guests that not only meets nutritional requirements but is served at the proper temperature, and is attractive and tasty, while at the same time attempting to minimize the costs of those meals. *(B) Subsidiary objectives of the maintenance department might consist of:* Attempting to minimize the cost of maintaining the facility and, whenever possible, ensuring that equipment citical to the care of patients does not break down. *(C) Subsidiary objectives of the medical records department might be:* To provide and maintain an efficient system in which patient records are kept safe from loss or destruction, protected from unauthorized perusal, adequately indexed, and rapidly available to authorized personnel, while also seeking to continuously assist the medical staff in their provision of patient care by updating the record format to meet their needs and ensuring that medical record practices and procedures comply with legal requirements. *(D) Subsidiary objectives of the purchasing department might be:* To procure materials, supplies, and equipment at the lowest possible cost, consistent with the quality necessary to meet the required standards of the using department and attempt to minimize costs by maintaining as low an inventory level as possible, yet ensuring that adequate supplies are always on hand.

Table 6–2 Examples of Primary, Secondary, and Departmental Objectives, and their Strategies

PRIMARY OBJECTIVES:	*A hospital may have primary objectives of:* Maximizing the level of patient care using the resources available and providing a wide range of services to meet the needs of the whole community. *An organization strategy might be:* *To attract the most qualified staff in the area, keep the physicai plant up to date, acquire the most modern equipment, and solicit philanthropic contributions.*

Table 6-2 Examples of Primary, Secondary, and Departmental Objectives, and their Strategies *(Continued)*

SECONDARY OBJECTIVES:

Secondary objectives could consist of:
    Providing a sound medical education program, being a responsible employer and a cost efficient organization, and conducting medical research.
An organization strategy might be:
    To actively recruit residents and apply for research grants.

DEPARTMENTAL OBJECTIVES:

(A) Objectives of the Dietary Department, for example, that would be subsidiary to the primary and secondary objectives of the organization might be:
    To serve food to patients, personnel, and guests that not only meets nutritional requirements but is served at the proper temperature and is attractive and tasty, while at the same time attempting to minimize the costs of those meals.
A departmental strategy might be:
    To use a premeasured portion system that will decrease costs and waste, to use frozen foods when possible in order to reduce labor content, and to use disposable plates and utensils.
(B) Subsidiary objectives of the Maintenance Department might consist of:
    Attempting to minimize the cost of maintaining the facility and, whenever possible, ensuring that equipment critical to the care of patients does not break down.
A departmental strategy might be:
    To develop a preventive maintenance schedule rather than to repair equipment as it breaks down.
(C) Subsidiary objectives of the Medical Records Department might be:
    To provide and maintain an efficient system in which patient records are kept safe from loss or destruction, protected from unauthorized perusal, adequately indexed, and rapidly available to authorized personnel, while also seeking to continuously assist the medical staff in their provision of patient care by updating the record format to meet their needs and ensuring that medical record practices and procedures comply with legal requirements.
A departmental strategy might include:
    Installing a mechanical storage and retrieval system and providing physicians with dictating equipment.
(D) Subsidiary objectives of the purchasing department might be:
    To procure materials, supplies, and equipment at the lowest possible cost, yet consistent with the required standards of quality, and to attempt to minimize costs by keeping the inventory level as low as possible, yet ensuring that adequate supplies are always on hand.
A departmental strategy might consist of:
    Developing a computerized information system which would monitor inventory levels, notify Purchasing when the safety stock level has been reached, and calculate the most economical order quantity. Another strategy might consist of pooling purchasing agreements with other area facilities in order to take advantage of quantity discounts.

---

reproduces the information contained in Table 6–1, along with examples of department strategies.

POLICIES

Policies are officially expressed or implied guidelines for behavior and decision-making within the organization. McFarland has stated that policies are the "planned expressions of a company's official attitudes toward the range of behavior within which it will permit or desire its employees to act."[4] In the performance of their duties and the execution of organization activity, the administrator, supervisor, and employee should act in a manner consistent with the policies of the organization. Viewed in a negative sense, *policies define the area of freedom for organization participants in regard to their behavior and the decisions they make when performing their duties.* In an extended sense, policies may be viewed as the specific delineation of permissible activity that will enable organized effort to result in the accomplishment of the organization's objectives.

In this sense, policies emanate from objectives, and their purpose is to provide the guidelines for people to follow while working. They are designed to help organizations attain objectives, and they should therefore be consistent with and supportive of them.

For example, if a primary objective of a health care organization is to provide quality patient care, a policy (guide to employee behavior and decision-making) might be to provide in-service training in order to maintain a staff able to give quality care in the future. This general policy serves as a guideline for how the organization wants its employees to behave. It indicates to supervisors that they should ensure that their personnel are continuously trained.

Hierarchy of Policies. Policies, like objectives, are arrayed in a hierarchy. Those that would affect the whole organization and are designed to assist in the accomplishment of the organization's overall objectives can be called general policies. They are usually broad in scope and are typically formulated by the administration. Operational policies, on the other hand, are usually designed to apply to a specific department or unit, can be quite narrow in scope, and are usually formulated by the department manager to facilitate the accomplishment of the department's subsidiary objective(s). In all instances, operational policies should be subsidiary to and consistent with general policies. Their purpose is to provide guidelines for behavior and decision-making for the given department. The Admitting Department, the Maintenance Department, the Central Supply Department, Nursing Services, the Out-patient Department, the X-ray Department, the Emergency Department, and the Pharmacy may each have departmental policies of their own which should be consistent with the overall general policies of the organization.

Given that the primary objectives of a health care organization are to *maximize the level of patient care using the resources available, to provide the range of*

---

[4]Dalton E. McFarland, *Management: Principles and Practice.* New York: The Macmillan Company, 1974, p. 369.

services required by the community, and to provide care to all who seek it, various general policies can be formulated to serve as guidelines for the accomplishment of those objectives. A general policy might be *to provide care for all those who have a need for services, including those unable to pay, so long as it is within the financial capability of the organization.*

This becomes a guideline for behavior and decision-making for the personnel in, for instance, the Admitting Department and the Emergency Department. Furthermore, each department may formulate operational policies within that general policy to guide its specific activities. For example, the Business Office may formulate the policy that those in emergent need will be charged according to their ability to pay, while all others are expected to render full payment of all hospital charges at time of discharge.

If one of the organization's secondary objectives is "to be responsible to its employees," the following general policies could be formulated: adequately compensate employees, promote from within and on merit whenever possible, and provide stability of employment. These general policies serve as a guide for the behavior of, for example, the Personnel Department, department heads of other services, and supervisors. The Personnel Department policy that would be subsidiary to the general policy might be to continuously update the compensation system's pay grades and rate ranges in order to remain competitive with similar facilities in the area. A Business Office operational policy that would be consistent with the general policy might be to transfer and train employees to perform cashiering, credit and collection, or third-party insurance billing duties should one area within the department become overstaffed because of a reduced workload.

In the hierarchy of policies in health care organizations, operational policies have been described as those concerned with departmental activities, while general policies are those that encompass the whole organization. The former exist within the scope of the latter and must be consistent with them.

FORMULATION AND LINKAGE

In the previous section we described objectives, strategies, and policies, indicated that they exist in a hierarchy, and alluded to the fact that they are interrelated. In order to clarify this interrelationship, this section will refer to the formulation model and its number cells, which can be found in Figure 6–1. Our discussion will be limited to the formulation of the organization's overall objectives, basic strategies, and general policies. Since the formulation of subsidiary departmental objectives, strategies, and operational policies would be much the same, we will leave it to the reader to apply the model.

As can be noted by viewing Figure 6–1, strategy and policy formulation are linked to, are supportive of, and flow from objectives. Both strategies and policies occur independently of each other and must be consistent. Therefore, any strategy that is formulated to represent a broad set of current and planned activities must be congruent with the prescribed areas of permissible behavior and activity as expressed by policies.

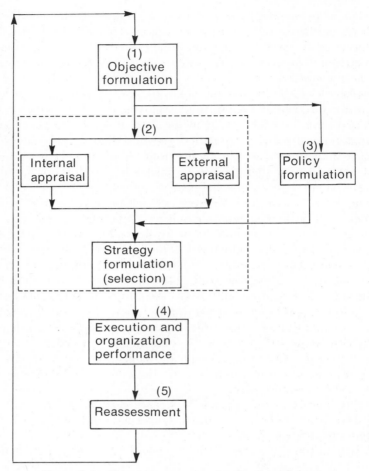

Figure 6–1   Objective, strategy, and policy formulation.

OBJECTIVE FORMULATION (1)

Objective formulation is the determination of the organization's primary and secondary objectives. Once established, these objectives become the targets toward which activity is directed. Their formulation is influenced by several factors.

One factor affecting the determination of the organization's objective(s) is its basic charter. A state mental hospital would have the objective of caring for the mentally ill to the exclusion of others. A nursing facility might have the objective of caring only for geriatric patients. A community general hospital would have the objective of servicing the wide range of medical needs for those residing in the community.

The values of those responsible for establishing the objectives become a second and very important factor affecting their formulation. These people would include the governing board, and in some cases the administrator, along with interested parties who can influence both, such as the medical staff who can make their values known in an attempt to influence the objectives of the organization. Founders may also have some influence, as in the case of the Mayo clinic. Because of the values of the Doctors Mayo, the clinic's primary objective is to be an outstanding medical facility with a specialty orientation. Another example of value influence is the Johns Hopkins Hospital. In the 1880's philanthropist Johns Hopkins donated a great deal of money toward the establishment of a medical school and hospital. The objective of the latter was to support the former in terms of training physicians and conducting research, as well as caring for private and indigent patients.

A third factor affecting objective formulation is the organization's constituency, which is composed of its patients, employees, and the community.[5] Obviously, the health care organization must have some specific objective relative to its patients which it seeks to accomplish. We could call it "quality patient care at reasonable costs." This primary objective can be further defined in terms of the type of patient (long-term or short-term) or the geographic area involved (local or national). If the facility is a community general hospital in a rural area, its objective may be to provide a wide range of services and to offer quality care to the total community, whereas one in an urban area may specialize.

The external environment is the fourth factor that influences the formulation of objectives, usually in a restrictive sense. For example, if the objective being considered is to become a renowned research center, a lack of community and governmental resource support would make it impractical. Or, if the objective of the organization is to be the area's largest in terms of the number of beds, planning agencies may serve as an environmental restraining force, particularly if there is an excess of hospital beds in the area.

STRATEGY FORMULATION (2)

The determination of the *means* by which organization objectives can be accomplished necessitates certain activities.[6] The answers to the questions "How can we achieve our objectives and what should be done to accomplish this?" entail (a) an appraisal of the internal strengths and weaknesses of the organiza-

---

[5]Thomas J. McNichols, *Policy Making and Executive Action.* New York: McGraw-Hill, 1967, p. 11.

[6]For a number of views on strategy formulation see C. Roland Christensen, Kenneth R. Andrews, and Joseph L. Bower, *Business Policy: Text and Cases.* Homewood, Illinois: Richard D. Irwin, Inc., 1973, pp. 107–119.

Frank F. Gilmore, "Formulating strategy in smaller companies." *Harvard Business Review, 49*:71, May-June, 1971.

William F. Glueck, *Business Policy: Strategy Formation and Executive Action.* New York: McGraw-Hill Book Company, 1972, pp. 94–113, 180–199.

Thomas J. McNichols, *Policy Making and Executive Action.* New York: McGraw-Hill Book Company, 1972, pp. 1–27.

Frank T. Paine and William Naumes, *Organizational Strategy and Policy.* Philadelphia: W. B. Saunders Company, 1974.

Seymour Tilles, "How to evaluate corporate strategy." *In* John W. Bonge and Bruce P. Coleman, Eds., *Concepts for Corporate Strategy: Readings in Business Policy.* New York: The Macmillan Company, 1972, pp. 148–163.

Karl H. Vesper and Yutaka Sayeki, "A quantitative approach for policy analysis." *California Management Review, 15*:119, Spring, 1973.

tion, (b) an examination of external environment and the limitations it might impose, and (c) the evaluation of and selection from among alternative courses of action (strategies) those that are feasible.

As noted, the present and planned activities (strategies) that are identified have the purpose of accomplishing objectives. To determine how or what *must* be done to accomplish those objectives, it is necessary to evaluate the organization's ". . . existing set of resources and skills"[7] and thereby identify the strengths and weaknesses of the organization. By taking an inventory through self-appraisal, deficiencies that will have to be rectified can be identified. Furthermore, the internal appraisal will indicate if certain courses of action are feasible, and whether the organization has the manpower, finances, buildings, and other resources to enable proposed activities to be carried out successfully.

Coupled with internal appraisal is an external appraisal which will identify the environmental limitations that may be imposed on the organization. Any strategy developed as a means for accomplishing objectives will have to take those limitations into account. Subsequent to internal and external appraisal, a number of strategies may be identified that would serve as the means for accomplishing objectives. After an evaluation of each strategy, one or several can be selected, usually by the administrator, for *execution*. At this time, the selected strategy serves as the set of planned activities for the organization.

POLICY FORMULATION (3)

As guidelines for behavior within the organization, policies give direction to the manner in which activities are to be carried out. Basically, general policies are established by the administrator. Their purpose is to facilitate the fulfillment of objectives by defining acceptable behavior, action, and activity. In this sense, they emanate from objectives and can limit the array of strategies. Any strategy adopted should be consistent with existing policies. A strategy that represents behavior or action inconsistent with present policy would not be appropriate. For example, to pay all personnel only the minimum wage required by law in order to reduce costs may be inconsistent with the policy of compensating employees on a par with other employees in the community, in addition to the fact that it would probably result in employee turnover.

EXECUTION (4)

Given the objectives and policies of a health care organization, and once a strategy has been selected as the means to accomplish those objectives, the strategy selected is then implemented or executed. As the planned activities occur, organization performance will be the result.

REASSESSMENT (5)

Upon execution, performance will follow and may then be compared to predetermined objectives to ascertain whether or not they are being accom-

---

[7]Germain B. Boer, "Extending the hospital planning horizon." *Hospital Administration*, *17*:54, Winter, 1972.

plished. If not, then a re-examination of the previously implemented strategy is called for to determine if another would be more effective.

Although our presentation of this complex subject—objective, strategy, and policy formulation—has been rather general, our intent has been to reinforce the following facts: first, objectives, strategies, and policies are interrelated. Second, the model presented in Figure 6–1 should enable the observer to identify the "what and how" related to organized activity. Finally, to the individual who is responsible for formulating objectives, strategies, and policies, we hope this discussion provides a methodology that can be expanded as circumstances dictate and will improve performance.

POLICIES REVISITED

Have you ever encountered the statement "You can't do that" or "It can't be done because it is against policy"? It is possible to think of numerous examples. Among them might be

1. You can't go to Mr. Smith's room now because it is against policy for more than two visitors to be in a patient's room at any one time.

2. You can't walk through here because it is against policy for unauthorized personnel to be in this area.

3. You can't leave work early because it is against policy for employees to leave before the end of a shift without supervisor approval.

4. You can't have a pay increase because it is against policy to change an employee's compensation except during the annual review period.

Have you ever encountered the statement "We will do it this way because it is the policy"? Examples might be

1. We will have our lunch period between 11:30 and 12:30 because it is the policy.

2. We will consider merit before seniority when evaluating people for promotion because it is the organization's policy.

3. We schedule this way because it is a policy that employees have two consecutive days off.

Because policies permeate organizations and affect all employees' activities and decisions, they require elaboration. Probably no other phenomenon affects so many. Furthermore, the narrow extension of policies results in procedures and rules with which we are constantly confronted. As a result, this chapter will conclude with (1) a section describing the characteristics of good policies, (2) a section devoted to procedures, and (3) a section on rules.

CHARACTERISTICS OF GOOD POLICIES

Good policies are not easily established. For a policy to be truly effective and stand the test of time, it must be clearly thought out, it must be appropriate, and it must serve to guide the ways in which the activities of the organization are carried out. Good policies will typically have a number of common characteristics.

First, policies must be *well thought out* before they are formalized. Policies made hastily and without consideration of their impact can be very detrimental. For example, a medical staff policy that requires "a full laboratory work-up for all newly admitted patients" may have a noble (or perhaps defensive) purpose, yet have adverse ramifications ranging from overworking the Laboratory Department to being extremely costly for those patients who may not require the tests. The policy that "meals will be served to hospital visitors" may seem at first glance to be a good policy; however, it may be very costly to the organization without contributing to its objective of patient care.

Second, policies must have enough *flexibility* so that they can be applied to not only normal but abnormal situations.[8] Inflexible policies can often distort their intended purpose of providing guidelines for behavior and decision-making. Situations may be encountered by a supervisor, department head, or employee that would require atypical action on his or her part.

Rigid and inflexible policies interfere with the employees' freedom to use judgment and may result in action contrary to what was intended. A policy which states that "all maternity patients *must be* (rather than *should be*) conveyed to their rooms by wheelchair (unless extenuating circumstances are present)" is designed to safeguard the welfare of the patient, minimize risk, and decrease the organization's liability by its reasonable attempt to prevent injuries. However, if an inflexible policy were to be applied religiously and without deviation, undesirable results could occur. When time is a critical factor, such as with a patient in labor, and there are no wheelchairs available in the Admitting Department, inflexibility and adherence to policy would in fact be construed as negligence. In this instance, reason and judgment should prevail in guiding behavior and decision-making. The decision to use another means of conveyance should have been made. Perhaps the best way to convey the fact that policies should be flexible is with the statement that "there is an exception to every policy."

In health care organizations, more so than in other types, policies relative to which employees participate in the care of patients and to what extent must necessarily be more rigid. There is a fine line between policy flexibility and inflexibility. There can be an inherent conflict between employee discretion and the requirements of patient welfare. The nurse cannot administer drugs at her own discretion; she must be directed to do so by a physician. As a result, policies that apply to employee behavior relative to patient care require rigidity. However, as pointed out in the maternity example, situations will arise wherein policy inflexibility would be dysfunctional.

The solution to this dilemma may lie in the establishment of criteria. Some policies, such as those dealing with direct patient care, may be formulated in a rather rigid tone, while others, such as personnel policies and purchasing policies, may incorporate greater flexibility.

---

[8]Edward C. Schlea, "Policy—A vital force." *SAM—Advanced Management Journal, 33*:26, July, 1968.

Third, for a policy to be effective it must be *acceptable* to those to whom it will apply. Acceptability implies that the organization's members consider the policy to be legitimate and fair. Policies that display favoritism to certain employee groups without a valid and legitimate reason or those which appear to be arbitrary will be resisted. For example, the two policies, "promotions will be made from within whenever possible" and "employees may switch off-days as long as they inform their supervisor and the service area is adequately manned," are valid, are sound reasoning, and should be accepted by those to whom they apply. However, policies stating that "all employees must clock in one-half hour before starting time without pay" and "bereavement leave will not be granted for attending the funeral of a next of kin" would not appear to be reasonable.

Fourth, for policies to serve their intended purpose they should be consistent with each other.[9] Inconsistency among policies not only is confusing but can also cause disharmony, competing activities, and employee dissatisfaction and frustration within the organization, and will detract from objective accomplishment. Inconsistencies generally occur between the operational policies of the various departments. For example, the Pharmacy Department policy of "filling outpatient prescriptions from 8:00 A.M. to 5:00 P.M." may be inconsistent with the Outpatient Department's policy of "providing service from 8:00 A.M. until 9:00 P.M.."

Fifth, policies should be as objective as possible. Specifically, they should not contain favorable provisions for one employee classification and not another except for legitimate reasons. The policy that "physicians will be assigned preferred parking" can be easily justified. However, the granting of assigned parking to business office employees and not to other members of the organization, who may have a more legitimate claim, would not be an objective policy.

Sixth, for policies to be *useful*, they should be clear and communicated to all individuals to whom they apply. It is the responsibility of the manager to ensure that his personnel are aware of how they should behave and what guidelines they have for making decisions while performing their jobs.

Finally, to serve their intended purpose, policies must be continuously *reevaluated* and changed if necessary.[10] The health care organization exists in a dynamic environment. As a result, it is necessary for it to continuously adapt to internal and external environmental changes. As changes occur, whether in terms of reformulated objectives and strategies, newly introduced medical techniques and knowledge, or laws, policies should be reformulated if necessary, and periodically examined to determine if they still contribute to objective accomplishment. Today the policy of not recognizing a union, in light of current law, is no longer appropriate. In a similar respect, some hospitals are changing policies covering the composition of the medical staff so that osteopaths are now granted staff privileges. Policies that were appropriate, well thought out, and acceptable ten years ago, or last year, may not be appropriate today.

---

[9]McFarland, op. cit. p. 372.
[10]John B. Miner, *The Management Process.* New York: The Macmillan Company, 1973, p. 154.

BUSINESS OFFICE

"Discharge Procedure"

Cashier

1. Floor Attendant notifies Cashier that a patient is ready to be discharged. Sends down Discharge Form 4–0165.
2. Before patient arrives at window, Cashier computes bill and has all papers in readiness.
3. Computes bill. If Blue Cross or private patient, amount should be fairly accurate in the inpatient register. Necessary only to scan discharge forms for any additional or omitted charges. If commercial insurance:
    a. Looks up verification on back of IBM card. If none shown, checks Insurance Clerk to see what information she might have. If not notified yet, no coverage is allowed and patient is reminded of hospital policy as explained at time of admission or subsequent interviews.
    b. Mathematically computes room and board difference as one amount due from patient.
    c. Deducts total room and board from total bill to find total miscellaneous charges and computes how much allowed according to verified coverage. Balance is the second amount due from patient.
    d. Adds both amounts due from patient as the patient's total bill.
4. Places all papers pertaining to patient's discharge in black accordion discharge file pending arrival of patient.
    Includes:
    a. Tapes and computations of bill
    b. IBM card
    c. Discharge approval card, Form 4–0165
    d. Any assignment forms pertaining to the patient; if none in file, blank form to be signed for commercial insurance accounts. Must be signed by *insured only.*
    e. Any other note for the patient
5. When patient arrives at window, explains bill to him and accepts payment.
    a. If credit problems arise regarding payment, refer to Credit and Collection Supervisor, Chief Clerk-Credit, or Director, Business Office — in that order.
    b. Cashiers are not to involve themselves in making credit arrangements, or signing of guarantees, except when the credit personnel are not available.
6. If no verification, and bill must be collected, suggests patient might file own claim. If patient prefers hospital to file and collect and then make a refund, this is allowed.
    a. Also asks patient to sign any claim and assignment form that might need his signature for insurance purposes.
7. When satisfactory payment is made, writes name of patient on discharge approval card and gives to patient or representative for presentation on floor.
8. Advises patient that an itemized statement will follow in approximately ten days, whether bill paid in full or not.
9. Advises patient that settlement being made is *not* final billing. Explains possibility of additional charges which are not down from the various service areas yet.
10. Stamps discharge date and writes case number on assignments or any other forms left and places in proper tray for the Insurance Department.
11. Stamps discharge date on IBM card and places in back of in-house box.
12. Makes call for taxi or ambulance for discharged patient if requested.

Figure 6–2 (Source: Mount Carmel Mercy Hospital and Medical Center, Detroit, Michigan. Used by permission.)

PROCEDURES

Procedures, like policies, guide behavior and activities. They are much narrower in scope than policies and tend to cover actions for specific situations. Typically, procedures consist of the itemized sequence of steps involved in performing a particular task. They are a prescribed way of doing something and become a standard method for performance. In a sense, they are a narrow reflection of policy.[11]

In a hierarchical array, procedures are subordinate to policies whether they are general or operational.[12] The purpose of established procedures is to give specific direction to employees for the carrying out of their duties. As an example, the procedural steps followed by the cashier when a patient is discharged are presented in Figure 6-2. Note that the steps are specific and also allow for a range of contingencies such as whether or not the patient has hospitalization insurance (and what type).

There can be occasions when situations warrant deviation from a prescribed procedure. In that case, the matter is referred to, or authorization to deviate is obtained from, the supervisor. The Purchasing Department procedure presented in Figure 6-3 allows for deviation in emergency situations.

---

[11] Schlea, op. cit. p. 30.
[12] McFarland, op. cit. p. 372.

PROCEDURE FOR PURCHASE:

When a department head has approved a decision that a certain item (or items) is necessary for purchase, a purchase request is made out and signed by the issuing department. This request is sent to the Purchasing Department, and this department then issues a Purchase Order after deciding upon which vendor to purchase the item from if competitive bids were obtained. Whenever possible, competitive bids should be obtained. This will have to be judged in individual cases based upon the situation.

When the item is delivered, the copy of the purchase order and receiving slip will be noted as received and sent to Accounting for authorization of payment.

In case of extreme emergencies, and only in such cases, an exception to the above procedure may be made with the understanding that the head of the department placing the emergency order personally assumes the responsibility of immediately following up the verbal order, given by himself or his representative, with proper department requisition. In no event will purchase orders be given to the departments via telephone. Purchase requisitions shall be sent to Purchasing for placement.

Figure 6-3 Purchasing Department Procedure. (Source: Mount Carmel Mercy Hospital and Medical Center, Detroit, Michigan. Used by permission.)

RULES

As was pointed out, procedures consist of the specific series of steps to be followed when performing routine tasks. They describe "how" something is to be done. In contrast, rules are specific statements requiring mandatory behavior and permit virtually no deviation. One writer has observed that rules are usually ". . . stated in such a way as to leave no doubt about what is to be done. They are specific and permit a minimum of flexibility and freedom of interpretation."[13]

Rules are required for organization stability. Without them, consistent behavior will not occur and it would be extremely difficult to achieve objectives. They denote the minimum behavior necessary to ensure coordination of activities and the maintenance of patient and employee safety.

Imagine a situation in which employees reported for work whenever they felt like it. Obviously, a rule relative to reporting time is necessary. Or picture what would happen to patient welfare if surgical personnel were not required to follow sterile techniques. The rule prohibiting smoking in specific areas, such as those where oxygen is present, is necessary for the welfare of both the patient and the employee.

Generally, rules are expressed in a negative fashion and carry sanctions which can be used to enforce compliance. The degree of sanction (punishment) will vary with the seriousness of the rule that has been broken. For example, the first infraction of the rule that "employees will not leave the premises without authorization" might result in counseling. After repeated offenses, the employee might be discharged.

In order to be effective, rules must be communicated to all employees who must abide by them. Rules are planned expressions of expected behavior. In order for the organization to adequately fulfill its objectives, rules must be formulated, be consistent, and reflect the intent of procedures and policies.

SUMMARY

This chapter, "Objectives, Strategies, and Policies," is an extension of the previous chapter on planning. In discussing objectives, strategies, and policies, we examined the formulation of each and, through the formulation model, demonstrated how they are interrelated.

We considered objective formulation to be the determination of the *desired output* of the health care organization. The types of objectives identified were primary, secondary, and subsidiary. Linked to objectives is strategy, representing the broad set of present and planned activity which constitutes the *means* by which the organization seeks to accomplish its objectives. Strategies, like objectives, are arrayed in a hierarchy in health care organizations.

---

[13]George A. Steiner, *Top Management Planning.* New York: The Macmillan Company, 1969, p. 267.

Policy formulation was also examined. It involves defining the area of freedom for organization participants in regard to their behavior and the decisions they make while performing their duties. Policies, whether broad or operational, are designed to help attain organization objectives. Subsidiary to policies are procedures and rules. The former indicates specific steps to accomplish a task, while the latter narrowly defines acceptable conduct.

DISCUSSION QUESTIONS

1. Discuss the difference between an organization's primary and secondary objectives and subsidiary departments' objectives. Give examples of each. How are they related? What would happen if they were inconsistent with each other?

2. Strategy has been identified as the means by which objectives can be accomplished. What is meant by *means*? How does strategy relate to planning? Give examples of strategies with which you are familiar.

3. Discuss the purpose of policies. What is meant by hierarchy of policies, and how would you relate procedures and rules to them?

4. Using Figure 6–1, describe how objectives, strategies, and policies are related to each other. What factors are considered in the formulation of each?

5. In Table 6–2, examples of objectives and strategies were given. Examples of policies were given in the text of the chapter. Identify and describe several sets of objectives, strategies, and policies in your present situation.

INCIDENTS

1. CLOSING PEDIATRICS

Your hospital has a Pediatric Department consisting of 35 beds. For the past several years the occupancy has varied between 40 per cent and 60 per cent with a definite downward trend which appears to be leveling off at about 45 per cent occupancy. The low level occupancy has caused quite a financial strain for your hospital. Other hospitals in the area are experiencing a similar situation. As a result, several of them have proposed forming a loosely knit association to study the situation in order to determine whether or not one or several of them should give up their Pediatric Department to enable the rest to have a higher occupancy rate. Hopefully, the results of this proposed action would be a reduction in costs for all concerned.

Although this particular proposal would be beneficial to the community as a whole, there are a number of policy and strategy questions that must be answered. Specifically, given that two objectives of your hospital are to provide a full range of quality services and to support residency programs, what would be the effect of the proposal on your hospital if it were decided that you should phase out your Pediatric Department? Among the things that should be considered are the following:

A. What effect would it have on the objectives?

B. Who are the organization participants and constituents who would influence the reshaping or reformulation of the objectives?

C. What would be their likely reaction?

D. What means would you employ to ensure that the proposal to close the department would be carried out effectively? What factors would you have to consider?

E. What would be the disadvantages of such a proposal?

F. How could you use the formulation model presented in Figure 6–1 to organize your thinking?

2. A PROPOSAL FOR AMBULATORY SURGERY

For many years at your large hospital, all surgeries were performed with the patient being admitted for a minimum of two days. Recently, in hospitals across the country, there has arisen the concept of ambulatory surgery in which, for certain procedures, patients can be discharged the same day that they are admitted. Your hospital does about 12,000 surgical procedures per year and perhaps as many as 1000 of them could be done on a "same day" basis. Your hospital's occupancy is 85 per cent and if the administration of the hospital promoted ambulatory surgery, this would probably have the effect of reducing the occupancy slightly.

Since this major decision would affect the means by which the hospital accomplishes its objectives, the board of trustees will vote on the proposal at its next meeting. Among the questions to be considered are:

A. Will this proposal enable the hospital to accomplish its objectives?

B. What impact will it have on costs, quality of care, and the hospital's personnel?

C. Should other organization participants be asked to give their opinion? If so, who?

3. VIOLATION OF POLICY

Bill Richardson, Purchasing Department storeroom clerk at Parks Memorial, a 200-bed hospital, spotted a fire in a difficult to reach air shaft. He ran to the nearest call box turned in the alarm, and asked a nearby woman to stay at the box until the hospital fire-protection crew arrived so she could tell them it was in the No. 2 shaft. After grabbing a soda-acid fire extinguisher, he crawled into the air shaft and at considerable risk to himself, because the fire was near electrical wiring, put out the fire. When the fire crew arrived, a smoked-befuddled Richardson was crawling out of the shaft.

He was congratulated and his department head wrote a commendation report to be attached to his personnel record. The ink was scarcely dry on the department head's signature when another fire broke out in the vicinity of the air shaft. Acidulated water from the extinguisher had seeped down into a high-voltage junction box, and within moments a severe electrical fire, *worse* than the one Richardson had put out, was raging. With some difficulty, the fire was brought under control.

Richardson was severely censured by the Director of Maintenance for using the wrong type of fire extinguisher. On the clip that held the soda-acid extinguisher to the wall was a large, color-coded placard that stated that the extinguisher was not to be used on electrical fires. A carbon dioxide extinguisher, approved for electrical fires, was located near the one Richardson had used. "You should leave things to personnel trained in their use," exploded the Maintenance Director. "There is a policy which states that in case of fire hospital personnel are to notify their supervisor, activate the closest fire alarm, see to the safety of the patients, and not to attempt to extinguish the fire themselves unless specifically trained to do so. Now you have created a real mess."

A. Should Bill Richardson have been reprimanded?

B. Is there anything wrong with the policy?

C. What action should the Maintenance Director take?

Part III

ORGANIZATIONAL DESIGN AND STRUCTURE

The first part of the book, *THE SETTING AND FRAMEWORK,* described the health care setting in the United States and fully developed the concept of management. Furthermore, a management model (Fig. 2–3) was provided and its basic components serve as the framework for the subsequent parts of this book.

In the second part, *OUTPUT—INPUT DETERMINATION*, attention was given to that particular component of the model. Managerial decision-making was presented and considered to be characteristic of all the other managerial processes. Furthermore, other integral components of output-input determination were presented in a chapter devoted to the planning process and in another devoted to objectives and strategies.

Using the management model presented in Figure 2–3 as the basic structure of the text, our next task is to discuss the organizing process. In Part III, *ORGANIZATIONAL DESIGN AND STRUCTURE,* we will focus on the activities that are characteristic of this process. In order for the health care organization to function effectively, care must be given to its design and *decisions made* relative to its structure. A manager is seldom able to build an organization setting from the beginning. He usually resides and exists within one which is already established. Even so, he must continuously examine ways to modify that setting in order to maintain it, improve it, and adapt it to external pressures and constraints.

This part will examine the organizing process in four chapters. The first chapter, Organizational Concepts, will offer an overview of classical and modern organization theory. It will serve to acquaint the reader with classical organizational concepts such as division of work, coordination, authority and responsibility, and delegation of work to name a few. In addition, modern organizational concepts such as matrix organizations and a portrayal of organizations from an open systems point of view will be presented. Finally, the informal organization, represented by emergent behavioral patterns, will be described and its particularly vital role within health care organizations will be emphasized.

The three succeeding chapters will focus on specific portions of health care organizations. Chapter 8, Structure of Health Care Organizations, will apply the concepts presented in Chapter 7 to health care organizations.

Chapter 9, Manpower Acquisition and Maintenance, will treat a major organizational activity—manpower acquisition (human resource-input). Subjects related to the maintenance of human resources such as wage and salary administration, employee development, and health and safety will be presented.

Finally, Chapter 10, Labor Relations, will focus specifically on the subject of unions. Included will be a history of unionization as it relates to health care organizations, an overview of the law, the impact unions have on health care organizations, some of the reasons why employees seek union representation, and an overview of collective bargaining.

This Chapter Contains:

- Introduction
- Classical Organization Theory
  The Bureaucratic Model
  Classical Principles of Organization
    Division of Work
    Coordination
    Unity of Command
    Authority–Responsibility
    Line and Staff
    Span of Control
    Delegation

- Modern Organization Theory
  Criticism of Classical Theory
  Project Organization
  Matrix Organization
  Organizations as Open Systems
    Systems Concept
    The Hospital as a System
    Types of Systems
    Special Characteristics of Organizational Systems

- The Informal Organization
  Nature of the Informal Organization
  Why People Form Groups
  Characteristics of Informal Groups
  Positive Aspects of Informal Organizations
  Negative Aspects of Informal Organizations
  Living With the Informal Organization

- Summary
- Discussion Questions
- Incidents

Chapter 7

ORGANIZATIONAL CONCEPTS

"When the acts of two or more individuals are
cooperative, that is, systematically coordinated, the
acts by my definition constitute an organization."

(Chester I. Barnard)[1]

INTRODUCTION

This quote expresses the heart of organization theory. The essence consists of people operating under a system of cooperation and coordination. Every health care organization fits this classic definition developed years ago by Chester I. Barnard. We will now describe the major concepts of organizational behavior that flow from this important framework.

The planning process entails making *decisions* concerning the formulation, modification, and reformulation of objectives (desired output), policies, and strategies. Concurrent with the ongoing reexamination of objectives, policies, and strategies is the continuous review of the organization setting in which activity is carried out and, if required, making decisions to change that setting. The *organization setting* includes the formal structure of roles and relationships designed (prescribed) for the organization's employees. It also includes an informal set of relationships within the formal structure.

The *organization process* embraces a multitude of activities that result in the establishment of authority-responsibility relationships and the interrelating of human and other resources in such a way that the work performed will lead to the fulfillment of the organization's objectives. These activities include the establishment of authority and responsibility relationships, the division of work, the delegation of that work, and the coordination of work effort. In addition, activities concerned with human resources — their acquisition and maintenance — are required so that work in the organization can be performed.

Essentially, the organizing process grows out of the human need for cooperation. When one considers the complexity of the work of health care organizations and the diversity of the professional and paraprofessional people who perform that work, it is clear that the need for cooperation exists; perhaps to a greater degree than in any other type of organization in our society.

Even in a single unit within institutional providers, such as the Nursing Service or the Radiology Department, there is such a wide range of work performed by people who have a multitude of skill levels that organizing their ef-

---

[1]Chester I. Barnard, *Organization and Management.* Cambridge: Harvard University Press, 1956, p. 113.

139

forts is vital to the overall effectiveness and efficiency of the organization. These two concepts although different must be considered together because they are both important. As we pointed out in Chapter 1, an organization's structure is effective (appropriate) if it facilitates individual contribution toward the attainment of the organization's objectives. An organization's structure is efficient if it facilitates this accomplishment of objectives with a minimum of cost. It is possible to be effective but not efficient and vice-versa. In view of the growing and concurrent demands for high quality services at the lowest possible cost, the health care manager must keep both concepts in mind when engaging in the activities of the organizing process.

This chapter will be devoted to a brief overview of organizational concepts. Specifically, we will present (1) classical organization theory, (2) modern organization theory, and (3) the informal organization. Since the subject matter is rather complex, the application of these concepts to health care organizations will, for the most part, be reserved for the following chapter.

ORGANIZATION DESIGN

As will be seen in this chapter, in spite of a great deal of attention from scholars and practitioners, there is no definitive, universally accepted theory about the way health care organizations should be designed. Consequently, health managers must choose from, adapt, and combine many theories of organization design. There are many reasons why this is necessary. First, the concerted effort to solve the problem of organization design that is evident today is relatively new. Second, it is very difficult to compare the relative effectiveness and efficiency of various designs. Finally, the solution to the problem of optimum organization design has been sought by a wide range of interested groups who do not always understand one another's language. The diverse and largely uncoordinated efforts of practicing managers, anthropologists, engineers, sociologists, psychologists, social psychologists, and other interested persons have produced many theories and conceptualizations that conflict. March and Simon say it best when they suggest, "The literature leaves one with the impression that after all not a great deal has been said about organizations, but it has been said over and over in a variety of languages."[2]

We shall attempt to provide both the latest and the best information about organization design. However, the reader should keep in mind that the thinking about organization is part of an evolutionary process and constant adaptation to organizational dynamics in health care delivery is necessary. It is helpful to divide organization theory into the classical approach and the modern approach.

CLASSICAL ORGANIZATION THEORY

What has come to be called classical organization theory emerged in the literature during the period 1890 to 1940, more or less coinciding with the

---

[2] James G. March and Herbert A. Simon, *Organizations*. New York: John Wiley and Sons, 1958, p. 5.

growth of scientific management literature. The concepts of scientific management and classical organization theory are not the same thing, and it is important to make a distinction between them. Scientific management, as developed and expounded by F. W. Taylor and the Gilbreths primarily in the early 1900's, dealt with work done at the lowest level of the organization. In contrast, classical organization theory was focused on the total organization and treated broader and more complex problems such as departmentation, span of control, and delegation of authority. The classical theorists viewed the problem of designing the structure of an organization as one including such managerial tasks as planning, directing, and controlling. They were also interested in developing general truths that would guide the manager in performing his tasks. The results of their efforts have come to be known as the "classical principles of organization."

One of the major developers of the classical organization theory was Max Weber (1864–1920), a German sociologist who is most often associated with the organizational concept of bureaucracy. His work is a logical beginning point in the analysis of organizations because Weber thought that bureaucracy, in its pure form, represented an ideal or completely rational form of organization.

THE BUREAUCRATIC MODEL

The term bureaucracy, usually associated with governmental organizations, stimulates a negative image in the minds of many people. It has come to represent the undesirable characteristics of "red tape," found in many large organizations: duplication, delay, and general frustration. The term originally meant something entirely different. Weber used it to describe an ideal organization structure based on the sociological concept of rationalization of collective activities.[3] Weber's concept of bureaucracy was an "ideal" type because he abstracted the concept from observations of actual organizations, yet no organization exactly follows the Weber model.[4]

Bureaucratic Characteristics.   Weber believed that to achieve the maximum benefits of an ideal bureaucracy, an organization must adopt several concepts. Among them were the following:

1. *Specialization and division of labor.* The tasks necessary to accomplish goals are divided into highly specialized jobs. The advantage in this is that jobholders can become expert in their jobs and can be held responsible for the performance of their duties. Another aspect of this concept is that the bureaucrat must know the precise limits of his sphere of competence in order to avoid infringing upon the spheres of others.
2. *Positions arranged in a hierarchy.* According to Weber, "The organization of offices follows the principle of hierarchy of positions; that is, each lower office is under the control and supervision of a higher one."[5] The authority of a supervisor is based upon expert knowledge. Authority, granted from the top, diminishes with each succeeding position below it and results in a chain of command.

---

[3]Max Weber, *The Theory of Social and Economic Organization*, trans. A. M. Henderson and Talcott Parsons. New York: Oxford University Press, 1947.

[4]Peter M. Blau, *Bureaucracy in Modern Society.* New York: Random House, Inc., 1966, p. 34.

[5]Weber, op. cit. p. 341.

3. *A consistent system of abstract rules.* Weber saw the need for "a continuous organization of official functions bound by rules."[6] A system of rules ensures a rational approach to organization and a degree of uniformity and coordination that could not exist without such a system. The basic rationale for rules is that the manager can use them to eliminate uncertainty in the performance of tasks due to the differences between various individuals. Beyond this, Weber believed that a set of rules and regulations provides the continuity and stability that an organization needs.

4. *Impersonal relationships.* Weber believed that the manager should possess "a spirit of formalistic impersonality, without affection or enthusiasm."[7] It should be remembered that Weber was speaking of an "ideal" situation. The rationale of this practice was to ensure that the bureaucrat did not permit emotional attachments or personalities to interfere with completely rational decisions.

5. *Technical competence.* "Employment in the bureaucratic organization is based on technical qualifications and is protected against arbitrary dismissal."[8] Promotions in the bureaucracy are made on the basis of seniority and achievement.

CLASSICAL PRINCIPLES OF ORGANIZATION

Although they are often treated separately, many of the classical principles of organization are inherent in the bureaucratic model. For example, the bureaucratic concepts of hierarchy, specialization, rules, and impersonality are at the top of the list of classical principles.

The major writers associated with the classical principles are Henri Fayol,[9] Luther Gulick and Lyndall Urwick,[10] and James Mooney and Alan Reiley.[11] Most of these early writers used organization and management principles interchangeably because of the importance classical theorists placed on organization. The following sections on the classical principles are not complete (for example, Urwick[12] lists 29 classical principles of organization) but these principles are the ones most commonly known and most widely used.

Division of Work.   Originally noted by Fayol as the first of his 14 principles of management, the division of work, or specialization of labor, is a natural means "to produce more and better work with the same effort."[13] This concerns what has been termed the primary step in organization, the determination and establishment of "the smallest number of dissimilar functions into which the

---

[6]*Ibid.* p. 330.

[7]*Ibid.* p. 340.

[8]Blau, op. cit. p. 30.

[9]Henri Fayol, *General and Industrial Management,* trans. Constance Storrs. London: Sir Issac Pitman and Sons, Ltd., 1949.

[10]Luther Gulick and Lyndall Urwick, eds., *Papers on the Science of Administration.* New York: Institute of Public Administration, 1937. Also see: Lyndall Urwick, *The Elements of Administration.* New York: Harper and Brothers, 1943.

[11]James D. Mooney and Alan C. Reiley, *Onward Industry?* New York: Harper and Brothers, 1931. Also see: James D. Mooney, *The Principles of Organization.* New York: Harper and Brothers, 1947.

[12]Urwick, op. cit. p. 119.

[13]Fayol, op. cit. p. 20.

work of an institution may be divided."[14] Implicit in this is departmentation with a natural division of labor. It is desirable to determine the activities necessary for the accomplishment of overall organizational objectives and then to divide these activities into the departments that perform the specialized functions. Departmentation has been developed beyond what the early classicists envisioned although Gulick and Urwick noted four possible bases for departmentation: purpose, process, persons and things, and place.[15]

The only significant change that has occurred in this concept is the addition of other bases for departmentation, such as time, service, customer, and equipment, in addition to the fact that product is now substituted for purpose, functional has replaced process, and territorial or geographical are now used instead of place.

Almost without exception in health care organizations, departmentation is made on the basis of function, such as administration, nursing service, ancillary services, and housekeeping services. Furthermore, a subsidiary form of functional departmentation is the use of the customer as a basis, specifically, in-patient or out-patient. The single most important advantage of functional departmentation is that it incorporates the benefits of specialization. Of course, any method of departmentation carries with it the possible dysfunction that departmental empires may build up and conflict to the point of detracting from overall goal attainment for the organization. Also, the problems of coordination become more complex as the number of departments multiplies.

Coordination. Coordination is the conscious activity of assembling and synchronizing differentiated work efforts so that they function harmoniously in the attainment of organization objectives.[16] The literature indicates that coordination and integration are used interchangeably. Integration has been defined as "The process of achieving unity of effort among the various subsystems in the accomplishment of the organization's tasks."[17] Clearly, these two terms have the same meaning.

According to Fayol the act of coordinating pulls together all the activities of the enterprise to make possible both its working and its success. The well-coordinated enterprise bears the following marks: each department working in harmony with the other departments; each department, division, and subdivision knowing the share of the common task it must assume; and finally, all departments and subdivisions having their working schedules attuned to circumstances. However, these requirements are not always fulfilled. Three reasons may be found to account for this lack of coordination. First, each department may know nothing and want to know nothing of the others; second, water-tight compartments exist between different departments; and third, no one thinks of the general interest. "This attitude on the part of the personnel,

[14]H. A. Hopf, *Organization, Executive Capacity and Progress.* Ossining, New York: Hopf Institute of Management, 1945, p. 4.

[15]Gulick and Urwick, op. cit. p. 15.

[16]Theo Haimann and W. G. Scott, *Management in the Modern Organization.* 2nd edition. Boston: Houghton Mifflin Company, 1974, p. 126.

[17]Paul R. Lawrence and J. W. Lorsch, "Differentiation and integration in complex organizations." *Administrative Science Quarterly, 11*:3, June, 1967.

so disastrous for a concern, is not the result of preconcerted intention but the culmination of non-existent or inadequate coordination."[18]

The classical organization theorists viewed coordination in a number of different ways. Ralph C. Davis saw coordination primarily as a vital phase of control.[19] L. A. Allen considered coordinating a managerial function along with planning, organizing, motivating, and controlling.[20] James D. Mooney viewed coordination as "the orderly arrangement of group effort, to provide unity of action in the pursuit of a common purpose."[21] He called coordination the first principle of organization, since coordination embraces all the principles of organization. Ordway Tead indicated coordination to be "the effort to assure a smooth interplay of the functions and forces of all the different component parts of an organization in order that its purpose will be realized with a minimum of friction and a maximum of collaborative effectiveness."[22]

Coordination relates to the synchronization of the actions of people within an organization and achieving this synchronization or coordination is one of the important goals of management. Chester I. Barnard even went so far as to say that under most circumstances "the quality of coordination is the crucial factor in the survival of the organization."[23]

Coordination is not easily attained. Each special departmental interest in an organization stresses its own opinion of how the organization's purposes should be accomplished, and each tends to favor one policy or another depending upon its function and viewpoint. The problem of different viewpoints applies both in and among the several levels of a managerial hierarchy. It takes thoughtfulness, the ability to be a good listener, and good will to see and understand a problem in work relationships with the group above or below. In spite of cooperative attitudes and self-coordination or self-adjustment by each member of a group, there will be duplication of action and conflicting efforts unless management synchronizes all of them. "Through coordination, management can bring about a level of accomplishment far greater than the sum of the individual parts."[24]

Coordination Mechanisms. As a rule, organizations establish several different mechanisms to achieve coordination. Litterer suggests three primary means: through the hierarchy, through the administrative system, and through voluntary activities.[25] In hierarchical coordination, the various activities are linked together by placing them under a central authority. In a simple organization, this form of coordination might be sufficient. Howev-

[18]Fayol, op. cit. p. 104.
[19]Ralph C. Davis, *The Fundamentals of Top Management.* New York: Harper and Brothers, 1951, p. 19.
[20]Louis A. Allen, *Management and Organization.* New York: McGraw-Hill Company, Inc., 1958, p. 24.
[21]James D. Mooney, *The Principles of Organization.* New York: Harper and Brothers, 1947, p. 5.
[22]Ordway Tead, *Administration: Its Purpose and Performance.* New York: Harper and Brothers, 1959, p. 36.
[23]Chester I. Barnard, *The Functions of the Executive.* Cambridge: Harvard University Press, 1938, p. 256.
[24]Haimann and Scott, op. cit. p. 128.
[25]Joseph A. Litterer, *The Analysis of Organizations.* New York: John Wiley and Sons, 1965, pp. 223–232.

er, in complex health care organizations, such as hospitals, that have many levels and many specialized departments, hierarchical coordination becomes more difficult. Although the administrator is a focal point of authority, at least for the administrative hierarchy of the hospital, it would be impossible for him to cope with all the coordinating problems that might arise throughout the hierarchy. Therefore, coordination through the hierarchical structure must be supplemented.

The administrative system provides a second mechanism for the coordination of activities. "A great deal of coordinative effort in organizations is concerned with a horizontal flow of work of a routine nature. Administrative systems are formal procedures designed to carry out much of this routine coordinative work automatically."[26] Many work procedures, such as memoranda with routing slips, help coordinate the efforts of different operating units. To the extent that these procedures can be programmed or routinized, it is not necessary to establish specific means for coordination. For nonroutine and nonprogrammable events, specific means such as committees may be required to provide integration.

A third type of coordination is through voluntary action when individuals or groups see a need for coordination, develop a method, and implement it.[27] Much of the coordination may depend upon the willingness and ability of the individuals or groups to voluntarily find means to integrate their activities with other organizational participants. Achieving voluntary coordination is one of the most important yet difficult problems for the manager. Voluntary coordination requires that the individuals have sufficient knowledge of organizational objectives, adequate information concerning the specific problems of coordination, and the motivation to do something on their own.

Another approach to coordinating activities is through the committee. Typically, committees are made up of members from a number of different departments or functional areas and are concerned with problems requiring coordination.[28] The use of committees for purposes of coordination is a well-established approach in health care organizations.

Additional means of integration have developed in many organizations. Lawrence and Lorsch have studied six organizations operating in the chemical processing industry to determine how they achieve integration. These organizations use a technology which requires not only differentiated and specialized activities but also a major degree of integration. The study was concerned with how organizations achieve both substantial differentiation and tight integration when these forces seem paradoxical. Results showed that successful companies use task forces, teams, and project offices to achieve coordination. There is a tendency to formalize coordinative activities which have developed informally and voluntarily.[29] In the most successful organizations, the influence of the integrators (those people who seem to hold the key to successful integration) stems

---

[26]*Ibid.* p. 230.
[27]*Ibid.* p. 223.
[28]Ernest Dale, *Organizations*, New York: American Management Association, 1967, Chapter 10, pp. 163–178.
[29]Lawrence and Lorsch, op. cit. pp. 1–47.

from their professional competence rather than from their formal position. They are successful as integrators because of their specialized knowledge and because they represent a central source of information in the organization. In the hospital, the individual physician, who may be one of many members of the medical staff and may not hold an important position of authority, plays a key role as an integrator, especially when the integration of activities around his patient is concerned. This integrative role relies almost totally on his specialized knowledge.

Others have recommended new structural forms to help with the problems of coordination. Likert feels that one mechanism for achieving integration could be to have people serve as "linking pins" between the various units in the organization.[30]

Horizontally, there are certain organizational participants who are members of two separate groups and serve as coordinating agents between them. On the vertical basis, individuals serve as linking pins between their own level and those above and below. Thus, through this system of linking pins, the voluntary coordination necessary to make the dynamic system operate effectively is achieved. This forms a multiple, overlapping group structure in the organization. Likert says:

> To perform the intended coordination well a fundamental requirement must be met. The entire organization must consist of a multiple, overlapping group structure with *every* work group using group decision-making processes skillfully. This requirement applies to the functional, product, and service departments. An organization meeting this requirement will have an effective interaction-influence system through which the relevant communications flow readily, the required influence is exerted laterally, upward, and downward, and the motivational forces needed for coordination are created.[31]

The activities required for organizational performance are separated through the process of vertical and horizontal differentiation. Differentiation is defined as "The state of segmentation of the organizational system into subsystems, each of which tends to develop particular attributes in relation to the requirements posed by its relevant environment."[32] Vertical differentiation establishes the hierarchy and the number of levels in the organization.[33] Horizontal differentiation comes about because of the need to separate activities so that they may be performed more effectively and efficiently. This usually results in the formation of departments within the organization.[34] For instance, in a hospital horizontal differentiation accounts for departments such as Radiology, Pharmacy, and Pathology. Vertical differentiation accounts for an administrator, a second level of assistant administrators, a third level of department heads and continuing on down.

---

[30]Rensis Likert, *The Human Organization.* New York: McGraw-Hill Book Company, 1967, p. 156.

[31]*Ibid.* p. 167.

[32]Lawrence and Lorsch, op. cit. pp. 3–4.

[33]Fremont E. Kast and J. E. Rosenzweig, *Organization and Management: A Systems Approach,* 2nd edition. New York: McGraw-Hill Book Company, 1974, p. 214.

[34]*Ibid.* p. 215.

Once the activities of the organization have been differentiated, they must be coordinated. Of course, the requirements of the environment and technical system involved very often determine the degree of coordination required. In some organizations, it is possible to separate activities in such a way as to minimize these requirements. In other organizations, particularly those functionally departmentalized such as hospitals, coordination is more important. It is necessary to recognize the interaction between the need to specialize activities and the requirements for coordination. The more differentiation of activities and specialization of labor there is, the more difficult the problems of coordination will be.

Unity of Command. The classical principle of unity of command suggests that each participant in an organization should be responsible to, and receive orders from, only one superior. (This principle is not always applied in health care organizations as will be seen in Chapter 8.) Fayol stressed this principle more than any other, stating that if it is violated "authority is undermined, discipline is in jeopardy, order disturbed and stability threatened."[35] This principle is derived from the bureaucratic concept of hierarchy.

It should be noted that one of Frederick W. Taylor's principles of scientific management, functionalization, is at variance with the classical principle of unity of command. Taylor experimented (rather successfully at the time) with an organization structure that permitted eight functional foremen to give orders to individual workers in certain specialized functional areas. In "Shop Management," Taylor advocated the functional plan as follows:

> Throughout the whole field of management the military type of organization should be abandoned, and what may be called the "functional type" substituted in its place.... If practicable, the work of each man in the management should be confined to the performance of a single leading function.[36]

Fayol responded to Taylor's functional idea of management with these words:

> For myself I do not think that a shop can be well run in flagrant violation of [unity of command]. Nevertheless, Taylor successfully managed large-scale concerns. How, then, can this contradiction be explained? I imagine that in practice Taylor was able to reconcile functionalism with the principle of unity of command .... I think it dangerous to allow the idea to gain ground that unity of command is unimportant and can be violated with impunity.[37]

Some aspects of this disagreement have been worked out by the use of line-staff relationships in many organizations. As organizations have grown more complex, it has become necessary to integrate personnel with specialized knowledge and functions into the managerial system. In many ways, the line and staff concept can be viewed as a necessary compromise in terms of the unity of command principle. The line organization is invested with the primary source of authority. It performs the major functions of the organization, while

---

[35]Fayol, op. cit. p. 24.

[36]Frederick W. Taylor, *Shop Management.* New York: Harper and Brothers, 1947, p. 99. Original copyright held by Taylor, 1911.

[37]Fayol, op. cit. pp. 69–70.

the staff supports and advises the line. This relationship is, of course, not as simple as these statements imply. In regard to the staff concept, Hodgetts has stated: "Many organizations have found, to their dismay, that although staff authority can be advantageous, it can also lead to authority conflicts between line and staff executives."[38]

Since line and staff relationships are essentially authority relationships, the principle dealing with authority must be dealt with before a meaningful discussion of line and staff can take place.

Equal Authority and Responsibility. In the view of the classicists, the legitimatization of authority at a central source ensures that the superior has the *right* to command and that the subordinate person has the *duty* to obey.[39]

The classical principle states that there must be an equal relationship between the responsibilities of a manger and the authority that he exercises. Urwick has stated:

> To hold a group or individual accountable for activities of any kind without assigning to him or them the necessary authority to discharge that responsibility is manifestly both unsatisfactory and inequitable. It is of great importance to smooth working that at all levels authority and responsibility should be coterminous and coequal.[40]

This principle of co-equalness of authority and responsibility does not provide a formula by which one can equate authority and responsibility. In fact, no sure formula exists. Yet this does not negate the principle's basic premise that if one is given responsibility in the organization, the authority to go with it must also be given.

Line and Staff. The most basic and meaningful way to view line and staff as an organizational concept is to see it as a matter of relationships. A line relationship is one in which a superior exercises direct supervision over a subordinate—a direct authority relationship. The nature of the staff relationship is advisory. As Mooney has stated, staff is auxiliary, and although "it may suggest that the structure of organization is like a double-track railroad, consisting of line and staff as two coordinate functions . . . there could be no more erroneous conception."[41]

Most of the problems created by line-staff conflicts stem from a failure to clearly define the operational difference between the two. Sometimes, managers are line managers within their own departments but become staff when dealing with outside departments (i.e., personnel manager or controller). As a result, personal conflicts and dual-authority situations can arise. The way to effectively counter this problem is to spell out each manager's functional authority in the organization.

It should be noted that the term "staff" has a different connotation in most

---

[38]Richard M. Hodgetts, *Management: Theory, Process, and Practice*. Philadelphia: W. B. Saunders Company, 1975, p. 174.

[39]John M. Pfiffner and Frank P. Sherwood, *Administrative Organization*. Englewood Cliffs, New Jersey: Prentice-Hall, 1960, p. 75.

[40]Urwick, op. cit. p. 46.

[41]Mooney, op. cit. pp. 34–35.

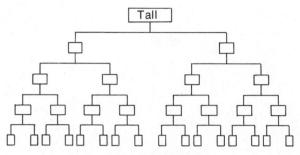

Figure 7–1 Tall structure.

health care organizations than it does in business and industry. In the health facility the term is used to describe the physicians and dentists who make up the *medical staff*. However, health care organizations also have the same line-staff relationship that exists in other organizations within the administration.

Limited Span of Control.   Span of control may be defined simply as the number of subordinates reporting directly to a superior. The classicists were in general agreement that there should be a limited number of subordinates reporting to a superior. Some even went so far as to specify numbers for the optimum span. More recent thinking suggests that there is no specific number of people a manager can effectively supervise.

A number of factors enter into the issue of the appropriateness of span of control. The level in the organization has a great deal to do with determining a suitable span. At the top level, five or six subordinates may be all that should exist. At a lower level, where work tends to be more standardized and rou-tinized, 15 may not be too many. Another factor is the nature of the work being performed. It may be easier to supervise 10 file clerks than five head nurses. The abilities and availability of managers should also be taken into ac-count. Obviously, the training and personal qualities of some managers permit them to handle more subordinates than others, thus facilitating a broader span. Similarly, the better the training, the higher the potential and self-direction of subordinates, the less they will need to have relationships with management and the more subordinates a given manager can have under supervision.

Many of the classicists, including Weber,[42] Urwick,[43] and Gulick[44] felt that the most efficient organization was one with a small span of control. The result-ing organization pattern was a "tall" structure, as presented in Figure 7–1. In a tall structure the small number of subordinates assigned to each superior allows for tight controls. The classical bureaucratic structure is very tall. Conversely, if an organization possesses wide or large spans of control it takes on a "flat" pat-tern, as depicted in Figure 7–2. Both Figures have the same number of person-

[42]Max Weber, "The essentials of bureaucratic organization: An ideal-type construction." *A Reader in Bureaucracy*, ed. Robert K. Merton et al. Glencoe, Illinois: The Free Press, 1952, pp. 18–27.

[43]Lydall F. Urwick, "The manager's span of control." *Harvard Business Review*, 34:41, May–June, 1956.

[44]Gulick and Urwick, op. cit. p. 9.

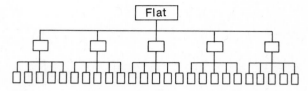

Figure 7–2   Flat structure.

nel. The difference is that the tall structure has four levels of management and the flat one has only two.

Most health care organizations (as we shall see in the next chapter) have a tall pattern. This is a result of the extreme differentiation and specialization of numerous and quite varied (i.e., laundry compared to nursing) departments. A rather limited span of control is required in most health care organizations and this is reflected in their tall rather than flat patterns.

Delegation of Routine Matters.   The classicists, almost without exception, felt that decisions should be made at the lowest level in the organization that would be accordant with good decisions. This meant that top management should not make decisions on routine matters that could be effectively handled at a lower level. Mooney and Reiley stated that "One of the tragedies of business experience is the frequency with which men, always efficient in anything they personally can do, will finally be crushed and fail under the weight of accumulated duties that they do not know and cannot learn how to delegate."[45]

The concept of delegation, as expounded by the classicists, has come to be treated as an integral part of the centralization and decentralization issue. Although closely related to delegation, decentralization is more: it has become a philosophy of organization and management. It requires considerably more than the simple handing of authority or responsibility to subordinates. As organizations discover when they begin to decentralize, a careful selection of which decisions to push down into the organization structure and which to hold at or near the top is required. Furthermore, specific policies to guide the decision-making are needed.

Decentralization of authority and decision-making is a fundamental phase of delegation. Where authority is not delegated, the organization is centralized. Of course, there cannot be absolute decentralization.[46] Dale has formulated some objective criteria that can be very helpful in measuring the extent of decentralization. He states the degree of decentralization is greater when used in relation to the following:

1. The greater the number of decisions made lower down the management hierarchy.
2. The more important the decisions made lower down the management hierarchy. For example, the greater the sum of capital expenditure that can be approved by the plant manager without consulting anyone else, the greater the degree of decentralization in this field.

---

[45]Mooney and Reiley, op. cit. p. 39.
[46]Hodgetts, op. cit. p. 179.

3. The more functions affected by decisions made at lower levels. Thus, companies which permit only operational decisions to be made at separate branch plants are less decentralized than those which also permit financial and personnel decisions at branch plants.
4. The less checking required on the decision. Decentralization is greatest when no check at all must be made; less when superiors have to be informed of the decision after it has been made; still less if superiors have to be consulted before the decision is made. The fewer people to be consulted, and the lower they are on the management hierarchy, the greater the degree of decentralization.[47]

In a study at General Motors, Peter Drucker discovered that executives who worked under a decentralized philosophy gave the following advantages of decentralization:

1. Speed and lack of confusion in decision-making.
2. Absence of conflict between the top management and the divisions.
3. A sense of fairness in dealing with executives, confidence that a job well done would be appreciated, and a lack of politics in the organization.
4. Informality and democracy in management.
5. Absence of a gap between the few top managers and the many subordinate mangers in the organization.
6. The availability of a large reservoir of promotable managerial manpower.
7. Ready visibility of weak managements through results of semi-independent and often competitive divisions.
8. Absence of 'edict management' and the presence of thorough information and consideration of central management decisions.[48]

The reader should not draw the conclusion that decentralization is intrinsically better than centralization. In general, decentralization is much more compatible with the modern behavioral aspects of management. It provides many advantages, such as those suggested by Drucker above. On the other hand, centralization (1) results in uniformity of policy, (2) enables others to use the skills and services of centralized staff, and (3) fosters better control of the organization's activities.[49]

The operational question faced by managers in deciding what amount of centralization or decentralization is desirable can only be answered by saying that it depends on the individual situation. Newman, Summer, and Warren suggest seven questions that should be considered in determining the degree of decentralization that is desirable in a particular situation:

1. Who knows the facts on which the decision will be based, or who can get them together most readily?
2. Who has the capacity to make sound decisions?
3. Must speedy, on-the-spot decisions be made to meet local conditions?
4. Must the local activity be carefully coordinated with other activities?

---

[47]Ernest Dale, *Planning and Developing the Company Organization Structure.* New York: American Management Association, 1952, Research Report No. 20, p. 107.
[48]Peter F. Drucker, *Concept of the Corporation.* New York: The John Day Company, Inc., 1972, pp. 47–48.
[49]Edwin B. Flippo, *Management: A Behavioral Approach,* 2nd edition. Boston: Allyn and Bacon, Inc., 1970, p. 162.

5. How significant is the decision?
6. How busy are the executives who might be assigned planning tasks?
7. Will initiative and morale be significantly improved by decentralization?[50]

It is fair to say that there is a wide discrepancy between the theory and the practice of decentralization. Nevertheless, its wide adaptation has greatly aided managerial acceptance of behavioral concepts in organization. Although the classicists never really addressed the behavioral issue, their principle of delegation was the most forward-thinking of the classical principles, and from it grew much of what is now called modern organization theory.

MODERN ORGANIZATION THEORY

In recent years, the classical principles have been criticized. Particularly cogent criticism of classical organization theory has come from Herbert A. Simon, who has pointed out the contradictions between many of the classical principles. He has even gone so far as to suggest the classical principles "cannot be more than proverbs" which have neither empirical validity nor universality of application.[51]

CRITICISM OF CLASSICAL THEORY

In general, most criticism of the classical organization theory has come from the behaviorally oriented organization theorists. Perhaps their criticism can be presented as a conviction that the classical approach is much too simplistic and too mechanistic to adequately deal with the complex human component of organization. This does not mean that the classicists are wrong, but that their theories are incomplete. March and Simon summarize five basic limitations of classical organization theory from a human standpoint:

1. The motivational assumptions are incomplete and inaccurate.
2. Intraorganizational conflict is generally ignored.
3. Constraints placed on the human as a complex information-processing system are given little consideration.
4. Little attention is given to the role of cognition in task identification and decision.
5. The phenomenon of program elaboration receives little emphasis.[52]

A great mass of research has been done to show that there is a more effective organizational structure substantially different from that contained in the classical design theory. Perhaps the most important recent research was done by Rensis Likert of the University of Michigan. He argues that effective organiza-

---

[50]William H. Newman, Charles E. Summer, and E. Kirby Warren, *The Process of Management,* 3rd edition. Englewood Cliffs, New Jersey: Prentice-Hall, Inc., 1972, pp. 54–56.

[51]Herbert A. Simon, *Administrative Behavior,* 2nd edition. New York: The Free Press, 1965, pp. 20–36.

[52]James G. March and Herbert A. Simon, *Organizations.* New York: John Wiley and Sons, Inc., 1958, p. 33.

tions encourage supervisors to "focus their primary attention on endeavoring to build effective work groups with high performance goals."[53]

In contrast, less effective organizations encourage supervisors to

1. Break the total operation into simple component parts or tasks.
2. Develop the best way to carry out each of the component parts.
3. Hire people with appropriate aptitudes and skills to perform each of these tasks.
4. Train these people to do their respective tasks in the specified best way.
5. Provide supervision to see that they perform their designated tasks, using the specified procedure and at an acceptable rate as determined by such procedures as timing the job.
6. Where feasible, use incentives in the form of individual or group piece rates.[54]

In classical design theory, these six points are the responsibilities of the manager. Likert's findings that these points do not result in effective organizations substantiate the earlier findings of Merton,[55] Gouldner,[56] Selznick,[57] and the Hawthorne researchers.[58]

Likert describes organizations in terms of eight dimensions, each of which is a continuum, with classical design organizations being at one extreme and what Likert calls "System 4" organizations opposite. System 4 organizations encourage greater utilization of the human potential by using practices which tap the full range of human motivations. These organizations, according to Likert, "ensure a maximum probability that in all interaction and in all relationships within the organization, each member, in light of his background, values, desires, and expectations, will view the experience as supportive and one which builds and maintains his sense of personal worth and importance."[59]

While the behavioralists have not solved the organizing problem, they have helped shape new structural models designed to meet some of the shortcomings of the classical theorists. Two such models are briefly presented here.

PROJECT ORGANIZATION

Highly technical industries (most notably the aerospace industry) may use *project organization* as a structural means for focusing a large amount of talent and resources for a given period on a specific project. The project "team" of various specialists is put together under the direction of the project manager.

---

[53]Rensis Likert, *New Patterns of Management*. New York: McGraw-Hill Book Company, 1961, p. 7.

[54]*Ibid.* p. 6.

[55]Robert K. Merton, "Bureaucratic structure and personality." *Social Forces*, 18:560, 1940.

[56]Alvin W. Gouldner, *Patterns of Industrial Bureaucracy*. New York: The Free Press of Glencoe, 1954.

[57]Philip Selznick, *TVA and the Grass Roots*. Berkeley: The University of California Press, 1949.

[58]T. N. Whitehead, *The Industrial Worker*. Cambridge, Massachusetts: Harvard University Press, 1938; Fritz J. Roethlisberger and William J. Dickson, *Management and the Worker*. Cambridge, Massachusetts: Harvard University Press, 1947; Fritz J. Roethlisberger, *Management and Morale*. Cambridge, Massachusetts: Harvard University Press, 1941; and Elton Mayo, *The Human Problems of an Industrial Civilization*. New York: Macmillan, 1933.

[59]Likert, op. cit. p. 103.

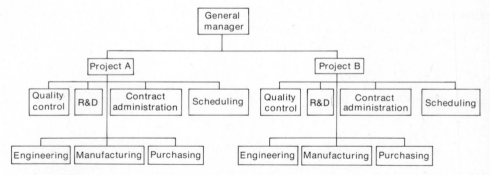

Figure 7–3 Project organization. (From Fred Luthans, page 173: *Organizational Behavior.* Copyright © 1973 by McGraw-Hill, Inc. Used by permission of the McGraw-Hill Book Company.)

In contrast to classical organization structures there is a strong emphasis on direct horizontal relations between specialists; communication rarely goes up a scalar chain and back down. Figure 7–3 represents a typical project organization approach.

Project organization offers greater flexibility and response to innovative ideas as opposed to the traditional functional organization structure. However, associated with its use are problems such as role ambiguity for members of the team and the fact that the project manager must adopt a new approach to his job. As Cleland and King point out,

1. He must become reoriented away from the purely functional approach to the management of human and nonhuman resources.
2. He must understand that purposeful conflict may very well be a necessary way of life as he manages his project across many vertical, organizational lines.
3. He must recognize that project management is a dynamic activity where major changes are almost the order of the day.[60]

These considerations make it clear that the project concept is not only a form of structural organization but also a philosophy of management. The project viewpoint is quite different from the functional viewpoint, as Figure 7–4 suggests.

MATRIX ORGANIZATION

When project organization is superimposed on a functional, hierarchical organization the result is *matrix organization*. This provides a horizontal, lateral dimension for the traditional vertical orientation of the functional organization.

Duncan Neuhauser has suggested that hospitals are matrix organizations: "The existence of both hierarchical (vertical) coordination through departmentalization and the formal chain of command and simultaneously lateral (horizontal coordination) across departments (the patient care team) is called a ma-

---

[60]David I. Cleland and William R. King, *Systems Analysis and Project Management.* New York: McGraw-Hill Book Company, 1968, p. 152.

Comparison of Functional and Project Viewpoints

Phenomenon	Project Viewpoint	Functional Viewpoint
Line-staff organizational dichotomy	Vestiges of the hierarchal model remain, but line functions are placed in a support position. A web of authority and responsibility relationships exists.	Line functions have direct responsibility for accomplishing the objectives; the line commands, staff advises.
Scalar principle	Elements of the vertical chain exist, but prime emphasis is placed on horizontal and diagonal work flow. Important business is conducted as the legitimacy of the task requires.	The chain of authority relationships is from superior to subordinate throughout the organization. Central, crucial, and important business is conducted up and down the vertical hierarchy.
Superior-subordinate relationship	Peer to peer, manager to technical expert, associate to associate relationships are used to conduct much of the salient business.	This is the most important relationship; if kept healthy, success will follow. All important business is conducted through a pyramiding structure of superiors-subordinates.
Organizational objectives	Management of a project becomes a joint venture of many relatively independent organizations. Thus, the objective becomes multilateral.	Organizational objectives are sought by the parent unit (an assembly of suborganizations) working within its environment. The objective is unilateral.
Unity of direction	The project manager manages across functional and organizational lines to accomplish a common interorganizational objective.	The general manager acts as the head for a group of activities having the same plan.
Parity of authority and responsibility	Considerable opportunity exists for the project manager's responsibility to exceed his authority. Support people are often responsible to other managers (functional) for pay, performance reports, promotions, and so forth.	Consistent with functional management; the integrity of the superior-subordinate relationship is maintained through functional authority and advisory staff services.
Time duration	The project (and hence the organization) is finite in duration.	Tends to perpetuate itself to provide continuing facilitative support.

Figure 7-4 A comparison of the project versus the functional organization. (Source: David I. Cleland, "Understanding project authority," *Business Horizons*, *10*:66, Spring, 1967. Reprinted by permission of the publisher.)

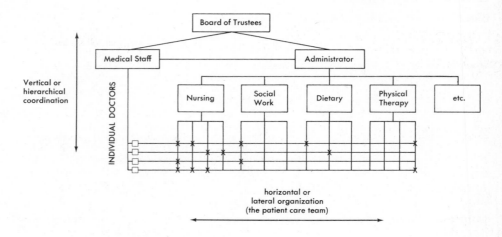

(x) Indicates both a member of a department and a patient care team.

Figure 7–5   The hospital as a matrix organization. (Source: Duncan Neuhauser, "The hospital as a matrix organization," *Hospital Administration, 17*:20, Fall, 1972. Used by permission of the publisher.)

trix organization."[61] Neuhauser's diagram of this may be seen in Figure 7–5.

At this point it is enough to say that matrix organization incorporates some of the best aspects of project organization and functional organization. Cleland and King summarize its advantages as follows:

1. The project is emphasized by designating one individual as the focal point for all matters pertaining to it.
2. Utilization of manpower can be flexible because a reservoir of specialists is maintained in functional organizations.
3. Specialized knowledge is available to all programs on an equal basis; knowledge and experience can be transferred from one project to another.
4. Project people have a functional home when they are no longer needed on a given project.
5. Responsiveness to project needs and customer desires is generally faster because lines of communication are established and decision points are centralized.
6. Management consistency between projects can be maintained through the deliberate conflict operating in the project-functional environment.
7. A better balance between time, cost, and performance can be obtained through the built-in checks and balances (the deliberate conflict) and the continuous negotiations carried on between the project and the functional organizations.[62]

ORGANIZATIONS AS OPEN SYSTEMS

The application of system theory to modern organization theory is very important. According to Scott, the qualities of modern organization theory are "its conceptual-analytical base, its reliance on empirical research data, and,

---

[61]Duncan Neuhauser, "The hospital as a matrix organization." *Hospital Administration, 17*:19, Fall, 1972.

[62]Cleland and King, op. cit. p. 172.

above all, its integrating nature."[63] Systems theory makes its greatest contribution to the understanding of organizations by stressing the interrelatedness and interdependency among the elements of all components of the organization.

Systems Concept. Basically a system is a set of interrelated and interdependent parts which form a complex whole, and each of those parts can be viewed as a subsystem with its own set of interrelated and interdependent parts. A few moments of thought about this definition will lead one to the conclusion that just about anything can be viewed as a system. In the health field we hear constant reference to the nervous system or to the circulatory system. An automobile is a system; it consists of parts arranged in a manner that produces a unified whole. Relationships of all kinds can be described as systems. We have, for instance, economic systems, transportation systems, communication systems, number systems, social systems, governmental systems, and legal systems.

Any discussion of systems must include the concept of subsystems. Systems are composed of parts which are systems themselves. For example, the human body is a system composed of various subsystems, such as the nervous or cardiovascular. These subsystems are composed of cells, each of which is also a system. Thus, systems usually exhibit a structure in which there are subsystems embedded within overall systems.

The Hospital As A System. An organization chart of a hospital shows how subsystems can be embedded in other subsystems to form a hierarchy of subsystems or the overall system, which is the hospital. Furthermore, the hospital, along with other health-care organizations, can be viewed as one component part of the health-care delivery system. Figure 7–6 illustrates the subsys-

---

[63]William G. Scott, "Organization theory: An overview and an appraisal." *Academy of Management Journal, 4*:15, April, 1961.

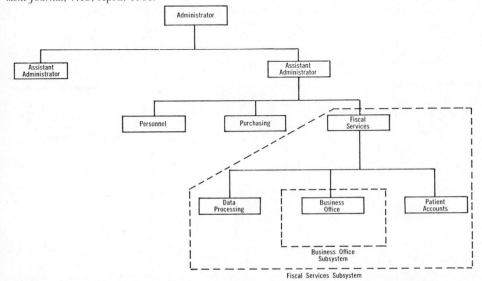

Figure 7–6 The hospital as a system with subsystems. (Source: Beaufort B. Longest, Jr., *Principles of Hospital Business Office Management.* Chicago, Hospital Financial Management Association, 1975, p. 61. Used by permission of the publisher.)

tems of a typical hospital. The fiscal services subsystem is enclosed in a broken line. It includes the business office subsystem. The hospital itself is the next system level shown. It entails the fiscal services subsystem along with other subsystems. The hospital itself can be thought of as a subsystem of the hospital industry, which can be thought of as a subsystem of the health services industry, and on and on. For our purposes, we will concentrate primarily on the hospital and one of its basic subsystems, the Fiscal Services Division, and one of the division's basic subsystems, the Business Office. The key point for the reader to understand is that the essential element of the systems viewpoint is a perspective of the hospital as a conglomerate of interrelated and interdependent parts. No one part (subsystem) can perform effectively without the others, and any action taken on or by one will have effects that can be traced throughout the organization, and in some cases throughout the organization's complex environment. As a result, there is an overwhelming need for coordination among the subsystems.

Types of Systems. Systems can be considered to be either closed or open and in interaction with their environment. Closed-system thinking stems primarily from the physical sciences and is applicable to mechanistic systems. Closed systems are seen as being self-contained. The open system is a more realistic view of the systems concept as it applies to management, since it recognizes that the system is constantly in dynamic interaction with its environment. Management systems should be open not only in relation to their environment but also in relation to themselves; internal interaction between components of a system affects the entire system.

To be completely functional, management systems should include feedback mechanisms, as noted in Figure 7–7. Through the process of feedback, the system continually receives information from its environment which helps it to adjust. (Note the similarity of Fig. 7–7 to the management model presented in Fig. 2–3, page 22.) Although feedback can be either positive or negative, for our purposes the most important is negative. Negative feedback is informa-

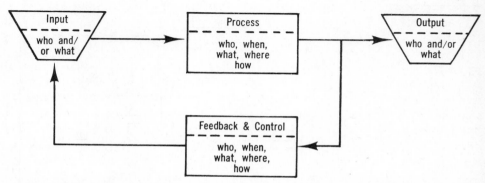

Figure 7–7 An open system (with a feedback mechanism). (Source: Beaufort B. Longest, Jr., *Principles of Hospital Business Office Management.* Chicago, Hospital Financial Management Association, 1975, p. 63. Used by permission of the publisher.

tion indicating that the system is deviating from a prescribed course and should readjust.

From Figure 7–7 one can see that a system is indeed an assemblage of parts forming a unitary whole. The dynamic nature of the parts of the system as they interrelate can be envisioned as well. The inputs into a system can be almost anything and what they are will depend largely on what outputs are desired. In fact, when one is designing a system, the desired outputs should be determined first. This means that before a suitable Business Office system can be developed, the objectives (desired outputs) must be determined. With the objectives in mind, the necessary inputs of people, things, and ideas can be obtained and processed to produce the desired outputs. The control mechanism exists to make certain that the desired outputs are obtained.

Importance of the Systems Point of View. Viewing organizations as systems provides a frame of reference or a viewpoint and permits the manager to see the organization as a whole with interdependent parts (a system composed of subsystems). Regarding a health care organization as a system has several far-reaching implications. For the administrator, it means that the larger system (health care delivery) must be identified and understood, and that the relationship of his organization to this larger system must be defined. Each health care organization is composed of many subsystems, and each subsystem has its own goals and objectives. *The systems concept stresses the dynamic nature of an organization and prevents the manager from viewing his job as one of managing static, isolated elements of the organization.* It makes each manager, regardless of what level he manages, realize that he contributes to some larger whole by meeting the objectives for which he is responsible. This is the key contribution of the systems viewpoint. Each manager realizes that he affects and is affected by everything that goes on inside the organization and, to a large extent, outside the organization.

Special Characteristics of Organizational Systems. Several characteristics of organizational systems apply directly to any health care organization. They are *contrived systems,* designed, built, and operated by human beings. The importance of this fact should never be overlooked. Human imperfections can cause a system to come apart at the seams. On the other hand, contrived systems can outlast those who created them many times over.

The concept of *boundaries* is important in organizational systems. The fact that health care organizations are open systems and therefore in dynamic interaction with their environment is very important. To a large extent, their success depends upon how well they cross the boundaries of the system and interact with outside systems such as consumers or patients, suppliers, state, local, and federal government agencies, physicians, and the other systems making up the external environment of the health care organization. Internal boundaries are also important. One of the key purposes of management is to ensure smooth coordination of the various subsystems which make up the organization. Boundaries, if the organizing process is to be accomplished, must not become walls, but should merely be reference points for authority and responsibility relationships.

Another important characteristic of organizational systems is that they strike a *balance between adaptive and maintenance mechanisms,* two mechanisms often in conflict. Organizational systems must have maintenance mechanisms which ensure that the various subsystems are in balance and that the total system is in accord with its environment. Maintenance mechanisms tend to be conservative; their purpose is to prevent the system from changing so rapidly that the subsystems or the total system become unbalanced. In contrast, adaptive mechanisms are necessary to provide a dynamic equilibrium which changes over time and allows the system to respond to variations in internal and external demands. It would appear that most health care organizations are organizational systems which place more emphasis on maintenance mechanisms than on adaptive mechanisms. In the long run, this may lead to stagnation.

One of the most obvious characteristics of some health care organizations (particularly hospitals) is their tendency, as organizational systems, to grow through *internal elaboration.* This tendency is evident in the movement of hospitals toward greater differentiation and a higher level of organization. The increased number of specialized departments and operational units within hospitals is largely due to mushrooming medical and scientific technology. Other support units are then developed to serve these departments. Although no one wants to stop or slow advances in technology, managers must realize that the natural tendency toward internal elaboration is responsible, in part, for increasing organizational complexity. As a result the organization is more complex and more difficult to manage.

One final but very important characteristic of organizational systems is the concept of *equifinality.* This means that the same, or similar, final results may be achieved by different organizations with different initial conditions and in different ways. In other words, the organizational system can accomplish its objectives with varied inputs and internal activities. The manager can introduce diverse inputs, transform them in a number of ways, and still achieve satisfactory output. If this view is extended further it could be suggested that management is not necessarily a process of seeking a rigid optimal solution to problems but rather one of having available a variety of satisfactory solutions from which to select.

THE INFORMAL ORGANIZATION[64]

Existing within the formal organization's pattern of authority-responsibility relationships is another equally important structure—the informal organization.[65] As we have seen earlier in this chapter, the formal organization is a planned-prescribed structure. It represents a deliberate attempt to establish patterned relationships among participants in the organization. A great deal of management time and effort goes into the establishment and maintenance of the formal organization. The results of these efforts include the development

---

[64]This section draws heavily on an article by Beaufort B. Longest, Jr., "Institutional politics." *Journal of Nursing Administration,* 5:38, April, 1975. (Adapted by permission of the publisher.)
[65]Chester I. Barnard, op. cit. p. 115. Barnard states: "By informal organization I mean the aggregate of the personal contacts and interactions and the associated groupings of people."

of an organization structure as depicted by the organization chart, job descriptions, formal rules, operating policies, work procedures, control procedures, compensation arrangements, and many other devices used to guide employee behavior. However, there are many interactions between members of an organization which are not prescribed by the formal structure. *These relationships and interactions which occur spontaneously out of the activities and interactions of members of the organization, but which are not set forth in the formal structure, make up the informal organization.* They are the emergent relationships among people.

One of the things which distinguish the classical organization theorists from the modern theorists (especially the behaviorists) is that the classical thinkers concentrated on the formal organization and the behaviorists have concentrated primarily on informal relationships. Formal and informal organizations coexist and are inseparable. They are totally intermeshed. It has been pointed out by Blau and Scott:

> It is impossible to understand the nature of a formal organization without investigating the networks of informal relations and the unofficial norms as well as the formal hierarchy of authority and the official body of rules, since the formally instituted and the informally emerging patterns are inextricably intertwined. The distinction between the formal and the informal aspects of organization life is only an analytical one and should not be reified; there is only one actual organization.[66]

NATURE OF INFORMAL ORGANIZATION

Actual awareness and interest in the informal organization stemmed from the famous *Hawthorne studies* of the 1930's.[67] These studies showed that informal organization is an integral part of the total work situation. Since the informal organization arises from the *social interaction* of participants in an organization, it has come to represent small groups and their patterns of behavior. Most of what managers know about the informal organization has come from the work of sociologists and social psychologists.

The formal organization and the informal organization together constitute the organizational setting within which work is carried out to accomplish objectives. The formal organization can be characterized by such items as the prescribed authority-responsibility relationships, the organization's hierarchical structure, the line-staff arrangement, and the planned division of work and departmentation: the planned manner in which people, things, and activities are interrelated.

On the other hand, the informal organization is characterized by the dynamic emergent behavior and activity patterns that occur within the formal organization structure as a result of people working with other people—their interaction and fraternization across formal stuctural lines. For example, the Director of Nursing Services occupies a formal organization position providing inherent authority and responsibility which prescribe her relationships to superiors, subordinates, and other organizational units. Because of personality,

---

[66]Peter M. Blau and W. Richard Scott, *Formal Organizations.* San Francisco, California: Chandler Publishing Company, 1962, p. 6.

[67]For a complete account of these studies, see F. J. Roethlisberger and W. J. Dickson, *Management and the Worker.* Cambridge, Massachusetts: Harvard University Press, 1939.

technical skill, leadership abilities, managerial capabilities, or any of a number of other reasons, it is possible for the Assistant Director of Nursing Service to have greater influence. In this situation the informal emergent behavior relationships supersede the planned design. This can create many problems for the health care facility but can also have a highly positive impact on patient care. Health care managers need to be familiar with the intricate involvements that make up the theory of informal organization. Many of these are described in this chapter.

Three facts about informal organization which the manager should accept from the outset are stated below.

1. *The informal organization is inevitable.* Management can eliminate any aspect of the formal organization because it is created by management. The informal organization is not created by management and cannot be canceled by management. As long as there are people involved, there will be an informal organization.

2. *Small groups make up the central component of the informal organization,* and group membership strongly influences the overall behavior and performance of members. Many sociologists now believe that the social unit (group), rather than the individual, is the basic component of the human organization.

3. *Informal organization has both positive and negative consequences for the organization.* Later, we shall examine the advantages and the disadvantages in depth. To capitalize on the advantages and to minimize the disadvantages, the manager should understand the informal organization and, therefore, must understand groups in the organization.

WHY PEOPLE FORM INFORMAL GROUPS

Needs.   When one considers why another human being does anything, the obvious starting point is with motivation. Motivation theory, presented in Chapter 11, has taught us that people are motivated by things which satisfy their needs. Informal groups most usually come into being in response to their members' *needs* that are not fully met in the context of the formal organization alone. The interpersonal contacts within the small group provide some relief from the boredom, monotomy, and pressures of the formal organization. An individual in a group is usually surrounded by others who share similar values and thus reinforce the individual's own value system. The group itself can be a power force which will minimize any threats to its members.

A second reason why people join small informal groups is that informal *status* (which may be brought about by nothing more than belonging to a distinct, more or less exclusive little unit) can be accorded by the group.

Third, informal group membership provides a degree of personal *security*. A group member knows that he is accepted as an equal by his peers and feels secure in their company. As a result of membership, an individual can express himself before generally sympathetic listeners and satisfy his recognition, participation, and communication needs. One may even find an outlet for leadership drives. These important forms of satisfaction are available in the group to a greater degree than in the formal organization.

Information.   Another very important reason for group membership is to secure information. The grapevine is a phenomenon familiar to all organization participants. Technically, it is the organization's informal communication channel. We will treat this topic more completely in Chapter 13; suffice it to say here that informal group membership provides members with an inside track to the flow of informal communication.

The common attribute all these reasons share is that each meets specific needs that are not fully met by the formal organization. Informal groups arise and persist in the organization because they perform the functions desired by their members.

CHARACTERISTICS OF INFORMAL GROUPS

It has been suggested that informal groups tend to possess the following characteristics: (1) a tendency to remain small, (2) the satisfaction of group member wants, (3) the development of unofficial leadership, (4) a highly complex structure of relationships, and (5) a tendency toward stability.[68]

The first two reasons have already been touched on. Since interpersonal relationships are the essence of informal organization, the informal group must remain small enough so that its individual members can interact frequently. We have seen that the motivation for forming informal groups is that the groups provide a mechanism to satisfy needs not satisfied by the formal organization.

Informal Leader.   The development of small-group leaders has been studied extensively. Some of the general conclusions about them can be summarized as follows:

1. The leadership role is filled by an individual who possesses the attributes which the group members perceive as being critical for satisfying their needs.
2. The leader embodies the values of the group from which he emerges. He is able to perceive these values, organize them into an intelligible philosophy, and verbalize them to nonmembers.
3. The leader is able to receive and filter communication relevant to the group, and effectively communicate the new information to the group. This role can be thought of as an information center.[69]

The informal group leader emerges from within the group because he can serve several functions for the group. He serves not only to initiate action and provide direction but also to compromise differences of opinion that exist on group-related matters. Furthermore, the leader serves to communicate group values and feelings to nonmembers, such as the representatives of the formal organization. Only as long as he is able to perform these functions can he maintain his leadership role.

Complex Relationships.   Another important characteristic of small groups is their tendency to develop a highly complex structure of relationships.

---

[68]Edwin A. Flippo, op. cit. p. 196.
[69]William G. Scott and Terrence R. Mitchell, *Organization Theory.* Homewood, Illinois: Richard D. Irwin, Inc., and The Dorsey Press, 1972, p. 97.

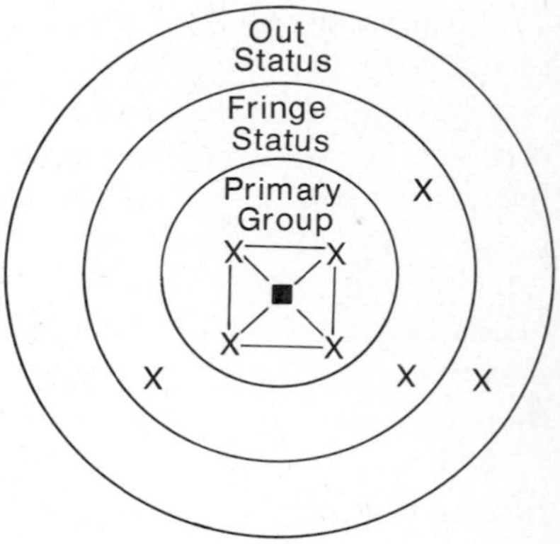

Figure 7–8 A model of informal organization.

Out Status
Fringe Status
Primary Group

In the informal organization, structure is determined by different status positions. Essentially, there are four status positions: (1) group leader; (2) primary group member; (3) fringe group member; (4) out of group.

Suppose, for example, that a manager wanted to analyze the structure of a group of nine people working in a section of the clinical laboratory where interpersonal problems existed. These people are located in a close general area with no artificial barriers (such as walls) to prevent their frequent association with each other. Experience tells us that each person will not associate with every other person with equal frequency. Instead, they will be selective in their association, regularly including some and excluding others.

Using sociometric techniques, which may be nothing more than observation, we can measure this phenomenon and obtain an accurate picture of the nature of the informal organization of the people in the laboratory (see Fig. 7–8).

The solid square in the center represents the leader of the group. Clustered around him are the other four members of the primary group. Their association is close, and is characterized by intense interaction and communication.

The three people in the fringe area are most likely newcomers. They are, in effect, being evaluated by the primary group and may in time become full members. If they are not accepted they will move to out status. In this case one person is already in out status. Although a part of the informal organization, this person is not accepted by the members of the primary group. Out status can have profound behavioral effects if the person wants to belong to the primary group. In some cases the rejection is mutual or may even be rejection of the group by the person in out status. Under these circumstances, the person in out status may get along quite well without primary group membership.

Informal organization interaction is not limited to group members. It also exists as people in the formal organization deal with each other in the accomplishment of work within the context of the formal organization. Figure 7–9 indicates the actual contacts between particular people in the organization. Observe that not all contacts go through formal channels; in some cases, certain levels of the organization are bypassed and in other cases, cross-contact is seen from one chain of command to another.

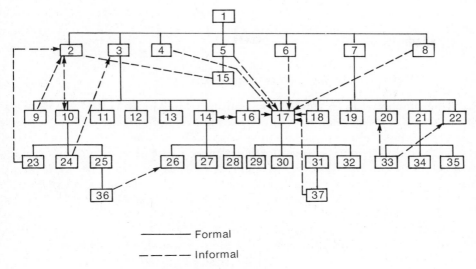

— — — — Formal

— — — — Informal

Figure 7–9   A contact chart.

Such charts do not show the reason for the informal relationships but they do serve to illustrate the complexity of the informal organization. It is quite possible that when the complexity of the formal organization and the informal organizations are considered together, a complete understanding of complex organizations cannot be achieved within the present state of the art of organization theory.

Stability.   The final characteristic of the informal group which we should examine is their tendency toward stability. As Keith Davis has suggested, "Although informal organizations are bound by no chart on the wall, they are bound by convention, custom, and culture."[70] To the manager it may appear that the informal organization resists all change. In truth, the informal organization resists only those changes that are interpreted as threats to the members' needs. It takes a great deal of time to establish the strong interpersonal ties that exist among people in the informal organization. Abrupt acts of management can break these ties instantaneously. For this reason, changes that are seen as a threat to established patterns within the informal organization will be resisted.

Let us assume that the Business Office of a hospital has been functioning for some time with a certain physical layout. The informal group and relationships that have evolved over time are probably deeply entrenched. Administration may decide, however, to rearrange the layout of the Business Office in the interest of efficiency. This decision could cause the break up of the patterns of social relations among the office staff and would quite likely be resisted. In many cases, changes of this type are countered by resistance in the form of complaining, work slowdown, reduction in quality, absenteeism, an increase in turnover, and so on. If administration is to effect the acceptance of

---

[70] Keith Davis, *Human Behavior at Work.* New York: McGraw-Hill Book Company, 1972, p. 256.

such change, it must be aware of and understand the dynamics of the informal organization, and possibly work with the informal group leader to implement the change.

POSITIVE ASPECTS OF INFORMAL ORGANIZATION

Complements the Formal Organization. The key benefit of the informal organization is that it blends with the formal organization to generate a workable system for the accomplishment of work. The formal plans and policies of the organization tend to be too inflexible to meet all the needs of a dynamic situation. At this time, the flexible and spontaneous characteristics of the informal organization can be of great advantage if they permit, or even encourage, deviations in the interest of material contributions toward the goals of the organization.

Dubin was among the first to recognize the necessary complementarity of the formal and informal organization when he stated: "Informal relations in the organization serve to preserve the organization from the self-destruction that would result from literal obedience to the formal policies, rules, regulations, and procedures."[71]

Provides Necessary Social Values and Stability to Work Groups. High turnover may be caused by a poor matching of man and job or for such pragmatic reasons as offers of better jobs or necessary moves. However, research has shown that many resignations occur because the new employee is unable to become a primary member of one or more informal groups. Group membership is a basic means by which employees achieve a sense of belonging and security. If an organization is so cold and impersonal that informal, interpersonal contacts are not encouraged or, in some cases, permitted then many employees will seek employment elsewhere. Of course, informal group membership can be carried to such an extreme that the place of work becomes a mere social circle. This has a detrimental effect on work output and, thereby, organization effectiveness and efficiency. Good management can avoid this extreme and provide an atmosphere in which workers, through informal relationships, can meet their needs.

Simplifies the Manager's Job. In a very real sense the informal organization can make things easier for the manager *if he or she remains in control of the situation.* It has been shown that when informal group support is available, the manager can supervise in a much more general way than when such support is not available. The manager can delegate and decentralize when the informal group is cooperative. Obviously, the converse of this is true as well. The task of the manager is to understand the informal organization and use it to his or her advantage. Flippo has stated,

Awareness of the nature and impact of informal organization often leads to better management decisions. Acceptance of the fact that formal relationships will

---

[71]Robert Dubin, *Human Relations in Administration.* Englewood Cliffs, New Jersey: Prentice-Hall, Inc., 1951, p. 68. This work has been revised in a 4th edition in 1974, but the point is how Dubin saw the complementarity in 1951.

not enable full accomplishment of organization tasks stimulates management to seek other means of motivation. If most of the work is done informally, the manager will seek to improve his knowledge of the nature of people in general and his subordinates in particular. If he realizes that organization performance can be affected by the granting or withholding of cooperation and enthusiasm, he will seek other means than the formal to develop desirable attitudes. He will not depend solely upon the authority of his position.[72]

Provides An Additional Channel of Communication. A well-known benefit of informal organization is that it provides an additional channel of communication for the organization. The grapevine can add to the administration's effectiveness if it will study and use it. The grapevine can relay certain information to employees and can be used to determine the feelings and attitudes of employees on various issues. However, the grapevine can cause problems if it is not understood by management. The free reign of unfounded rumors can be destructive. In a very real sense, all the advantages of the informal organization carry the seeds of trouble. Some potential disadvantages will be examined next.

NEGATIVE ASPECTS OF INFORMAL ORGANIZATION

Anyone who has had to deal with an informal organization realizes that the advantages outlined above are not always realized. In many cases, the disadvantages far outweigh the potential advantages. The formal organization deals with human behavior as we would like it to occur in the organization, whereas the informal organization deals with human behavior as it actually occurs.

Dissimilar Objectives. The most clear-cut disadvantage is that in many situations the individuals and groups that make up the informal organization can, and on occasion do, work at cross-purposes with the objectives of the formal organization. It is a basic fact of organization life that what is good for the employee is not always good for the employer, and vice-versa. Cost containment may be an objective of the organization but not of the informal group if it is translated into transferring group members or not awarding pay increases. The employee may want to meet the objectives of both his group and his employer, but often these are in conflict. The result is known as role conflict.

Role Conflict. Suppose we take the situation of the head nurse as an example. On the one hand, administration's expectations stress her role in the managerial system and the need for decision-making, planning, executing, and controlling activities in her area of responsibility. On the other hand, as a first-line supervisor she often has close ties with other nursing personnel in her unit who may be, in many cases, her former peers. Their expectations of her do not necessarily coincide with those coming from administration. Furthermore, she has many inputs from other head nurses and her own perception of the role to be played. Usually, it is not possible to simultaneously satisfy the expectations of two or more participants when compliance with one precludes compliance with the others.

A good bit of this role conflict can be avoided by recognizing that the more compatible the interests, goals, methods, and evaluation systems of the formal

---

[72]Flippo, op. cit. p. 202.

and informal organizations can be made, the more productivity and satisfaction can be expected.

It should be noted that even the potentially negative impact of conflict should be weighed against the constructive and positive function of conflict in fostering creativity and innovation. A relatively conflict-free organization tends to be static. Some conflict should exist as a condition for the generation of fresh ideas.

LIVING WITH THE INFORMAL ORGANIZATION

We have seen that the existence of the informal organization within the formal structure is a fact of organization life. The formal and informal aspects of the organization must be balanced if optimum performance and goal attainment (both for individuals and for the organization) are to be achieved.

If administration tries to suppress the informal organization it creates a situation in which the informal organization is strengthened in order to counteract the autocratic administration, and thus protect the employees, and make the work situation acceptable in their view. The opposing forces clash, and the result is reduced organization effectiveness and efficiency.

On the other hand, if the formal organization is too weak to accomplish its objectives, the informal organization can grow to be too strong, and this may lead to such undesirable abuses of power as work restriction, insubordination, disloyalty, and other manifestations of a generally anti-institution attitude.

The optimum situation is one in which the formal organization is strong enough to maintain a unified thrust toward attainment of the objectives of the organization but at the same time permits a well developed informal organization to maintain group cohesiveness and teamwork. In the words of one authority, "The informal organization needs to be strong enough to be supportive, but not strong enough to dominate."[73]

A relationship such as the one described above is at best difficult to achieve. There are, however, several steps which can be taken to move the organization in the direction of a properly balanced formal and informal relationship. Among them are the following:

1. Administration must understand the informal organization, and its actions must convince employees that it understands and accepts the informal organization. Of paramount importance here is the impact on the informal organization from any action taken by administration and the resultant implications.

2. Administration must integrate the interests of the informal organization with those of the formal organization to the maximum extent possible. While doing this, administration should prevent any actions of the formal organization from unnecessarily threatening the informal pattern of relationships, or it should at least involve the informal group in proposed changes. This participation tends to give the group a sense of control over their destiny, and fosters communication upward and downward, which will

---

[73]Davis, op. cit. p. 272.

minimize unfounded rumors, and thereby, enhance the likelihood of cooperation.

It must be remembered that the informal relationships which exist in any organization are among the most important. They deserve the attention of everyone concerned with the effectiveness of the organization.

SUMMARY

The organizing process was defined as the *establishment of authority-responsibility relationships and the inter-relating of human and other resources in such a way that the work performed will lead to the fulfillment of the organization's objectives (desired output)*. In other words, it deals with the setting in which work activity occurs. The formal organization and the informal organization *together* constitute the organizational setting. They coexist and are inseparable. Therefore, both were treated in this chapter.

The classical organization theory was presented, and the bureaucratic model was described along with the classical concepts of division of work, unity of command, authority and responsibility, span of control, and delegation.

Modern organization theory was also treated. Specifically presented as alternate ways to view health-care organizations were the concept of matrix organization, which superimposes a project organization over the traditionally functional, hierarchical organization, and the open-systems theory.

Those relationships and interactions which occur spontaneously out of the activities and interactions of members of the organization, but which are not set forth in the formal structure, make up the informal organization. The nature of small groups explains, to a large extent, the informal organization. If the health care manager is to fully utilize the positive benefits of the informal organization and at the same time minimize its negative impact, he must do two things: (1) understand the informal organization and accept it as a fact of organizational life, and (2) to whatever extent possible, integrate the interests of the informal organization with those of the formal organization.

DISCUSSION QUESTIONS

1. What are the major characteristics of the bureaucratic form of organization structure? What are its advantages and disadvantages?

2. Discuss the concept of departmentation and apply it to a hospital, a long-term care facility, and a government organization.

3. Why is "coordination" so important for health care organizations and what are some of the means available for coordination?

4. The classical principle of "unity of command" suggests that an individual should only be responsible to and receive orders from one supervisor. Discuss the implication of this in relation to the nurse.

5. Discuss the interrelationship among span of control, delegation, and centralization-decentralization.

6. Discuss the characteristics of a matrix organization and how it differs from the "classical" functional organization.

7. Adopting a systems point of view, indicate why health care organizations can be considered as open systems functioning within a broader system. Identify the components (subsystems) of a health care organization, and relate that organization to a broader system (i.e. the health care delivery system).

8. Examine the management model in Figure 2–3 (page 22) and discuss its similarity to the open systems section of this chapter.

9. Discuss the reasons why informal groups form and what their major characteristics are.

10. Weigh the positive and negative aspects of the informal organization.

INCIDENTS

1. THE MEDICAL STAFF

A health care spokesman recently declared that in a typical hospital the medical staff has authority without responsibility, and the administrators have responsibility without authority.

A. What is meant by this statement?

B. Do you agree with it? Why?

2. THE NEW ADMINISTRATIVE RESIDENT *

Jack Johnson, a new and ambitious administrative resident at St. Thomas Hospital, was very eager to get things done and was constantly on the lookout for departmental sections to streamline. One day he found a gold mine in the switchboard. He rolled up his sleeves on this one when he found out that while turnover was very low, there was a great deal of dissatisfaction among the switchboard operators. The eight of them who were very close in age (mid-40's), socialized with one another after working hours, and frequently discussed personal matters. Mr. Johnson regarded Mrs. Kelly, the chief operator, as being very personable. She got along well with the public but constantly complained that the employees were overworked and underpaid.

Mr. Johnson checked area hospitals and found that among switchboard operators St. Thomas had one of the lowest rates of pay in town. When he approached the administrator on the matter of higher pay, he was told that it would be impossible to increase the pay for the operators at the present time.

Mr. Johnson set about to do what he could to help the operators. He found that they were working split shifts, and since in his opinion this obviously was not practical, he changed their working schedule. To his surprise, the chief operator reacted very unfavorably to the change in schedule. He then rearranged the work activities by hiring a receptionist so that the operators would be able to concentrate on running the switchboard. The receptionist was not given any cooperation by the switchboard operators, and the first two new employees who occupied the position resigned. Mr. Johnson felt that the chief operator was responsible for the operators' not accepting the new receptionist. He requested that the administrator terminate the chief operator. The administrator refused to do this. Mr. Johnson suddenly found himself in the position of having the switchboard department in worse shape than when he started "reforming" it.

---

*Adapted with permission of the publisher from James A. Hamilton, *Decision-Making in Hospital Administration*, University of Minnesota Press, 1960, pp. 278–280.

    A. What do you think about the behavior of Mr. Johnson?
    B. Why did the telephone operators react the way they did?
    C. Why did the operators not extend help to the receptionists?
    D. What problems do you see in the behavior of the chief operator?
    E. If you were the administrator, what would you do about this set of events?

3. LAUNDRY INCIDENT

Shortly after his graduation with a technical degree from a junior college, Mr. James Jones accepted a position with the 150-bed Jefferson Memorial Hospital, located in a small town in one of the Eastern States.

He stated that, "It was a fine opportunity for someone like myself who was only 23 years old. I was the assistant to Mr. Smith, who was manager of the hospital's laundry. I was anxious to learn the laundry business and since I was living alone it was not long before I literally lived in the laundry. We had many technical problems. The work was intensely interesting and my boss was a very fine man.

"The seven laundry workers were a closely knit group and in the main they were older men. Several had spent a lifetime in the laundry. Many of them were related. They felt that they knew the laundry business from A to Z and they were inclined to 'pooh-pooh' the value of a technical education. The manager had mentioned to me when we discussed the duties and responsibilities of the position that no graduate of a technical institute had ever been employed in the hospital's laundry. He added, 'You will find that the men stick pretty well together. Most of them have been working together for more than ten years which is rather unusual in a laundry, so it may take you some time to get accepted. But, on the whole, you will find them a fine group of men.'

"At first, the men eyed me coldly as I went around and got acquainted. Also, I noticed that they would clam up as I approached. A bit later, I became aware of cat-calls when I walked down the main aisle of the laundry. I chose to ignore these evidences of hostility because I considered them silly and childish. I believed that if I continued to ignore these antics the men would eventually stop, come to their senses and realize the ridiculousness of their behavior.

"One Saturday, about a month after I had started, I was down in the Sorting Room. As I entered it I observed a worker who was busy cleaning the floor with a hose from which flowed water at pretty good pressure. It was customary to 'hose down' the Sorting Room every so often. I was busy near one of the linen carts when, all of a sudden, I was nearly knocked down by the force of a stream of water. The worker had deliberately turned the hose on me. I knew that he had intended to hit me by the casual way in which he swung around as though he had never seen what he had done."

    A. Why was Mr. Jones "hosed down"?
    B. Did Jones' behavior contribute to the event?
    C. What did Smith do and what should he have done when Mr. Jones first started his employment?
    D. If you were Mr. Jones, how would you have conducted yourself during your first several weeks of employment?
    E. What should be done with the employee who "hosed down" Mr. Jones?

This Chapter Contains:

- Introduction
- The Hospital as a Health Care Organization
  The Hospital Defined
  Functions of the Hospital
- Organizational Problems Faced by the Hospital
  Organizational Coordination
  Managing Organizational Conflict
  Innovative Organizational Change
  Bringing about Organizational Change
- Hospital Organization
- Organizational Triad
  Governing Body
  Administrator
  Medical Staff
  Hospital–Medical Staff Relations
- Contingency Theory and the Hospital
- The Long-Term-Care Facility
- Summary
- Discussion Questions
- Incidents

Chapter 8

THE STRUCTURE OF HEALTH CARE ORGANIZATIONS

"One of the most critical concerns of modern society is how to create and maintain organizations which are rational and adaptive (so as to minimize unpredictability of behavior and uncertainty of outcomes while taking full advantage of the benefits of an advanced technology), economically efficient, and satisfying to their members, clients, and communities."

(Basil S. Georgopoulos)[1]

INTRODUCTION

In his comments on health care organizations (quoted above), Basil Georgopoulos makes several major points. First, the purpose of these organizations is to efficiently provide health care. Second, in order to accomplish that purpose they must (a) be rationally structured and (b) be able to adapt to both internal and external changes. These are the tasks of the health care manager. The question is, "How does he create and maintain such organizations in order to accomplish these tasks?" In this chapter we will endeavor to answer that question. The wide range of health care organizations existing in the delivery system were presented in Chapter 1. In the preceding chapter, Organizational Concepts, classical and modern organization theories were presented. In this chapter, we will devote our attention to the application of those theories to health care organizations.

In view of the wide range of organizations in the health care delivery system, it will not be possible to describe them all in detail. The reader may find the excellent treatment of this subject in Neuhauser and Wilson, *Health Services in the United States* (published by Ballinger Publishing Company of Cambridge, Massachusetts in 1974), to be of assistance in gaining a better understanding of the complexities of the various components of the health delivery system.

Two of the basic health delivery organizations will be described—the hospital and the long-term-care facility. Many of the principles and concepts that will be presented here apply to all types of health organizations regardless of their size or purpose. To illustrate this point, consider the similarities in the or-

---

[1]Basil S. Georgopoulos, *Organization Research on Health Institutions.* Ann Arbor, Michigan: Institute for Social Research, 1972, p. 3.

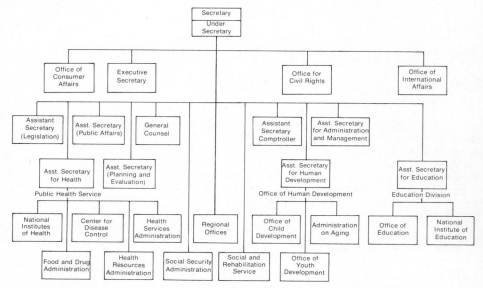

Figure 8-1 The U. S. Department of Health, Education, and Welfare. (Source: Office of the Federal Registrar, as of January, 1975.)

ganization charts of the U. S. Department of Health, Education, and Welfare, the Illinois State Department of Public Health, and the Advisory Council on Health and Social Services Planning of the Atlanta Regional Commission (the official planning agency for all state and federal programs carried out in the seven county Metropolitan Atlanta region) which are presented in Figures 8-1, 8-2, and 8-3.

HEW, created in 1953, has undergone almost constant reorganization since its inception. Similarly, state departments of health and local health planning and delivery organizations have a history of evolutionary organizational

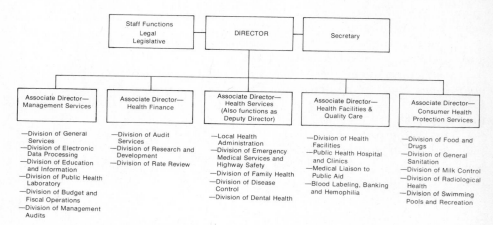

Figure 8-2 State Department of Public Health, Illinois. (Source: Illinois Department of Public Health, as of January, 1975.)

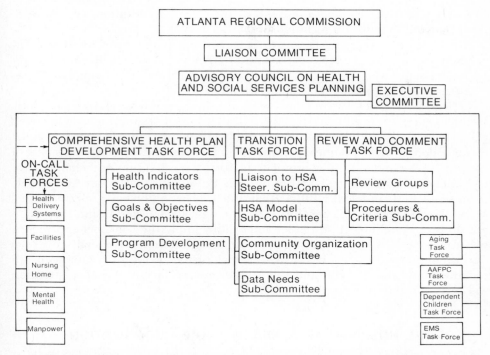

Figure 8–3 Advisory Council on Health and Social Services Planning, Atlanta Regional Commission. (Source: Atlanta Regional Commission, as of January, 1975).

changes. The passage of the 1974 National Health Planning and Resources Development Act (PL 93–641) ensures that the structure of federal, state, and local health agencies will continue to change in the years ahead.

The purpose of PL 93–641 is stated in its preamble: "to facilitate the development of recommendations for a national health planning policy, to augment areawide and state planning for health services, manpower, and facilities, and to authorize financial assistance for the development of resources to further that policy." Public Law 93–641 is the most important health legislation since the enactment of the Medicare and Medicaid programs in the mid 1960's. Some view it as a forerunner of national health insurance.[2] Among its provisions are the following:[3]

1. Local health system agencies (HSA's), state health planning and development agencies (SHPDA's), and statewide health coordinating councils (SHCC's) are to be created and will be responsible for planning and resource development at their respective levels.
2. Local health planning is emphasized and the agencies have review authority for federal funds and are to conduct periodic reviews of the appropriateness

---

[2]William Skerry, "PL 93-641: Beyond planning toward control." *Hospital Progress*, 57:10, March, 1976.
[3]Eugene J. Rubel, "Implementing the National Health Planning and Resources Development Act of 1974." *Public Health Reports*, 91:3, January–February, 1976.

of existing organizational providers in their area. In addition, certificate of need requirements are included in the Act.

3. Furthermore, the agencies are to have consumer and provider represent- ation and are charged to incorporate all segments of the health care delivery system (consumers, providers, third-party payers, and educational and gov- ernmental institutions) into their planning.

Clearly, PL 93–641 mandates significant changes in federal, state, and local health agencies. It is quite likely, however, that health organizations at all levels will remain basically bureaucratic pyramids. They are and will continue to be divided along functional lines. They have and will continue to have set spans of control. There are and will continue to be formal mechanisms and channels for communication and control, and so on. The differences that exist result largely from scope and complexity rather than the application of basic organizational principles and concepts. Therefore, after we describe selected health care orga- nizations in detail here, the reader can readily apply the concepts and princi- ples to all types of health care agencies and organizations. We shall now turn our attention to the organizational structure of the two most common health care facilities—the hospital and the long-term-care facility. Primary attention will be given to the former.

THE HOSPITAL AS A HEALTH CARE ORGANIZATION

THE HOSPITAL DEFINED

One of the important steps to take when analyzing something is to define what is being analyzed. The problem with defining an institution such as the hospital is the existence of a number of different definitions. To the patient it is a place to receive medical care; to the physician it may be a workshop in which he can practice his profession; to the medical or nursing student it may seem to be an educational institution. Perhaps most useful would be to define the hospi- tal as a *health team*. Such a definition emphasizes the human interrelationships in the organization. This does not mean that the hospital does not need a phys- ical plant, equipment, and supplies in order to function. Nor does it explain the complex social, political, and economic relationships that the hospital has with the external environment. From this definition it follows that the hospital is largely a human endeavor. Consequently, a brief description of those who are a part of this health team is presented here.

A logical beginning point for our description is to consider the *community to be served* as members of the team. The community to be served is composed of those people who may at some time use the hospital's facilities. The hospital is directed by a *governing board* who should be considered members of the health team. In addition, there are over three million hospital workers (a very diverse group) who cover the range from unskilled and semi-skilled labor to highly trained professionals. Usually, there are two to three such employees for each hospital bed. A. F. Wesson, in his study of one hospital, identified 23 different occupations represented in a single hospital ward.[4] All these *employees* must be

---

[4]A. F. Wesson, "The social structure of a modern hospital." Ph.D. dissertation, Yale University, 1951.

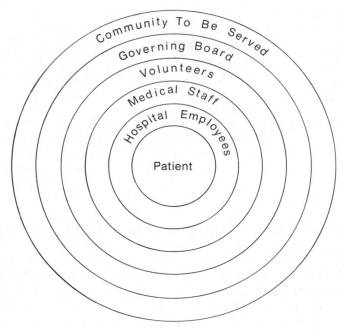

Figure 8–4. The hospital as a health team.

considered members of the health team. The *medical staff*, consisting of those physicians and dentists who use the hospital's facilities, are members of the health team as well. This nation's hospitals receive a tremendous amount of time and energy from *auxiliaries and volunteers*. They, too, must be considered members of this team. Finally, it is necessary to think of the *patient* as a member of this team. After all, it is the patient who is the focal point of the activities that are the work of the hospital. This is indicated in Figure 8–4.

FUNCTIONS OF THE HOSPITAL

Historically, the hospital has been a place for the care of the sick and dependent, usually the poor. Today, however, a broader view of the hospital allows for its use as a center for all technical services required by both the bed-bound and ambulatory patient; as a place for basic and post-graduate training of personnel; as a laboratory for medical and administrative research; and as a center for preventive services and health promotion among the general population. Roemer and Friedman have said that the modern hospital has a full range of important functions:

First, there are diagnostic and treatment services to inpatients. Within this broad function are many subdivisions of medical, surgical, obstetrical, pediatric, and other special forms of care. Psychiatric service and rehabilitation may be included. Involved in all of these inpatient services are various modalities, including nursing, dietetics, pharmaceutical skills, laboratory and x-ray services, and varying refinements of diagnosis and therapy. Second, there are services to outpatients, with an equally wide range of specialties and technical modalities. A third hospital function concerns professional and technical education, for many classes of health personnel must work in hospitals and thereby receive training. A fourth function is medical research, since the accumulation of patients in hospitals provides the basis for scientific investigation into the causes, diagnosis, and treatment of diseases. A fifth function concerns prevention of diseases or health promotion in the surrounding population; there are many ways that hospitals, as centers for technical skill, can offer services to people before they are sick or can protect patients from the hazards of disease beyond that for which they have come to the hospital.[5]

Hospitals vary primarily in the amount of emphasis they give to each of these functions. The difference will depend largely upon the basic objectives of the particular hospital. For example, a large medical center will usually emphasize education and research to a much greater extent than a small general hospital will.

ORGANIZATIONAL PROBLEMS FACED BY THE HOSPITAL

The hospital is a complex organization with various objectives and diverse participants. Thus, it has a number of organizational problems which are of considerable importance to the efficient and effective functioning of the organization. The following sections deal with three of these organizational problems: (1) coordination; (2) managing conflict; and (3) innovation.

ORGANIZATIONAL COORDINATION

In terms of differentiation of activities and specialization of labor, hospitals are among the most complex organizations in modern society. They are characterized by a detailed division of labor into a number of technical skills. The work of the institution is so specialized and performed by such a variety of workers that very significant coordination problems often arise.[6]

In Chapter 7, the subject of coordination was presented in depth. It was viewed as a means of synchronizing and pulling together different activities. As a result, the sum of work effort produces a meaningful and effective whole. Furthermore, the thinking of various writers on how to attain coordination was described. Included were such methods as hierarchy, administrative system, and voluntary coordination.

Although the coordination of diverse groups and activities is of critical importance in the modern hospital, it is not the only organizational problem. Another critically important problem, and one that is closely related to coordination in many ways, is organizational conflict.

MANAGING ORGANIZATIONAL CONFLICT

In addition to the problem of organizational coordination, the administration of a hospital must deal with a second major problem: managing organiza-

---

[5] Milton I. Roemer and J. W. Friedman, *Doctors In Hospitals*. Baltimore: The Johns Hopkins Press, 1971, pp. 1–2. Reprinted by permission of the publisher.

[6] Basil S. Georgopoulos and Floyd C. Mann, *The Community General Hospital*. New York: The Macmillan Company, 1962, pp. 270–271.

tional conflict. The tremendously complex structure of the hospital suggests that the institution is likely to have a fairly high level of conflict among the various participants. (In broad terms, conflict may be defined as all kinds of opposition or antagonistic interaction.) As Schultz and Johnson suggest,

> Evidence of conflict in hospitals is readily apparent. Nurse and nonprofessional hospital employee strikes receive wide publicity. Periodically, administrator-medical staff conflicts break into public view. Furthermore, hospital-client conflicts seem to be increasing as consumers of hospital service level charges of inefficiency and inattention to consumer expectations.[7]

Attitudes about the role of organizational conflict are diverse and, with the passage of time, are undergoing a transition. Early management theorists had a straightforward attitude. During the period prior to the mid 1940's, most management thinkers (with the notable exception of Mary Parker Follett) saw all conflict as destructive; management's role was to rid the organization of conflict.

This traditional approach was succeeded by the behavioral view, still the most prevalent view about managing conflict in modern organizations. Essentially, this approach reflects an *acceptance* of conflict as a fact of organization life. Conflict is unquestionably a part of the fabric of an organization as complex as the modern hospital. Disagreements over organization objectives can be found among administrators, trustees, physicians, nurses, and other participants. Departments and individuals compete for recognition, prestige, and power. Empires are often built at the expense of some other part of the organization.

The behavioralists seek to rationalize conflict. For example, Katz has said, "... it should be added that we are not assuming that all conflict is bad and that the only objective toward which we should work is the resolution of conflict. Group conflict has positive social functions...."[8]

The newest approach to conflict, which is not taken by very many managers, is a more positive one called the "interactionist philosophy" by Stephen P. Robbins.[9] He suggests that the interactionists' philosophy differs from the behavioral viewpoint since it (1) recognizes the absolute necessity of conflict, (2) explicitly encourages opposition, (3) defines conflict management to include stimulation as well as resolution methods, and (4) considers the management of conflict as a major responsibility of all administrators.[10]

The interactionists accept, and sometimes encourage, conflict by recognizing that not only may the level of conflict be too high and require reduction, but it may also be too low and need increased intensity. The interactionists believe organizations that do not stimulate conflict increase the probability of

---

[7]Rockwell Schulz and Alton C. Johnson, "Conflict in hospitals." *Hospital Administration*, *16*:36, Summer, 1971.

[8]Daniel Katz, "Approaches to managing conflict." In *Power and Conflict in Organizations*, Robert L. Kahn and Elise Boulding (eds.), New York: Foundation on Human Behavior, Basic Books, Inc., 1964, Chapter 9.

[9]Stephen P. Robbins, *Managing Organizational Conflict*. Englewood Cliffs, N. J.: Prentice-Hall, Inc., 1974, p. 13.

[10]*Ibid.* pp. 13–14.

stagnant thinking, inadequate decisions, and, in extreme cases, organizational demise.

The problem with the existence of conflict in hospitals and other types of health care organizations is that it can affect the quality of patient care. Georgopoulos and Mann, for instance, have found a higher quality of care in hospitals where physicians and nurses have a greater understanding of each other's work, problems, and needs.[11] Results from studies done in mental hospitals show that patients are adversely affected by staff conflict.[12]

The administration's task is to balance the level of conflict so that the positive benefits (chiefly, innovative organizational change, which is discussed next) can be achieved without disrupting the quality of patient care. As one might expect, this is extremely difficult.

INNOVATIVE ORGANIZATIONAL CHANGE

The American hospital, and to a somewhat lesser extent the Canadian hospital, is under unprecedented pressure to change both its goals and its methods of operation. These pressures stem from consumers and their advocates, government, leaders in the medical establishment, and the public's growing awareness that as an institution the hospital is not as efficient as it should be. The force of these pressures is exacerbated by the fact that the continuing progress being made in medical science and technology is outstripping the system for delivering health services. It is clear to the knowledgeable observer that the institutional role of the hospital is being redefined.

There are many types of changes that can occur within organizations. A very important way to differentiate between these changes is to see whether the change is imposed on the organization (a government regulation, for example) or whether the change is made without direct, coercive, external pressure. Managers in health care organizations are quite familiar with imposed change. They face a large and growing barrage of new regulations which require that they change one aspect or another of their operations. In this discussion, however, we are more concerned with innovation than with imposed change. The open system view of organizations which was presented in Chapter 7 suggests that hospitals interact with, react to, and influence their environments. The hospital that only reacts to its environment (where changes are literally forced by external pressures) cannot be thought of as an innovative organization. To be innovative, conscious planning and decision-making are required before the event which forces change occurs.

If one observes a number of organizational changes in hospitals, a variety of objectives seem to be present. These objectives might be such things as higher performance, greater motivation, reduced turnover, or any one of an almost limitless number of possibilities. However, in hospitals, organizational changes usually fit into one of two broader objectives: (1) changes in the hospital's level of *adaptation* to its environment, or (2) changes in the internal *behavior*

---

[11]Georgopoulos and Mann, op. cit. p. 400.

[12]Alfred H. Stanton and Morris S. Schwartz, *The Mental Hospital.* New York: Basic Books, Inc., 1954, pp. 342–365.

patterns of participants. Hospitals are constantly struggling to adapt themselves to their external environment. The administrator cannot control the hospital's environment; therefore, he must introduce organizational changes which will allow the hospital to deal with the challenges imposed from outside the organization as a result of consumer demands, government regulation, medical and scientific advances, planning agencies, third-party payers and so forth. For the most part, hospitals make organizational changes in response to these environmental pressures. In some cases, however, changes are made without outside pressure or in anticipation of future pressures. This innovative behavior characterizes hospitals that lead their industry instead of follow it. It can be said that such hospitals are attempting to change their environments as well as themselves.

Obviously, if a hospital's level of adaptation is to be improved, the behavior patterns of a number of employees must be modified in terms of their relationships to each other and to their jobs. Thus, the second basic objective of organizational change is to alter the behavior patterns of organization participants.

BRINGING ABOUT ORGANIZATIONAL CHANGE

Change, whether it represents an innovation or is merely imposed by pressures external to the organization, can be introduced by a number of approaches. A useful way to divide the various approaches is to look at those that emphasize *what* is to be changed and those that emphasize the process of *how* change is introduced.

One of the most widely used delineations of the *what* approaches is made by Harold J. Leavitt.[13] He describes three approaches to organizational change: structure, technology, and people. Structural approaches to the introduction of change include utilization of the organization chart, budgeting methods, and rules and regulations. Technological approaches stress changes introduced by new physical layouts, job descriptions, work standards, or new work methods. People approaches stress alterations in attitudes, motivation, and behavioral skills. Changes of this type are made through training programs, selection procedures, and performance appraisal programs.

A good illustration of *how* approaches is contained in Larry E. Greiner's work, which identifies seven approaches most frequently used by managers.[14]

I. Unilateral Power
   A. *The Decree Approach.* A "one-way" announcement originates with a person of high formal authority and is passed on to those in lower positions.
   B. *The Replacement Approach.* Individuals in one or more key organization positions are replaced. The basic assumption is that organizational changes are a function of a key man's ability.

---

[13]Harold J. Leavitt, "Applied organization change in industry: Structural, technological, and human approaches." In *New Perspectives in Organization Research*, W. W. Cooper, H. J. Leavitt, and M. W. Shelly, III (eds.), New York: John Wiley and Sons, Inc., 1964, pp. 55–71.

[14]Larry E. Greiner, "Patterns of organization change." *Harvard Business Review, 45*:119, May–June, 1967.

C. *The Structural Approach.* Instead of issuing a decree or injecting new blood into work relationships, management changes the required relationships of subordinates working in the situation. When the structure of organization relationships is changed, behavior is also affected.

II. Shared Power

A. *The Group Decision Approach.* Group members participate in selecting from several alternative solutions specified in advance by superiors. This approach involves neither problem identification nor problem solving, but emphasizes group agreement to a particular course of action.

B. *The Group Problem Solving Approach.* Problem identification and problem solving through group discussion offer the group a wide latitude, not only in choosing the problems to be discussed but also in developing solutions to these problems.

III. Delegated Power

A. *The Data Discussion Approach.* Presentation and feedback of relevant data to the client system is accomplished either by a change catalyst or by change agents within the hospital. Members of the organization are encouraged to develop their own analyses of the data, presented in the form of case materials, survey findings, or data reports.

B. *The Sensitivity Training Approach.* Managers are trained in small discussion groups to be more sensitive to the underlying processes of individual and group behavior. It is assumed that changes in work patterns and relationships follow changes in relationships. The sensitivity approach focuses upon personal relationships first, then on improving work performance.

It should be noted that few changes can be introduced successfully by using only one of these approaches. A balanced approach carefully combining several elements is necessary. For example, an administrator may wish to encourage a more effective communication network among department heads. To accomplish this change, he will need to take a people approach and provide the department heads with a training program in communication skills. However, the full implementation of this change will also require structural changes encouraging more open communication among department heads.

Organizational change is a very complex process. The manager concerned with introducing, managing, and responding to organizational change needs a conceptual framework of the process. Recent research indicates that in order to see the process of change clearly and objectively it is necessary to think of organizational change as an *evolving series of stages*. It does not occur all at once. Instead, one phase sets the conditions necessary for moving into subsequent stages. Kurt Lewin identified three phases of change—unfreezing, changing, and refreezing.[15] The "unfreezing" stage is the first step necessary in stimulat-

---

[15]Kurt Lewin, "Group decision and social change." In *Readings in Social Psychology*, E. E. Maccoloy, T. M. Newcomb, and E. L. Hartley (eds.), New York: Holt, Rinehart, and Winston, Inc., 1958, pp. 197–211 (particularly pp. 210–211).

ing people to recognize the need for change. The "changing" stage involves the introduction and application of the change. Finally, the "refreezing" stage provides the necessary reinforcement to make certain that new behavior patterns are adopted on a permanent basis.

Lewin's basic model has stimulated intensive research into the various phases of change and into the relationships among them. Modern organization research has identified two major processes which seem to underlie all stages of organizational change. One is a "micro" process of social and personal learning in which managers unlearn old patterns of behavior and adopt new ones. The other is a "macro" process involving the question of power and its distribution within an organization. An important issue now before students of organizational change is that of "power equalization" versus "power expansion."[16] In essence, power equalization implies that power is a fixed quantity which requires that some managers gain and others lose power in an organizational change. Conversely, power expansion suggests that it is possible for all managers to increase their power. There is no consensus on the role of power in change, although recent research seems to support the belief that the power expansion theory most nearly reflects what actually occurs in an organizational change.[17]

We can now turn our attention to how the hospital organizes itself in order to carry out its functions and solve the problems outlined above (along with others such as resource allocation and goal attainment).

HOSPITAL ORGANIZATION

Max Weber has suggested that large-scale organizations need some way of dealing with the idiosyncrasies of individuals in the organization so that they do not interfere with the organization's ability to accomplish a specific task.[18] One way of doing this is to set up a bureaucracy in which each person has a place and a set of tasks. The typical bureaucratic structure is a pyramid (see Fig. 8–5). This structure is based on a chain of command through which authority and responsibility are delegated logically.[19]

---

[16]For example, see Arnold Tannenbaum, *Control in Organizations.* New York: McGraw-Hill Book Company, 1968 (especially chapter 21).

[17]Greiner, op. cit. pp. 125–126.

[18]Max Weber, *The Theory of Social and Economic Organizations.* Translated by A. M. Henderson and Talcott Parsons. New York: The Free Press, 1947, pp. 151–157.

[19]George R. Wren, "Can business benefit from new organizational patterns?" *The Atlanta Economic Review,* 21:14, January, 1971.

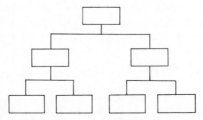

Figure 8–5   Typical bureaucratic pyramid.

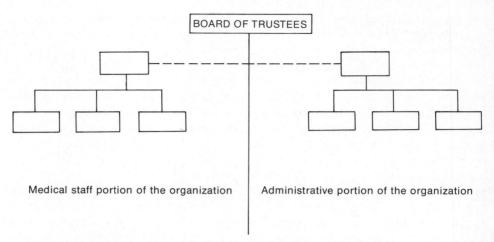

Medical staff portion of the organization | Administrative portion of the organization

Figure 8–6 Dual pyramid of the typical hospital.

The organizational structure of the typical community general hospital differs substantially from the bureaucratic model of many other large-scale organizations. This difference is a result of the unusual relationship that exists between the formal authority of position represented by the administrative hierarchy and the authority of knowledge possessed by the medical professionals in the hospital. The hospital would be much less complicated if it fit the general organizational pyramid. This, however, is not the case. In the typical community hospital, the medical staff does not fit into the pyramid, as those people who work for the hospital (i.e., have their salaries paid by the hospital) do. (The medical staff does fit into the basic bureaucratic pyramid in hospitals such as those of the Veterans Administration.) The medical staff consists of those physicians and dentists who have been authorized by the governing board to admit and attend patients in the hospital. Generally they are paid by their patients, not by the hospital. That they do not fit into the pyramid of the hospital is not an exclusion since most physicians relish the independent nature of this relationship. As a result, the organizational pattern is literally a dual pyramid with the administration hierarchy and the medical staff hierarchy existing side by side (see Fig. 8–6).

Harvey L. Smith has described this pattern as the basic duality of hospitals.[20] He maintains that two lines of authority—lay and professional—exist within the hospital. One line of authority is that hierarchy which extends from the trustees through the administrator and the department heads to the various employees of the hospital. The second is composed of the various professional persons in the organization, especially the physicians. Although the physician may have little formal authority in the organization, his actual authority is very great indeed.[21]

---

[20] Harvey L. Smith, "Two lines of authority–the hospital's dilemma." In *Patients, Physicians, and Illness*, E. Gartly Jaco (ed.), New York: Free Press, Inc., 1958, pp. 468–478.
[21] *Ibid.* p. 59.

Alan D. Bauerschmidt has stated:

> The physician and his agents including the nurses and other ward personnel have the capability to exert power throughout the hospital structure. Some areas appear to be reserved for administrative rule, others are reserved for professional rule, while still other areas of the organization are best described as hybrids. It is in this last area that the many conflicts of jurisdiction arise.[22]

The complexity of this pattern becomes evident when one considers that although people in the organization have just one immediate superior (a highly desirable attribute of bureaucratic organizations), employees such as nurses take orders from their own head nurse, who is a member of the administrative hierarchy, as well as from the medical chief of their respective service, and individual physicians on the medical staff in regard to individual patients. For these orders to be contradictory is not unheard of, since each group of participants interprets the means for attaining objectives in terms of its own value systems and requirements.

The hospital is a very complex social system with substantial conflict among the participants—the patients, physicians, trustees, administrative staff, and paramedical personnel. The diversity of the institutional organization creates major problems. The governing board has the legal authority over, and responsibility for, the institution. The medical staff possesses the technical knowledge to make the decisions regarding questions of patient care and treatment. The administrative staff is responsible for the day-to-day operation of the hospital. These three elements, sometimes referred to as the organizational *triad*, share the same basic objectives. However, they interpret the means for meeting these objectives in terms of their own values and personalities. These values and personalities, unfortunately, are not the same for each element of the triad. This makes the hospital perhaps the most complex institution in American society.

Figure 8–7 represents a "typical" organizational pattern for a medium-sized voluntary hospital. Only the most common departments are shown here. This figure provides us with the opportunity to view the organizational complexity of the typical hospital. The administrative portion of the organization, including the administration, nursing division, professional services, support services, and the controller, is shown with the medical staff portion of the organization. The reader can see clearly the "dual pyramid" aspect of hospital organization. The Board of Trustees makes up the third component of the organizational triad of the hospital.

The triad (governing body, administrator, and medical staff) will be described in some detail in the following section. Although it was written more than a decade ago, the reader will find Paul J. Gordon's classic article on the top management triangle in hospitals very informative and interesting. In it, Gordon suggests that the relationships within the organizational triad

> ...stem from the power relationships, the control relationships, and the alternatives available to each group in what can here best be seen as a negotiated rela-

---

[22] Alan D. Bauerschmidt, "The anomalies of hospital organization: The implications for management." Ph.D. dissertation, University of Florida, 1968, pp. 142–143.

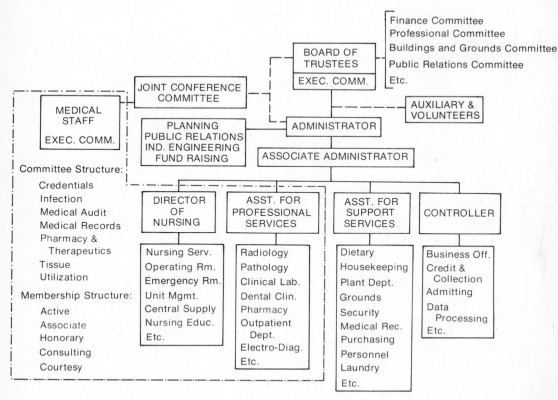

Figure 8–7 Organization chart of a medium-sized, voluntary general hospital. (Source: A Primer for Hospital Trustees. Washington, D.C., United States Chamber of Commerce, 1974. Used by permission.)

tionship and one constantly subject to renegotiation. They stem out of the alternative means of leverage and the amount of power behind that leverage that is available to each party involved in the negotiation. . . . Stated baldly, on a day-to-day basis, the voluntary hospital corporation and its agents have no legal or organizational means of controlling the service that the hospital has been set up to render.[23]

ORGANIZATIONAL TRIAD

GOVERNING BODY

Hospitals derive their legal status from state-granted charters or from their parent body. The powers to maintain and operate a hospital that are a result of its legal status are vested in and exercised by the governing body, a group of people authorized by law to conduct, maintain, and operate the hospital. The governing body may be called Board of Trustees, Board of Directors, Board of

---

[23]Paul J. Gordon, "The top management triangle in voluntary hospitals. I and II." *Journal of the Academy of Management*, 4:205, December, 1961; 5:66, April, 1962. This quote is from 1962, p. 72. This material may also be found in *Hospital Administration*, 9:46, Spring, 1964.

Governors, Board of Councilors, Commissioners, or some comparable designation.

Legally and morally, the governing board has the ultimate responsibility and authority for operation of the hospital. McGibony has described their function as follows:

1. The governing authority determines policies with relation to community needs;
2. maintains proper professional standards through direct legal responsibility for the exercise of due care in the appointment and review of activities of the medical staff;
3. coordinates the clinically professional interests of the hospital with the administrative, financial, and community needs;
4. provides adequate financing and control of expenses;
5. keeps fully informed on hospital matters and abreast of the hospital literature.
6. selects an administrator for the hospital, delegates to him responsibility with corresponding authority and lets him function without undue interference.[24]

The American Hospital Association (AHA) describes the role of the governing body (board) as follows:

The governing board must define goals and objectives to meet community health care needs and establish policy to meet those goals and objectives. In addition, the board must accept the moral and legal responsibility for the quality of services provided by the health care institution and for ensuring quality of service provided by others within the institution. The assumption of these responsibilities by the governing board constitutes "acts of governance."[25]

The governing board accomplishes its work primarily through a committee structure. Committees vary from hospital to hospital but normally there will be the following, as noted by the AHA:

1. The Executive Committee, composed of the officers of the board and the chairmen of other standing committees, is empowered by the bylaws to assume the authority and responsibility of the governing body in the interim between meetings, especially in emergency situations. It reviews and evaluates all other committee reports before action is taken by the whole board.
2. The Professional Committee, made up of selected board members, oversees professional care in the hospital. Working closely with the medical staff and administration, this committee establishes and reviews policies that ensure the highest quality of patient care possible. An important function of this committee is to recommend appointments to the medical staff. They cooperate closely with the credentials committee of the medical staff in this regard.
3. The Finance Committee, a very important committee, is responsible for reviewing such issues as budgets, financial statements, appointments of hospital auditors, and related financial matters, and for offering their recommendations to the whole board.

---

[24]John R. McGibony, *Principles of Hospital Administration*, 2nd ed. New York: G. P. Putnam's Sons, 1969, p. 148.

[25]American Hospital Association, "Governance of health institutions." Developed by the AHA, Chicago, Illinois, 1974.

4. The Personnel Committee evaluates and recommends policies in the area of the hospital's relationship to its employees.
5. The Joint Conference Committee, made up of equal numbers of board members and members of the medical staff, provides liaison between the governing board and physicians in order to promote mutual understanding and to provide a forum for the exchange of information and ideas. The administrator usually sits in as an *ex officio* member. This committee often represents one of the best mechanisms available in the hospital for consideration of issues having both clinical and administrative aspects.[26]

There may be other standing committees of the board (such as Public Relations, and Building and Grounds) and, in addition, there may be special or *ad hoc* committees appointed at various times to meet specific needs such as a fund raising program or searching for a new administrator.

ADMINISTRATOR

The administrator or hospital director (sometimes called the president when the hospital is organized along the lines of the corporate model) is the chief executive of the hospital. His or her basic function is to manage the inputs of the organization (manpower, material, technology, information, and capital) in order to achieve the desired outputs established for the hospital. The administrator's staff may include assistants to whom he or she delegates authority. However, the burden of designing, changing, and operating an effective organizational structure to meet the hospital's objectives falls mainly on the administrator's shoulders.

The way in which administrators spend their time varies depending on the type of hospital and its size, among other things, but a general description of the percentage of time they allocate to various activities is contained in Table 8–1.

---

[26] Adapted with permission from, "Governance of health care institutions." Developed by the American Hospital Association, Chicago, Illinois, 1974.

Table 8–1 Percentage of Administrator's Time Spent on Various Activities

ACTIVITY	TEACHING HOSPITALS	ALL GENERAL	400 BEDS OR MORE	1–99 BEDS
Planning	25.8	25.5	31.2	23.3
Directing and coordinating	4.5	24.6	20.7	23.6
Controlling	16.5	11.4	8.6	10.9
Organizing	12.9	3.9	3.1	4.1
Operating*	(negligible)	1.9	0.3	8.0
Extramural	36.9	20.9	22.7	16.2
Personal	3.4	11.8	13.5	13.9

*As used here, Operating means routine paper work such as filling out reports and signing papers. The implication is that in larger hospitals, these tasks are delegated to subordinates.

(Source: The figures for teaching hospitals come from E. J. Connors and J. C. Hutts, "How administrators spend their day." *Hospitals,* 45:45, February 16, 1967. The figures for all general hospitals and those for 400 beds or more and 1–99 beds are from R. T. Murray et al., "How administrators spend their time: a research report." *Hospital Progress,* 49:49, September, 1968.)

In essence, the function of the administrator is to *manage* the hospital. We have defined management as an interactive set of social/technical processes occurring within a formal organizational setting with the purpose of accomplishing predetermined objectives through the utilization of human and physical resources. Inherent in this definition are four specific criteria which define the role of the hospital administrator. The first of these is the creation of and the adherence to a set of objectives. Activity must be directed toward some end — the objectives of the hospital.

Second, there must be input resources. Economic resources are by definition scarce. As a result, the hospital administrator is responsible for their allocation. The administrator is concerned with attaining goals (effectiveness) with the best allocation of the scarce resources (efficiency).

A third criterion which helps to define the role of the hospital administrator is that there must be other people in the organization. It is with people and through people that hospital administrators perform their work.

Finally, the organizational necessity to change with time helps to define his role. Kovner has said: "The administrator, because of his training, position, and responsibilities, is for many hospitals the person most qualified and most likely to act as change agent."[27]

It should be obvious to the reader that the hospital administrator faces one of the most demanding management jobs in modern society. The training for this complex administrative function is provided by a number of major universities in the United States and Canada which offer graduate degrees in health and hospital administration. These programs consist of one to two years of full-time academic study and may include an administrative residency of up to one year in a hospital or other health-related organization under the preceptorship of an administrator. Most programs are members of the American Association of University Programs in Health Administration located in Washington, D.C.

The basic curriculum in these graduate programs covers three principal areas. The first is the study of administrative theory, concepts, and skills. Health administration encompasses organization theory, financial management, economic systems, quantitative skills, human relations, behavioral science, and law. The second area is the study of the elements of health services and medical care, encompassing environmental and personal health services, with special regard for their major components, their stable and unstable characteristics and interrelationships (including planning), the patterns of their organization, the principles of their administration, and their basic economics. Third is the study of hospital functions, organization, and management, which involves the role of the hospital in the delivery of health services, research and education, history of hospitals, financing, planning of services and facilities, forms of organization and operation, evaluation of services, staffing, and legal aspects.

[27]Anthony R. Kovner, "The hospital administrator and organizational effectiveness." *In:* Basil S. Georgopoulos, ed. *Organization Research on Health Institutions,* Ann Arbor, Michigan: Institute for Social Research of the University of Michigan, 1972, p. 373.

MEDICAL STAFF

The third component of the organizational triad is the medical staff. By definition, the medical staff of a hospital is the organized group of physicians and dentists who have been authorized by the governing board to attend patients and participate in related duties, functions, and programs of the institution.

The key word in this definition is *organized*. The Joint Commission on Accreditation of Hospitals, (J.C.A.H.), which sets the criteria by which hospitals are accredited, states as a basic principle of hospital organization that

> There shall be an organized medical staff that has the overall responsibility for the quality of all medical care provided to patients, and for the ethical conduct and professional practices of its members as well as for accounting therefore to the governing body.[28]

The variation among hospitals in terms of size and organizational complexity makes it impossible for the J.C.A.H. to set forth specific instructions on how the medical staff is to be organized. However, the medical staff is generally classified into the following categories:

1. Active staff deliver most of the medical services within the hospital and perform all significant organizational and administrative duties pertaining to the medical staff. Active staff members may vote and hold office.
2. Associate staff are members who are being considered for advancement to the active medical staff. They may not vote and, in most cases, may not hold office on the medical staff. However, they can admit their patients to the hospital.
3. Consulting staff, (when this category exists) are top medical practitioners who are not members of another category of the medical staff but who wish to make their services available as consultants to contribute to improved patient care. Consulting staff neither vote nor hold office.
4. Courtesy staff are given the privilege to admit an occasional patient to the hospital. They neither vote nor hold office.
5. Honorary staff are former members honored with emeritus positions or other outstanding practitioners whom the medical staff desires to honor.

Medical Staff Officers.   The officers of the medical staff are usually the president, vice-president or president-elect, secretary-treasurer, and immediate past-president. The title chief of staff is often used in lieu of that of president. This person is the key to the medical staff organization. According to the J.C.A.H., his duties include the following:

> • Serving as the presiding officer at medical staff meetings;
> • Serving as the chairman of the medical staff executive committee and as an ex officio member of all medical staff committees;
> • Appointing medical staff committee members (except when membership is specified in the medical staff bylaws);
> • Enforcing medical staff bylaws, rules and regulations;

---

[28]Joint Commission on Accreditation of Hospitals, *Accreditation Manual for Hospitals, 1970.* Chicago: JCAH, 1971, p. 33.

- Serving as an ex officio member of the governing body, where organizationally permitted;
- Presenting, if chairman of the executive committee, the views, policies, needs and grievances of the medical staff to the chief executive officer and the governing body;
- Serving, if chairman of the executive committee, as the responsible representative of the medical staff to receive and interpret policies from the governing body, and to report on and interpret to the governing body the performance and maintenance of the medical staff's responsibility for providing good medical care; and
- Acting as medical staff spokesman for the staff's external professional and public relations.[29]

Committees of the Medical Staff.   Because of the diverse responsibilities of the medical staff, a committee structure is necessary to ensure adequate attention to the various areas. Once again, size and organizational complexity will dictate the extent of the committee structure but the committees which will usually be found to be desirable are the five that follow.

1. The Executive Committee is the only medical staff committee *required* by the J.C.A.H., which states that

There must be an executive committee that represents the medical staff, has responsibility for the effectiveness of all medical activities of the staff and acts for the medical staff. The executive committee is the mechanism for providing a clearly defined formal relationship between the medical staff organization and the chief executive officer of the hospital.

The executive committee ordinarily will be composed of the president, the president-elect, the immediate past-president, the secretary-treasurer, department heads and one or more members at large from the active medical staff; it may vary in size and composition, however, in accordance with the needs of the hospital. The chief executive officer of the hospital should attend all meetings of this committee.

The executive committee must be empowered to act on behalf of the medical staff, as well as to coordinate the activities and general policies of the various departments and services, under such limitations as may be imposed on the committee by the medical staff bylaws, rules and regulations. The committee should meet at least monthly, and must maintain a permanent record of its proceedings and actions. Further functions and responsibilities of the executive committee should include at least the following:

- To receive and act upon the reports of medical staff committees;
- To consider and recommend action to the chief executive officer on all matters of a medico-administrative nature;
- To implement the approved policies of the medical staff;
- To make recommendations to the governing body;
- To take all reasonable steps to ensure professionally ethical conduct on the part of all members of the medical staff and to initiate such prescribed corrective measures as are indicated;
- To fulfill the medical staff's accountability to the governing body for the medical care rendered to the patients in the hospital; and
- To ensure that the medical staff is kept abreast of the accreditation program and informed of the accreditation status of the hospital.[30]

---

[29] *Ibid.* pp. 39–40. Reprinted by permission of the Joint Commission on Accreditation of Hospitals.

[30] *Ibid.* p. 41. Reprinted by permission of the Joint Commission on Accreditation of Hospitals.

2. The Credentials Committee has the important responsibility for assessing the qualifications for staff appointments and for recommendation of privileges, limitations, and departments. The committee makes recommendations for endorsement by the medical staff. (The governing board makes the final decisions regarding appointments to the medical staff.)
3. The Medical Audit Committee, or Medical Care Evaluation Committee, has the important responsibility of ensuring clinical practice of the highest possible quality.
4. The Utilization Review Committee serves to ensure that the hospital's resources are used optimally and in the best interest of the patient. (For a complete treatment of this important hospital function, see *Quality Assurance Program for Medical Care in the Hospital,* published by the American Hospital Association in 1972).
5. The Joint Conference Committee has already been described under committees of the governing board. The reader should recall that this joint committee of the governing board and the medical staff (with the administrator acting ex officio) serves the critical function of medico-administrative liaison.

In larger, more complex hospitals, there are usually several other committees of the medical staff such as the Tissue Committee, Infections Committee, Blood Transfusion Committee, Pharmacy and Therapeutics Committee, and Medical Education Committee. These titles are descriptive; nothing more will be said about them.

Departmentation of the Medical Staff.   Departmentation of the medical staff along the lines of medical specialties (medicine, surgery, obstetrics-gynecology, pediatrics, and so on) usually occurs when the duties and functions become too complex to be handled by the staff as a whole. Competent chiefs or chairmen of clinical departments are appointed through a process that is outlined in each medical staff's bylaws.

> The clinical department chairmen are essential elements in the line of authority within the medical staff organization, and are accountable to the executive committee for all professional and medical staff administrative activities within their departments. They must be responsible for departmental implementation of actions taken by the executive committee. They also must maintain continuing surveillance of the professional performance of all members of the medical staff with privileges in their department, and must report regularly thereon to the medical staff executive committee.[31]

Medical Staff Bylaws.   There must be a blueprint for the organization and operation of the medical staff if it is to function. This blueprint is the medical staff bylaws. The J.C.A.H. states that

> The medical staff must establish a framework for collegial self-government, in order to accomplish effectively its functions and responsibilities. Therefore, the medical staff must develop and adopt, subject to the approval of the governing body, a set of bylaws, rules and regulations that create an atmosphere and framework within which each member of the medical staff can act with a reasonable degree of freedom and confidence. The bylaws, rules and regulations of the medi-

---

[31]*Ibid.* p. 40.

cal staff must state the policies under which the medical staff regulates itself. There should be a mechanism for and evidence of a periodic review and revision, as necessary, of the bylaws, rules and regulations. The bylaws, rules and regulations shall at least:

- Delineate the organizational structure of the medical staff.
- Specify qualifications and procedures for admission to and retention of staff membership, including the delineation, assignment, reduction, or withdrawal of privileges.
- Specify the method of performing the credentials review function.
- Provide an appeal mechanism relative to medical staff recommendations for denial of staff appointments and reappointments, as well as for denial, curtailment, suspension, or revocation of clinical privileges. This mechanism shall provide for review of decisions, including the right to be heard at each step of the process when requested by the practitioner. The final decision must be rendered by the governing body, within a fixed period of time.
- Delineate clinical privileges of nonphysician practitioners, as well as responsibilities of the physician members of the medical staff in relation to nonphysician practitioners.
- Require a pledge that each practitioner will conduct his practice in accordance with high ethical traditions, and will refrain from:
  - Rebating a portion of a fee, or receiving other inducements in exchange for a patient referral;
  - Deceiving a patient as to the identity of an operating surgeon, or any other medical practitioner providing treatment or service; or
  - Delegating the responsibility for diagnosis or care of hospitalized patients to another medical practitioner who is not qualified to undertake this responsibility.
- Provide methods for the selection of officers and department/service chairmen.
- Outline responsibilities of the medical staff officers and clinical department/service chairmen.
- Specify composition and functions of standing committees as required by the complexity of the hospital.
- Establish requirements regarding the frequency of, and attendance at, general and departmental meetings of the medical staff.
- Require that the evaluation of the significance of medical histories, authentication of medical histories, the performance and recording of physical examinations and the prescribing of treatment, be carried out by those with appropriate licenses and clinical privileges, within their sphere of authorization.
- Establish requirements regarding completion of medical records, including records of the emergency department or service, the outpatient department or service, and where one exists, the home care program.
- Provide for a mechanism by which the medical staff consults with, and reports to, the governing body. Because the governing body of the hospital, acting through the chief executive officer, has the overall responsibility for the conduct of the hospital, and the medical staff has the overall responsibility for the provision of medical care to patients, there must be full communication between these two bodies. Both must be informed adequately regarding hospital activities. Further, representatives of the medical staff should participate in any hospital deliberations that affect the discharge of medical staff responsibilities.[32]

---

[32] *Ibid.* pp. 40–48. Reprinted by permission of the Joint Commission on Accreditation of Hospitals.

HOSPITAL–MEDICAL STAFF RELATIONS

In the context of the highly specialized and complex hospital organization, one can see the difficulties faced by the governing board, administrator, and medical staff when developing policies and practices to simultaneously maintain the professional prerogatives of the physician and the integrity of the total organization.

Robert H. Guest has made an in-depth review of the literature pertaining to the structural relationships linking governing board, administration, and medical staff. His major conclusions have a great deal to say about the future directions of these relationships. For example, Guest has found that the main structural unit which links the individual doctors to both administration and the governing board is the executive committee of the medical staff. Guest also found that the literature strongly supports the notion that there should be medical representation on the governing board and that "reciprocal representation," with the administrator and board members present in staff meetings, is also useful. The literature suggests that "the dynamic links throughout the hospital organization are those forged through the informal day to day interactions, not by the periodic 'engineering' of structural arrangements."[33]

Perhaps no single organizational problem facing the hospital is more significant than that of developing a more effective working relationship between the hospital and its medical staff. Two prestigious national commissions (the Secretary's Advisory Committee on Hospital Effectiveness and the National Advisory Commission on Health Manpower) have called for greater involvement on the part of physicians in the management and decision-making aspects of hospitals.

Three major studies have dealt with the question of medical staff–hospital relationships. These are Georgopoulos and Mann's study of 41 community general hospitals, published in 1962,[34] Roemer and Friedman's study of the relationship between medical staff organization and hospital performance, published in 1971,[35] and Duncan Neuhauser's study of the relationship between administrative activities and hospital performance, also published in 1971.[36] Table 8–2 contains a summary of the principal approaches and findings of the three studies. In essence, these studies suggest the necessity for providing increased participation by physicians in the organization's management.

CONTINGENCY THEORY AND THE HOSPITAL

We have seen previously that there are divergent points of view about how all types of organizations, including hospitals, should be structured to ac-

[33] Robert H. Guest, "The role of the doctor in institutional management." *In* Basil S. Georgopoulos, ed. *Organization Research on Health Institutions*, Ann Arbor, Michigan: Institute for Social Research of the University of Michigan, 1972, p. 296.

[34] Georgopoulos and Mann, op. cit.

[35] Roemer and Friedman, op. cit.

[36] Duncan Neuhauser, *The Relationship Between Administration Activities and Hospital Performance*. Research Series, No. 28, Chicago: Center for Health Administration Studies, University of Chicago, 1971.

Table 8-2   Summary of Major Studies of Medical Staff Organization

	PRIMARY EMPHASIS	PRINCIPAL FINDINGS AND IMPLICATIONS
Georgopoulos and Mann	Focused on the relationship between type and extent of physician participation and quality of coordination	1. Those physicians more involved in hospital affairs (e.g., chief of staff) perceived greater degree of coordination 2. Greatest amount of tension existed among doctors themselves 3. Suggest that greater use of overlapping committee membership and coordinative roles results in less tension and better coordination of effort
Roemer and Friedman	Focused on the relationship between degree of structure of medical staff organization (e.g., per cent of physicians under contract) and scope, economy, and quality of services rendered	1. The more highly structured the staff the greater the scope and quality of services rendered and the lower the expenses per patient day 2. Tension and conflict highest in staffs with an intermediate degree of structure. Those highly structured have the necessary salaried physicians to provide the needed coordination and integration; in those with little structure the doctors can operate independently of administration as well as of each other
Neuhauser	Focused on the impact of rules and regulations and visibility of consequences on quality of care	1. Board chairman and administrators who are more aware of their hospital's activities (visibility of consequences) have higher quality of care 2. Rules and regulations not necessarily harmful to quality of care, especially where the rules and regulations are established by the physicians themselves 3. There is some suggestion that greater physician involvement in hospital affairs is associated with higher quality of care

(Source: Stephen M. Shortell, "Hospital medical staff organization: structure process, and outcome." Reprinted with permission from the quarterly journal of the American College of Hospital Administrators, *Hospital Administration* [retitled *Hospital and Health Services Administration*], *19*:104, Spring, 1974.)

complish their objectives. Some have taken the view that the organization functions best under centralized direction; others argue with equal strength that decentralized authority and responsibility are best. The hospital, with a range of activities from the relatively low skill production-type work in housekeeping, laundry, and maintenance to the highly specialized and professionalized activities of physicians, nurses, and technologists, presents a perplexing challenge to managers. The one thing that should be made clear at this point is that there is *no one correct way* to organize and manage a hospital. What works best for one group of participants in one hospital setting may not work best for another group in another setting. Several writers have formalized this concept and have called it the Contingency or Situational Theory of Management.[37]

The modern hospital may well be the best example of applied Contingency Theory, since it explains what otherwise would be a most peculiar organizational structure having a highly structured administrative hierarchy on the one hand and a comparatively loosely structured medical staff on the other. Duncan Neuhauser has suggested that "Contingency theory would suggest, and the empirical evidence supports the idea, that this is fundamentally a rational way to organize a hospital given the current technology and tasks involved. It also explains the persistence of this organizational form in thousands of independent hospitals."[38]

This does not mean that the hospital as it is now organized is perfect or, in many cases, even adequate. It simply means that the structure is rational and, if properly managed, can be effective.

The single most important adjustment in the hospital's organizational pattern — indeed, the only one that will make it as effective as it needs to be — is to provide the physician with a more integral role in the organization. There must be a basic integration of the administrative and clinical decision-making that goes on in the hospital.

Developments in the past decade have mitigated the traditional separation of medical and administrative activities in the hospital. Court decisions holding the hospital liable for medical practice within its walls, PSRO's, a more knowledgeable public, and reimbursement mechanisms are but a few of the factors which have served to erase many of the traditional distinctions between medical and administrative activities. As Stephen Shortell has stated, "Administrative activities increasingly touch upon the practice of medicine, and clinical practice, in turn, is heavily involved with issues of managerial efficiency and effectiveness."[39]

No one knows at this point *how* to bring about this integration. Perhaps emphasizing the role of the physicians as head of the patient care team under a matrix organization arrangement (see Chapter 7) will accomplish the adjust-

---

[37] George F. Lombard, "Relativism in organizations." *Harvard Business Review,* 49:55, March-April, 1971; and Robert J. Mockler, "Situational theory of management." *Harvard Business Review,* May-June, 1971.

[38] Duncan Neuhauser, "The hospital as a matrix organization." *Hospital Administration,* 17:15, Fall, 1972.

[39] Stephen M. Shortell, "Hospital medical staff organization: structure, process, and outcome." *Hospital Administration, 19:*105, Spring, 1974.

ment. With the appointment of full-time salaried chiefs of staff and chiefs of services some hospitals have moved in this direction. The inclusion of physicians on hospital governing boards has generally had positive effects. Whether these or other approaches will eventually bring about the desired results remains to be seen. It is encouraging at this point to observe that all three parts of the organizational triad—governing board, administration, and medical staff—recognize their interrelatedness and are searching for ways to make the organization more efficient and more effective.

THE LONG-TERM-CARE FACILITY

On page 12 we cited the American Hospital Association's definition of a long-term-care facility (nursing home) as being

> An establishment that provides—through an organized medical staff, a medical director or a medical adviser, permanent facilities that include inpatient beds, medical services, continuous nursing services, and health-related services—diagnosis and treatment for patients who are not in an acute phase of illness but who primarily require skilled nursing care on an inpatient basis.

The early role of these health care organizations was to provide custodial care. The modern role goes well beyond this and includes the provision of continuing care for those recovering from surgical procedures or medical problems, assisting the patient in achieving maximum physical and emotional health, and assisting the elderly in achieving an active participation in life.[40]

Long-term-care facilities in the United States are still largely sole proprietorships, with the owner also serving as administrator. Some are owned by partnerships; some (a rather small but growing proportion) are owned and operated as part of a chain; and some are owned and operated by a non-profit corporation. In comparison to the hospital industry, in which roughly 90 per cent of the institutions are non-profit, the long-term-care industry has only about 10 per cent of the facilities operated on a non-profit basis. This pattern of ownership accounts for the organizational difference between hospitals and long-term-care facilities at the level of the governing board. Below board level, the organizational pattern differs mainly in the sense that long-term-care facilities offer a much narrower range of services than hospitals and the medical staff is organized in a much less complex way. Figure 8–8 illustrates a typical organizational structure of a long-term-care facility.

Other Health Care Organizations

In Chapter 1, we described many different types of health care organizations. The reader may apply the principles and concepts in Chapter 7 to most of these organizations, just as we have done here with hospitals and to a lesser extent with long-term-care facilities.

---

[40]Florence L. McQuillan, *Fundamentals of Nursing Home Administration.* Philadelphia: W. B. Saunders Company, 1974, p. 3.

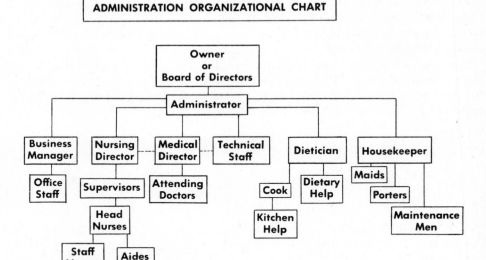

Figure 8-8 Long-term care facility organization chart. (Source: Florence L. McQuillan, *Fundamentals of Nursing Home Administration*, 2nd ed. Philadelphia, W. B. Saunders Co., 1974. Used by permission of the publisher.)

SUMMARY

In this chapter we have applied the principles and concepts of organization that were presented in the previous chapter to hospitals and long-term-care facilities. The hospital is seen as a complex organization providing the basic functions of patient care, research, education, and preventive medicine.

In carrying out these functions, the hospital faces several key organizational problems: coordination of the various participants and activities, managing organizational conflict, and achieving a suitable level of adaptation. The heart of the hospital as an organization is the organizational triad, consisting of the governing body, the administration, and the medical staff. There is no best way to organize the hospital. As we have seen, the hospital is an excellent example of the application of the contingency theory of organization.

The organization of the modern long-term-care facility is similar to that for hospitals except that the medical staff is neither as highly organized nor as complex and the range of services is not as broad.

DISCUSSION QUESTIONS

1. Discuss the similarities and differences in the structure of those organizations presented in Figures 8–1, 8–2, and 8–3.

2. In this chapter the hospital has been defined as a health team. What other definitions could be given?

3. What are the chief organizational problems faced by the hospital? What is the role of the administrator in dealing with each?

4. What functions does the hospital serve?

5. How does the typical hospital differ organizationally from the typical bureaucratic pyramid form of organization? Why?

6. What is the "organizational triad" of the hospital? What are the major functions of each component of the triad?

7. Alan D. Bauerschmidt, quoted on page 185, stated that portions of the hospital are ". . . reserved for administrative rule, others are reserved for professional rule, while still other areas of the organization are best described as hybrids." Viewing Figure 8–7 (shown on page 186), classify those portions of the hospital organization that fall within these three "areas of rule."

8. What is the nature of the medical staff-hospital relationship? What can be done to improve it?

9. What are the implications for the hospital administrator in the statement that "there is no one correct way to organize and manage a hospital"?

10. How does the long-term-care facility differ organizationally from the hospital?

11. What concepts and principles of organization would be useful in setting up a hospital laboratory; the nursing department in a long-term-care facility; the business office in a family planning clinic?

INCIDENTS

1. THE SECRETARIES

There are three secretaries in the Business Office of Memorial Hospital. The secretarial output proved to be a bottleneck in the smooth flow of work in the office. The secretaries had been assigned to various sections of the business office and the office manager discovered that when one secretary was overloaded with dictation, transcription, and related secretarial duties, one or both of the other secretaries had time on their hands. The peaks and valleys of the secretaries' work loads were usually in contraposition as follows:

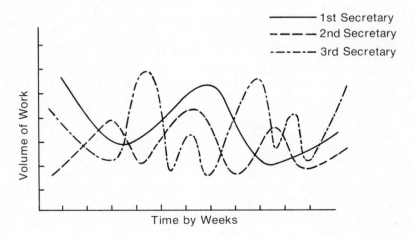

The business office manager decided to pool the work of the secretaries instead of assigning them to one section of the office. On Friday afternoon the business manager called the three secretaries into his office and explained the new idea. They made little comment. Over the weekend, however, one of the secretaries called the business office manager and told him that she was resigning effective the following Friday.

On Monday, the other two secretaries spoke to the business office manager and told him that they did not like the new plan. They felt that their job status would be lowered by the pooling arrangement. The business office manager pointed out that the secretaries would be performing exactly the same work as before, at the same rate of pay, with the same titles. The secretaries said that they had been aware of the overload situation but had not done anything about it because they had thought they were doing things the way the business office manager wanted. The two secretaries then asked if they could work out a plan on their own.

Realizing that the pressure of his regular duties required his full attention, the business office manager shrugged his shoulders and told the secretaries to make their own arrangements. A replacement for the departing secretary arrived toward the end of that week.

Within a few weeks the three secretaries had devised a plan for synchronizing and interchanging work during rush periods. While the plan looked very much like a pooled arrangement of work, the secretaries were satisfied that they had not lost status. The business office manager was also satisfied because there were no further secretarial work stoppages.

A. Discuss the relations between the content and structure of formal organization relative to small working groups.

B. Does small group behavior in itself represent a method of building cooperative organization, even though the area of organization may span only a small part of total facility activity?

C. How far should a health care facility structure its organization in detail? Should the details of organization be left to the interworkings of small groups rather than being spelled out in detail by management?*

2. THE NEW ADMINISTRATOR

You have recently been appointed administrator of the ABC Hospital, a 300-bed general acute hospital on the West Coast. The previous administrator of the hospital retired, and on taking over you find many problems existing. Because the previous administrator refused to delegate authority, you find that all 17 hospital department heads report directly to you, rather than to assistant administrators or an associate administrator. You have not been able to ascertain the quality of performance of the department heads, but you have a suspicion that the competency level of most of them is not going to be up to your expectations. One reason you feel this way is because the former administrator refused to delegate, and left very little room for the department heads to "develop themselves." As a result, you find them coming to you for every decision. You are bombarded day-in and day-out with requests for permission to do the smallest things involving minor decisions.

On the other hand, the medical staff has been allowed to go on with such a great deal of freedom that you are quite concerned that the hospital may not be able to pass the next inspection by the Joint Commission on Accreditation of Hospitals. Medical records are not up-to-date, committee minutes are very incomplete, and it looks as if most of the medical staff committees did not meet during the past two years. Your philosophy is that although the medical staff should have a great deal of leeway in self government, the board of trustees has the legal responsibility for conduct of the hospital, and there must be mutual teamwork set up between the board, the administration, and the medical staff in order that the objectives of the hospital can be met.

A. As a new administrator of this hospital, what are some of the things you would do?

B. What priorities would you establish?

C. What major problems do you feel you would face in making the changes you would like in this hospital?

---

*Source: Beaufort B. Longest, Jr., *Business Management of Health Care Providers*, a packaged training program published by the Hospital Financial Management Association, Chicago, Illinois, 1975. Used by permission of the publisher.

3. THE MEDICAL STAFF

You are the administrator of Bradley Hospital, a 400-bed general voluntary hospital. The chief of the medical staff has just told you that many members of the medical staff are unhappy because they feel you are trying to control their activities too closely. The chief of staff stated, "We feel that the hospital administration should take care of the non-medical areas and leave the practice of medicine where it belongs—in the hands of the physicians."

A. How would you respond to the chief of the medical staff?

4. THE EMERGENCY DEPARTMENT

You are the administrator of a hospital with a very active Emergency Department. Approximately 60,000 patients are seen annually. Traditionally the organization of this department has been like that of many hospital emergency departments. Nursing service employees report to Nursing Service; the registration clerks and the cashiers and other clerks report to the Admissions Department; the security officers report to the Security Department; the house staff physicians who provide medical services report to their various chiefs of the departments (such as Internal Medicine and Surgery); and the crisis intervention social workers report to the Department of Social Work.

You have just employed a full-time salaried physician as Director of the Emergency Department. The new Director has told you that he needs to make some changes so that he can carry out the job at hand. The basic change he wants to make is to organize the department so that all nursing service employees report directly to him instead of to the Nursing Service. He has considerable experience in emergency medicine, and has told you that this change will help the employees feel a greater esprit de corps, since they would all be in one department rather than having to divide their loyalty between the Emergency Department and their "home" department. The director feels this change will promote efficiency as well as boost morale and will make it easier to coordinate the work of the Emergency Department.

In discussing this, the Director of Nursing Services has said that if you approve this change, the new Emergency Department Director should not expect Nursing Service to provide any nurses for a shift even in an emergency. For example, if one or more emergency nurses do not come in owing to sickness, it will be up to the director to call in other emergency nurses from home to staff the Emergency Department, rather than expect the Nursing Service to take nurses from various floors of the hospital. (At the present time when the Emergency Department needs more nurses, either because of absenteeism or sudden increased activity in the Department, nurses are pulled from various floors to augment the staff.)

The Director of Nursing Services has also pointed out that in the past the Nursing Service (with help from the Personnel Department) has been responsible for recruiting and training all nursing personnel in the Emergency Department. If the change is made, she feels that this activity should then become the responsibility of the Director of the Emergency Department.

At the present time, all of the nurses in the Operating Room report to the Department of Nursing Service even though there is a salaried chief of surgery who heads up the Department of Surgery. The same is true in intensive care; here, the nurses report to the Nursing Service Department even though there is a salaried physician who is head of the Intensive Care Unit. It seems that these other physicians do not mind nursing employees reporting to Nursing Service, because they retain responsibility for directing the professional activities of nursing in their respective departments.

A. Why do you suppose the Director of the Emergency Department wants the nursing personnel to have a direct line relationship to him?

B. What advantages and disadvantages would this have in comparison to the pattern in the Operating Room and the Intensive Care Unit?

C. Will this change accomplish the things the Director of the Emergency Department claims (better esprit de corps, efficiency, morale, coordination)? Why? Why not?

D. What decision would you, as the administrator, make in this situation? Why?

This Chapter Contains:

- Introduction

- Obtaining Employees
  Manpower Planning
  Manpower Sources
  Job Analysis
  Recruitment
  Selection
  Orientation

- Maintaining Employees
  Employee Appraisal
  Training and Development
  Wage and Salary Administration
  Discipline
  Health and Safety
  Pension Programs

- Summary

- Discussion Questions

- Incidents

Chapter 9

MANPOWER ACQUISITION AND MAINTENANCE

"The human resources of most organizations are
properly viewed as their most important asset."
(Dale S. Beach)[1]

INTRODUCTION

The delivery of sound patient care can only be made possible with the acquisition and maintenance of adequate numbers of skilled personnel. Few other industries in the service field have as high a concentration of labor in their budget as health care systems do. It is axiomatic that health care can only be supplied through people, not only in hospitals but also in extended and long-term-care facilities, clinics, and doctors' offices. In this chapter, we will concentrate on the acquisition and maintenance of manpower as it applies particularly to health delivery organizations rather than private practices.

In Chapters 7 and 8, we described the principles and concepts of organization design and their application to the health care facility. In order to bring the organization to life it must be manned with competent people. This manning of the organization with people who are competent to fill various roles designed into the structure is called staffing, and is part of the organizing process. Organizing involves not only the work setting but also the acquisition and maintenance of necessary manpower (human resources). In this chapter we will present the activities that are characteristic of manpower acquisition and maintenance by following the time flow presented in Figure 9–1.

Staffing becomes important when we realize that health services are provided by people who are often in direct contact with the recipients of those services. For this reason, all managers have a responsibility for ensuring that the proper people are acquired, trained, and placed in positions commensurate with their abilities.

In staffing, the function of the governing board and top level administrators is largely to establish suitable personnel policies and acquire key executive personnel to see that the policies are carried out. Personnel policies are formal statements (which should be in writing and available to every employee) concerning the relationship between the organization and its employees. The chief executive of the organization is responsible for coordinating the implementation of the policies.

---

[1]Dale S. Beach, *Personnel: The Management of People at Work.* New York: Macmillan Publishing Co., Inc., 1975, p. 219.

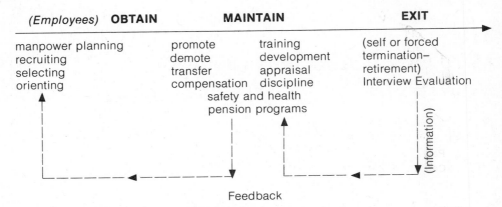

Figure 9–1   Manpower acquisition and maintenance flow chart.

Staffing is one of the central aspects of a manager's responsibility over a particular part of the organization. Of course, in most organizations the manager is aided substantially by the Personnel Department. Although it is true that in many health care organizations the staffing of a large department such as the Nursing Service is done by the Director, this trend is changing. We now find that many Personnel Departments are responsible for staffing and preparing the manpower budget as well as acting as in-house consultants.

Figure 9–2 illustrates the important relationships that the Personnel Director must establish and maintain. The Personnel Department has responsibility in several key areas: (1) employment, (2) employee relations, (3) manpower utilization, (4) compensation and employee services, (5) research, and (6) staff development and training.

It is important to remember, however, that the ultimate responsibility for the selection of personnel and the development of those currently employed rests with the line manager. Sometimes, in its eagerness to be of service or as the result of a manager's abdication of some of his responsibility, the Personnel Department may assume too large a role. This should be guarded against. If the manager permits the Personnel Department to select, train, promote, and make placement decisions, his or her relationships with subordinates will be weakened.

An effective manpower acquisition and maintenance program requires a coordinated and balanced effort on the part of the Personnel Department and the line managers in the organization. In most organization structures, the personnel executive's function is to manage his own department and act as an "in-house consultant" to the other executives and managers in the hospital. In this capacity, he gains the trust of the others and knows his material in order to offer suggestions to his "client population" (other managers) but does not take over the responsibility of running their functions.

One important aspect of staffing is the cost of the activities associated with acquiring and maintaining employees. These activities might include recruiting, interviewing, testing, placing, orienting, training, and supervising new employees until they reach a level of patient care quality and productivity that is

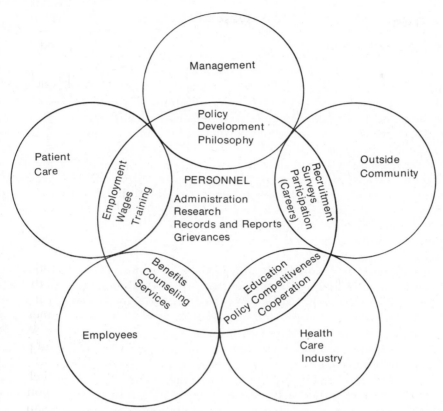

Figure 9-2 Personnel relationships. (Source: Internal records, Mount Carmel Mercy Hospital and Medical Center, Detroit, Michigan.)

commensurate with their salary. The most obvious impact of this cost is felt when a turnover occurs, but turnover means more than cost in dollars. It may mean additional work for other employees until a vacancy is filled. It usually means operating for a period of time with less than optimum effectiveness. It may even mean that work does not get done or is done poorly for a period of time. There are occasions, however, when planned turnover can show a cost saving for the health care institution. These occasions occur when a number of professionals, particularly nurses, leave the system when occupancy may be down because of the time of year and closing units (or at least reducing the staffing levels of these units) is appropriate. This may occur more frequently in university towns, where the population is reduced at the end of the school year.

Staffing has the dual objective of bringing personnel into the organization (acquiring) and keeping those who are effective in the organization (maintaining). This chapter is divided into two main sections. The first is concerned with obtaining employees, and the second is concerned with maintaining employees. Since the success of the health care organization is largely a reflection of the people who work in it, the organization's human resources are its most vital asset.

OBTAINING EMPLOYEES

MANPOWER PLANNING

Viewing the first activity in the time flow model presented in Figure 9–1, we can note that manpower planning precedes recruitment, selection, and the induction of new employees into the organization. Through manpower planning the health care organization determines its personnel needs. Because organizations are dynamic, these manpower needs change. Some of the principal factors contributing to the need for additional personnel are[2]

1. Employee turnover — a normal rate of turnover through resignation and retirement means that the organization must constantly seek new employees.
2. Nature of present work force — when considered in the context of the changing technology of the typical health care organization, it is apparent that extensive retraining for present personnel must take place constantly and new employees must be brought in from the outside to fill newly created positions.
3. Rate of growth of the organization — growth in health care organizations can be in terms of expansion of present size (the addition of 100 beds, for instance) or growth in the range of services provided (such as the addition of a Nuclear Medicine Department or a Rehabilitation Department). In either case, there normally is a demand for an increase in manpower.

Health care organizations can take one of two basic approaches as a way to handle their requirements for new employees: plan for future needs, or wait until specific openings occur and seek replacements then. For some types of organizations the latter approach may be acceptable, but in the dynamic health care organization, with its vital function of maintaining the continual provision of health services, it is absolutely essential to plan for both short-term and long-term manpower needs.

Manpower planning has been defined as "the process of determining manpower requirements and the means for meeting those requirements in order to carry out the integrated plans of the organization."[3]

Planning Activities. Sound manpower planning involves five basic steps.

Step One. An estimate must be made of the number and types of jobs to be filled at some point in the future. The only real difference between short-term planning and long-term planning is how far into the future one looks. Short-term planning is usually for one year in the future and long-term planning is for two to ten years. Whether the range of the plan is short or long, the initial step is to develop a picture of the organization at some future point and estimate the jobs that will exist at that time. This is often fairly subjective, but such factors as the objectives of the organization, planned organizational changes, and anticipated technological advances can be taken into account.

Step Two. Once the future structure of the organization is anticipated, it is necessary to develop an estimate of the manpower that will be required at that

---

[2] Adapted from Dale S. Beach, op. cit. p. 220.
[3] Bruce P. Coleman, "An integrated system for manpower planning." *Business Horizons, 13*:89, October, 1970.

time. Unless the organization is going to change drastically (such as a major change in patient mix), this step is straightforward for many categories of personnel. Hospitals and long-term-care facilities have well established staffing ratios for those involved in patient care, but the number and types of supportive and managerial employees are not so closely related to the number of patients served. Judgment and past experience usually serve as major guides in this step.

Step Three. Next, a careful analysis of the present manpower resources of the organization must be made to determine the quantity and the quality of the present manpower resources. The manpower audit or, as it is sometimes called, the skills inventory which is a result of this analysis is simply a compilation of facts concerning each employee's age, job title, amount of experience, length of service, education, special skills, and so forth.

Step Four. Once a complete picture of present manpower resources is obtained, the planner can turn his or her attention to forecasting the changes that will occur in the present work force in terms of entries and exits and movements within the organization. All organizations experience losses of manpower for such reasons as retirements, deaths, voluntary terminations, and discharges. The pattern of these losses in the past can indicate future patterns, unless some intervening factor comes into play. For example, a new hospital in the vicinity may draw away a sizable portion of an existing hospital's work force. These factors must be taken into account. Many losses will be replaced by entries from outside the facility, and this will be discussed later.

Also related to these losses will be the movement of people within the health care organization. One factor which distinguishes this type of organization from many others is the large proportion of the work force that has received specific training for specific jobs (RN's, medical technologists, and pharmacists, for example). This means that there is not as much movement as in some other types of organizations. Because of training and licensure requirements, upward mobility is blocked. (For example, the LPN cannot be promoted to RN without additional training and licensure.) Nevertheless, there will be some upward movement as a result of promotions, particularly in managerial positions, and some lateral movement in the form of transfers. These movements must be taken into account when forecasting changes in the present work force over any specified period of time.

It should also be noted that the skills inventory, factors of experience, and often education will have to be adjusted upward with the passage of time. State requirements for continuing education credits for continued certification (licensure) have existed in the field of education for many years. In recent years, there have been changes in this direction for the health care industry, with particular emphasis being placed upon administrators of long-term-care facilities and registered nurses. In some states, the continuing education units are required for license maintenance for physicians. In the future, hospitals will be faced with the necessity of making decisions in regard to what part they will play in the continuing education and training of all of their professional employees.

It can be seen that manpower planning deals with a dynamic situation in which the planner is trying to forecast the demand for employees at some point in the future *and* simultaneously forecast the changes that will occur in the present work force. The quality and effectiveness of manpower planning will be determined by how well this is done.

Step Five. Based on the conclusions reached in the four previous steps, the planner should be able to determine the needs of the organization at a particular point in the future, as well as the projected status of the work force at that time. The manpower plan consists of determining how these needs will be met.

MANPOWER SOURCES

A standard way to classify the sources of manpower supply is to separate the sources into two categories: (1) internal sources and (2) external sources. By utilizing internal sources, the health care organization can fill a vacancy by transferring or promoting from within. In order for the organization to be able to make the best use of its potential internal manpower, it is important that the skill inventories mentioned earlier include career ladder planning and the necessary training to upgrade personnel with potential for internal transfers. When people are trained and on tap for these promotions, it means that a vacancy will occur somewhere else in the organization and will need to be filled as well. Actually, using internal sources usually means a higher cost of staffing because two or more positions are involved. However, this is offset by giving the work force the confidence that the organization is interested in its employees and wants to give them the opportunity to advance and improve in their work situation.

In addition to the internal sources, the health care organization may bring new employees in from the outside. Advertising vacancies or relying on present employees to "pass the word" to potential employees often generates applications. Visits to schools and colleges or contacts with public and private employment agencies may also be useful.

There are other sources of supply for health workers, including those who simply walk into the organization to seek employment; however, the ones mentioned above are the most promising. There are significant supply problems in many areas (primarily rural and inner-city) which are exacerbated by fragmentation, specialization, maldistribution, and the increasing demand for health services. At this time, approximately 200 different positions are required to staff a general acute care hospital, well over the 300 mark for a large metropolitan teaching institution, and this number is growing. Attracting and maintaining a suitable manpower supply of this diversity is one of the major tasks facing management. The technical aspects of accomplishing this task make up the remainder of this chapter.

JOB ANALYSIS

Before it is possible to recruit, select, and introduce a new employee into the health care organization, there should be a guide to indicate what types of skills and training are required. The information needed to guide these activities generally results from *job analysis*. The Personnel Department is usually responsible for this analysis, which consists of observing and studying a job to determine its content (duties and responsibilities), the conditions under which the work is performed, its relationship to other jobs, and the skills, training, attitudes, and abilities necessary to perform the job.[4]

There are four basic ways by which job information can be gathered for analysis: (1) observation, (2) a questionnaire, (3) an interview, and (4) a combination of two or more of the first three. The information obtained through job analysis becomes the source for the development of *the job description* and *the job specification documents*.

The content and format of the job description and the job specification documents can vary among organizations. However, the more general practice is to include the listing of job title, summary, and duties in the "job description" document and to enumerate the employee qualifications necessary to perform the job satisfactorily in the "job specification" document.[5] In many health care organizations, there is an existing set of job descriptions and job specifications. Where they do not already exist, or where they need to be updated, the reader will find *Job Descriptions and Organizational Analysis for Hospitals and Related Health Services*, 1971, a publication of the U.S. Department of Labor, developed in cooperation with the American Hospital Association, very useful. This book contains excellent job descriptions for all types of hospital employees. With only minor adjustments, these descriptions can easily be used as models for job descriptions in other types of health care organizations. Figure 9–3 is a *sample* job description for a hospital nurse aide and Figure 9–4 is a sample job specification document.

Descriptions and specifications for each job should be maintained and updated whenever the content of the job or its performance requirements change. With this information available, the communication between the line manager and the Personnel Department can be greatly simplified. When a vacancy occurs, the Personnel Department is notified by means of a requisition, and recruitment for someone who meets the requirements set forth in the job specification document can begin.

Figure 9–5 depicts a good way to visualize the relationship between job analysis, job description, and job specification. The reader should keep in mind that the job analysis procedure is a method for obtaining (by interviews, observation, and so on) detailed information about the duties involved in each job and the qualifications an employee must have to perform them. This information is written up on the job description form from which the job specification can be abstracted.

Dale S. Beach has suggested that the following items are the principal ones covered in a job analysis program. After each item, a few brief comments are given to indicate why this information is important and what is included in the item.

---

[4]Leon C. Megginson, *Personnel: A Behavioral Approach to Administration.* Homewood, Illinois: Richard D. Irwin, Inc., 1972, p. 209.

[5]Beach, op. cit. p. 200.

Date: _____

Job Title: _____ NURSE AIDE _____ *Code Number:* _____

Department: _____ NURSING SERVICE _____ *Sub-Division of Sec.:* _____

Work Location: _____ *Shift:* _____

Scheduling Details (Days on or off, etc.): _____

JOB DESCRIPTION (The Job Itself)

Job Summary (1 or 2 sentences to identify the job) is responsible for performing specific basic nursing duties with the supervision of a registered nurse and after attending a required three-week orientation program. As a member of the nursing team, she assists in recognizing the personal needs of the patient. She cares for the assigned patients, their rooms, the work-rooms, and nursing equipment.

Tasks and Duties (Start with major responsibilities and proceed to minor ones.)
A. Is responsible for patient care as assigned.
　1. Receives report from Team Leader or Charge or Head Nurse on her patients.
　2. Assists patients with trays and feeding.
　3. Writes out assignment on Daily Sheet.
　4. Organizes the work for the shift. (Decides which patients or treatments need to be done first and which later.)
　5. Reports to Team Leader or Charge or Head Nurse.
　　On the assigned care given.
　　If there is a change in patient's condition or any special observations.
　　On leaving and returning to the floor.
　　Toward the end of the shift for the day.
　6. Carries out the nursing care and duties.
　· IS PREPARED TO DO THE FOLLOWING:
　　Answer signal lights.
　　Arrange patients' bedside units. (See that all equipment is clean.)
　　Make beds—unoccupied, occupied, and anesthetic.
　　Strip beds for baths or discharges.
　　Prepare patients for meals.
　　Assist in serving and removing meal trays.
　　Feed patients as necessary.
　　Place soiled linen in laundry bags and deposit same in laundry chute.
　　Give oral hygiene to patients and care for patients' dentures.
　　Give baths: complete, partial, tub, shower, and Sitz.
　　Give back rubs.
　　Give and remove bed pan or urinal.
　　Obtain specimens: Urine, stool, and sputum.
　　Strain urine for stones and examine A.C. urine specimens for sugar
　　Measure Intake and Output.
　　Empty Foley bags and Wagensteen bottles.
　　Give routine H.S. (Evening care).
　　Assist patient to move and accompany to another department.
　　Sit at bedside of restless patient.
　　Admit and discharge (by wheelchair) patients.
　　Assist with a physical examination.
　　Care for the body after death.
　　Apply binders, breast, abdominal, and scultetus.
　　Apply Ace bandages and T.E.D. stockings.
　　Comb, brush and wash hair.
　　Take temperature (oral and rectal), pulse, and respirations.

Give enemas, S.S. Fleets and oil.
Apply ice collars with supervision.
Do peri-care.
Dress newborns for discharge.
Assist patients on bedside commode.
Weigh patients.
Apply pelvic or cervical traction when muscular traction is ordered.
Clean utility room, linen room, C.S.R. cart, treatment room, etc.
Care for patients in Isolation as assigned.
7. Attends and participates in Team Conferences.
B. Attends In-Service programs and assists in orientation of new personnel as required.
C. Familiarizes herself with her job description.
D. Treats information about patients as confidential.
E. Performs other duties as assigned.

Equipment Used:
None

Responsibility for Money, Securities, Valuables:
None

Responsibility for Supervising and/or Training Others:
None

Figure 9–3 Sample job description (Source: Mount Carmel Mercy Hospital and Medical Center, Detroit, Michigan. Used by permission.)

JOB SPECIFICATIONS (The Person to Fill the Job)

Age Range: 18 or older

Education: High school graduation or equivalent recommended.

Experience: Previous experience desired but not mandatory.

Special Training, Knowledge or Skills: Reading, writing.

Physical Requirements (standing, lifting, walking, reaching, etc.): Good physical and mental health. (Pre-employment physical is done by staff physician.)

Special Requirements (tact, judgment, initiative, etc.): References: Personal and previous employment. Sincere desire to care for the sick.

Professional or Craft Affiliation, License, etc.: None.

Other: N/A.

Figure 9–4 Sample job specification document. (Source: Mount Carmel Mercy Hospital and Medical Center, Detroit, Michigan. Used by permission.)

```
┌─────────────────────────────────────────┐
│              JOB ANALYSIS                │
│                                          │
│     A process for obtaining all pertinent│
│                job facts                 │
└─────────────────────────────────────────┘
```

(Facts are written up in job description)

```
┌─────────────────────────────────────────┐
│            JOB DESCRIPTION               │
│                                          │
│    A statement containing items such as  │
│         Job title                        │
│         Location                         │
│         Job summary                      │
│         Duties                           │
│         Machines, tools, equipment       │
│         Materials and forms used         │
│         Supervision given or received    │
│         Working conditions               │
│         Hazards                          │
└─────────────────────────────────────────┘
```

(Those qualifications necessary to
perform the job are determined and
written up in job specification)

```
┌─────────────────────────────────────────┐
│           JOB SPECIFICATION              │
│                                          │
│   A statement of the human qualifications necessary│
│   to do the job usually containing such items as│
│        Education                         │
│        Experience                        │
│        Training                          │
│        Judgment                          │
│        Initiative                        │
│        Physical effort                   │
│        Physical skills                   │
│        Responsibilities                  │
│        Communication skills              │
│        Emotional characteristics         │
│        Unusual sensory demands such as   │
│           sight and hearing              │
└─────────────────────────────────────────┘
```

Figure 9–5 Relationship between job analysis, job description, and job specification. (Source: Adapted from Dale S. Beach, *Personnel: The Management of People at Work*. New York: Macmillan Publishing Co., Inc., 1975, p. 200. Used by permission of the publisher. Copyright © 1975 by Dale S. Beach.)

Job Title and Location—These properly designate and identify the job. Some standardization and consistency of job titling is considered advantageous.

Job Summary—This is included in most job descriptions to give the reader a quick capsule explanation of the content of the job. Usually one or two sentences in length.

Job Duties—Usually a comprehensive listing of the duties is included together with some indication of the frequency of occurrence or percentage of time devoted to each major duty. Always include what the job holder does as well as some indication of how he performs the tasks.

Relation to Other Jobs — This item helps to locate the job in the organization by indicating the job or jobs immediately below the one being analyzed, comparable jobs, and the one immediately above it in the hierarchy.

Supervision Given — For those jobs possessing a supervisory responsibility an explanation of the number of persons directly supervised and their job titles is given.

Mental Complexity — This and similar terms, such as initiative, ingenuity, judgment, resourcefulness, and analytical requirements, are used to cover the degree of mental difficulty and skill required by the job.

Mental Attention — This factor relates to the degree of mental concentration and alertness required.

Physical Demand — Commonly included under this heading is an enumeration of the types of physical activity and effort required. It may involve such actions as walking, lifting, bending, climbing, and sitting.

Physical Skills — Examples are manual dexterity, eye-hand-foot coordination, motor coordination, and color discrimination.

Responsibilities — There are many kinds of responsibility that may be assigned to a job holder. Examples of these are responsibility for the supervision of others, responsibility for product, process, and equipment, responsibility for safety of others, responsibility for confidence and trust, and responsibility for preventing monetary loss to the organization. For certain jobs, such as high-level management ones, the responsibility factors weigh heavily in establishing the pay and status of the work.

Personal Characteristics — For certain jobs such personality attributes as personal appearance, emotional stability, maturity, initiative and drive, and skill in dealing with others are important.

Working Conditions — This item pertains to the environment in which the job holder must work.

Hazards — The conditions of work may be such that the job holder faces certain hazards to life and limb. The nature of the hazards and their probability of occurrence must be considered.[6]

The information obtained through job analysis and written up in the job description and job specification documents has many uses for the health facility manager: organization and manpower planning, recruitment, selection, employee compensation, training, and performance appraisal. It should be clear that all activities encompassed by manpower acquisition and maintenance are based upon an effective job analysis program.

RECRUITMENT

Recruitment involves the searching for and the attracting of prospective employees, from either outside or within the health care organization. The major sources of manpower have already been described. This activity is primarily a responsibility of the Personnel Department, so it will not be covered at length in this book. However, health care managers should be aware of a major piece of legislation which has had a tremendous impact on recruitment policies. Under the provisions of Title VII of the Civil Rights Act of 1964,[7] it is

---

[6] *Ibid.* p. 210. Reprinted by permission of the publisher. Copyright 1975.

[7] Complete copies of the Civil Rights Act of 1964, Public Law 88–352, can be found in the government documents section of most university and public libraries. Individual copies can be obtained from the Superintendent of Documents, Government Printing Office, Washington, D.C. 20402.

unlawful for an employer (health care organization) to discriminate against employees with respect to their hiring, discharge, or conditions of employment because of such persons' race, color, religion, sex, or national origin.

The prohibitions of the law go even further. They restrain health care organizations from discriminating against an employee or applicant for employment because he or she has supported any lawful practice or because he has made a charge, testified, assisted, or participated in any way in an investigation, proceeding, or hearing in connection with it. It is also unlawful to indicate in advertising any preference or discrimination based on race, color, sex, or national origin except when these specifications are bona fide occupational qualifications for that employment.

The limitations imposed on employers do not stop with recruitment. A number of employment practices are prohibited if the actions taken result in discrimination because of race, color, religion, sex, or national origin. Included are the following: discharging a person, permitting segregation that limits an employee's advancement, the use of employment agencies in order to discriminate, and similar practices. If the actions taken are not meant to discriminate, the law does not forbid them. This would apply to actions resulting from seniority systems, merit performance systems, and different standards of compensation or terms of employment.

Affirmative Action. Another factor that must be taken into consideration in the recruitment process is Affirmative Action Planning, which, contrary to the belief of some persons, is neither defined nor required under Title VII of the *Federal Civil Rights Act of 1964* as amended. However, when the Equal Employment Opportunity Commission (EEOC), the administrative and enforcement agency for Title VII of the Civil Rights Act, finds an employer guilty of discrimination it may request that the employer take affirmative action. If the employer refuses to do so, the EEOC may appeal to the courts who, should the EEOC's decision be upheld, can order affirmative action to correct the deficiencies.

An affirmative action plan has been defined as an organization's *positive* remedy for problems that create inequality or lack of equal opportunity within its total employment picture. It is a *result-oriented* program designed to materially increase the non-discriminatory utilization of women and minority group members at all levels and at all segments of the employer's work force. Affirmative action as a concept and a policy is not new to the vast majority of health care organizations. Nondiscrimination in all facets of the employment relationship has long been a basic published personnel policy of these organizations. An affirmative action plan simply formalizes the development and implementation of an employer's policy of nondiscrimination by establishing goals to be accomplished within established time frames.

All aspects of the employer-employee relationship are defined, including employment, promotion, demotion, layoff, termination, recruitment, recruitment advertising, rates of pay, employee benefits, and selection for training. To date, the Office of Federal Contract Compliance (OFCC), which administers affirmative action planning, has not required affirmative action on the part of health care organizations solely because they participate in Medicare. The order applies to federal government contracts that include, but are not limited to, grants for research, education, training, and so forth. Part three of the order and the regulations implementing it require an affirmative action plan as a prerequisite to *construction contracts* paid for, in part or wholly, with federal funds. In addition to federal laws and executive orders relating to non-discrimination in employment, certain states have enacted legislation prohibiting discrimination in employment and requiring affirmative action. In some instances, state laws can be more stringent than comparable federal legislation.

SELECTION

Assuming that the recruitment activity is being effectively carried out, the organization will have applicants for the existing job openings. The next activity then is to select from among these applicants.[8] It should be remembered that job specifications serve as a guide when selecting applicants. The essence of the selection procedure is to determine whether a given applicant is suited for the job in terms of training, experience, and aptitude. Personal characteristics such as attitudes, age, health, sex, and marital status may be relevant to the performance of the job under consideration. However, a word of caution is in order. Care must be taken not to use any of these personal characteristics in any way that even suggests the possibility of discrimination on the basis of race, creed, color, age, or sex as outlined in the discussion of Title VII of the Civil Rights Act of 1964. Furthermore, no individual will possess *all* of the desired characteristics to the maximum extent. To determine the "best" applicant for a particular vacancy, the characteristics of each applicant must be considered and weighed against the others.

There are three basic sources of information that can be used in the selection process:
1. Historical and background information about the individual, such as education, training, and previous employment, can be obtained from the application form. Further, references and letters of recommendation can be useful.
2. Interviews can yield a great deal of information about an individual if they are properly carried out. There are two types of interviews widely used in the selection process. The first is the directed interview, which is planned and led by the interviewer. It is confined to objectively verifiable facts about which the interviewer expects to get information by asking specific questions. In staffing, this type of interview is most often used when employees are being selected and oriented, when job descriptions are being prepared, and at the time of an exit interview. The second type of interview is the nondirected interview which has the more ambitious purpose of achieving understanding and building confidence. In practice, these two approaches often merge, and the interviewer who is perceptive and flexible will change his approach as warranted by the situation.
3. Testing can be useful to measure a prospective employee's skills and aptitudes. However, a word of caution is indicated here regarding Civil Rights legislation. The use of employment tests—defined by EEOC as "any-paper-

---

[8]For a complete description of the selection process see Leon C. Megginson, op. cit. pp. 270–272.

and-pencil" or performance measure used as a basis for any employment decision and all formal, scored, quantified, or standardized techniques of assessing job "ability"—is the subject of considerable controversy in fair employment law. Title VII expressly states that it is not unlawful for any employer to give and to act upon the results of any professionally developed ability or psychological test provided that the test is not used to discriminate against women and minority group members.

There are two conflicting interpretations of this statement. Some say that it protects any test unless there is specific intent to use it for discriminatory purposes. However, the Supreme Court has ruled that any test which has an adverse effect upon women or minority group applicants must be validated as job related regardless of whether or not the employer's intent is discrimination.

The EEOC has set up testing guidelines to serve as a workable set of standards for employers, unions, and employment agencies in determining whether their selection procedure conforms with the obligations contained in Title VII. Under these guidelines, tests which purport to measure applicants for relevant personal characteristics probably will almost never be deemed valid for fair employment purposes. Even a test that seems to directly measure job related skills may not meet the guidelines. In order to ensure that a test does meet the EEOC guidelines, employers must conduct follow-up studies which demonstrate a correlation between the test performance and the job performance. A word of caution—the test must be validated in this way for each minority group taking it, if technically feasible to do so. Testing does provide one of the criteria for measuring selectivity of a potential candidate but the above-mentioned EEOC guidelines must be carefully followed to avoid possible charges of discrimination.

The most important thing to remember about these selection techniques is that they must be used together to be really effective; each provides some information to be used in the selection of employees.

ORIENTATION

This is the formal act of informing new employees about the organization and their place in it. A successful orientation program will build the employees' sense of identification with the health care institution, help them gain acceptance by fellow workers, and give them a clear and understandable picture of the many things they need to know as they assume their roles in the organization. Ideally, an orientation program will provide the employees with an environment and setting in which they can become familiar with the entire health care organization, either through a group tour or some form of pictorial description such as a slide program. They will meet in person, or perhaps on video tape, the administrative and executive group and have an opportunity to ask questions. The orientation program should include information about the physical plant, the structure of the organization, the fire and safety program, employee health service, and personnel services such as counseling and employee benefit programs. The employee benefit program should be explained in detail to help them identify those benefits they are entitled to and give them the opportunity to ask questions regarding these programs. The orientation program should include not only this organization-wide orientation but the individual department orientation for specific information regarding the job, policies, and procedures for that department.

MAINTAINING EMPLOYEES

Once the manpower needs of the health care organization have been determined, and manpower sources have been identified, the people who have been recruited and selected become employees of the organization. They have been acquired; however, these employees must now be maintained. Specifically, the continuous activities connected with appraising current performance, training and development, compensation, and discipline must be carried out as well as providing for the health and safety of employees (see Fig. 9–1). These activities will be discussed in this part of the chapter, which deals with "maintaining" the human resources of the health care organization.

EMPLOYEE APPRAISAL

The central component for maintaining employees is a complete understanding of their performance in the organization. This understanding comes from employee appraisal and can then lead to rational training and development based on needs and to the most equitable treatment in terms of compensation.

Employee appraisal means evaluation of the individual with respect to his or her performance on the job.[9] This is quite different from job evaluation or job appraisal, which will be described later. In one instance the job is being evaluated relative to other jobs and in the other, individual employees are being evaluated.

Appraisal Methods.   There are a number of different approaches to employee evaluation or appraisal. The four basic approaches are (1) Comparative-ranking or grading methods, (2) Person-to-person comparison method, (3) Rating-scale method, and (4) Check-list method or factor-comparison rating plan.

Whatever approach is taken, it is important that employee appraisal be performed in a systematic manner. The purpose of a formal rating system is to reduce to objective terms the performance, experience, and qualities of employees in comparison with the requirements indicated in the job description document. To accomplish this, job knowledge and job skill, desire to keep abreast, quality of work accuracy, thoroughness, quantity of work, initiative, ability to work with others, mental alertness, dependability in response to direction, neatness and work appearance, attendance, and punctuality must be taken into consideration.

Benefits of Systematic Appraisal.   A formal evaluation system helps the manager consider these factors more carefully, and reduces the chances that personal biases will distort the rating. It also forces the manager to observe and

---

[9]Wendell French, *The Personnel Management Process: Human Resources Administration.* Boston: Houghton Mifflin Company, 1970, p. 287.

scrutinize the work of subordinates not only from the point of view of how well the employee is performing the job, but also from the standpoint of what can be done to improve performance. An employee's poor performance and failure to improve may be due in part to the manager's own inadequate supervision. A formal appraisal may serve to evaluate and improve the manager's own performance.

A formal appraisal system serves another important purpose. Every employee has the right to know how well he or she is doing and what can be done to improve work performance. Most employees want to know what their supervisors think of their work. An employee's desire to know how he or she stands can be interpreted as a need for assurance that he or she has a future in the organization.

Regular appraisals are an important incentive, particularly to the employees of a large organization. Many workers have the feeling that because of the great amount of job specialization, the individual worker's contributions are lost and forgotten. Regular appraisals provide some assurance that the employee is not overlooked by his or her superior and the entire organization.

Regular appraisals of all subordinates should be made by the manager at least once a year, normally considered a sufficiently long period of time. If an employee has just started in a new and more responsible position, it is advisable to make an appraisal within three to six months. In some organizations, appraisals are made according to the dates each employee started; in others, all appraisals are made once or twice a year on fixed dates. As time goes on, periodic appraisals become an important influence upon an employee's morale. They help reaffirm the manager's interest in the employee and in his or her continuous development and improvement.

Appraisal Forms.   In order to facilitate and simplify the appraisal process, most health care organizations find it advisable to use performance appraisal forms. These forms stipulate various elements for appraisal in objective terms, and they typically are known as "performance appraisal" forms. For most managers, therefore, performance appraisal becomes primarily a matter of filling out these rating forms, which may have been prepared by the Personnel Department in conjunction with other elements of administration.

Although there are numerous types of forms for the evaluation or appraisal of workers, most include factors that serve as criteria for measuring job performance, intelligence, and personality. The following are some of the factors most frequently included in performance rating forms for workers: supervision required, attitude, conduct, cooperation, job knowledge, safety, housekeeping, adaptability, absenteeism, tardiness, judgment, quantity of work, and quality of performance. For each factor, the manager may be provided with a number of choices or degrees of achievement. Some appraisal forms will use a series of descriptive sentences, phrases, or adjectives to assist the manager in understanding how to judge or evaluate the various rating factors. Many forms are of a "check the box" type and are relatively easy to complete.

Figure 9–6 represents a simple but effective form that provides for evaluation based upon observable behavior on the job. The employee as well as the supervisor has the opportunity to comment on the evaluation.

Appraisal Problems.   In spite of the apparent simplicity of performance appraisal forms, a manager is often faced with a number of problems when completing them. First of all, not all raters will agree on the interpretation of what is meant by terms such as "excellent," "good," "average," or "poor." Descriptive phrases or sentences added to each of these adjectives are helpful in choosing the level that most adequately describes the employee.

Another problem is that one manager's appraisal of employees may be more severe than another's. Some managers do not give low ratings because they are afraid of antagonizing their subordinates, who will then be less cooperative. Low ratings may also negatively reflect on the manager's own ability, and suggest that employees have not been motivated to improve themselves.

The manager should also be cognizant of the problem of allowing a rating of one factor to influence the rating of the other factors. If he or she feels that an employee is weak in one area (production, for instance), the manager may tend to rate the employee low on most factors. One way to avoid this "halo" effect is to rate all employees on the same factor at one time before starting on the next.

It is important to let the employee see his or her rating (note the place for the employee's signature on the sample form in Figure 9–6) and to discuss it. One of the principal advantages of appraisal is the feedback it gives the employee. Promotions, demotions, and adjustments in compensation (except for cost of living or tenure increases) should be based on the objective information obtained from the employee appraisal. The reader may find the American Hospital Association's publication "Employee performance appraisal programs: Guidelines for their development and implementation" useful in applying this process in health care facilities.

TRAINING AND DEVELOPMENT

A second basic part of maintaining the human resources of the health care organization is training — *the process of changing the behavior of employees through an organized procedure by which they learn the skills, abilities, and attitudes needed by them to perform their work in the best manner.* In most health care organizations, the training effort can be broken down into staff training and line training. Staff training departments are usually found in large hospitals and governmental health care organizations. They incorporate a staff of educators who are responsible for in-service education. This function, if not designated as a separate departmental function, is often assigned to the Personnel Department. Another method of fulfilling this training and development need is that of cooperative effort, in which a group of organizations such as hospitals may share training staff responsibilities with each other, add the specialists needed to do the job, and split the cost equally. Line training responsibilities are typically assigned to individual department heads.

In addition to training as a part of maintaining the human resources of the health care organization, special mention of management development should also be made. Essentially, management development is a program that increases the capacities of managers to achieve desired objectives.[10]

---

[10] Michael J. Jucius, *Personnel Management.* Homewood, Illinois: Richard D. Irwin, Inc., 1971, p. 265.

HOSPITAL AND MEDICAL CENTER EMPLOYEE_____CLOCK NO. _____

PERFORMANCE APPRAISAL REPORT (PAR) DEPARTMENT_____JOB TITLE_____

3 mo._____ 6 mo._____ 1 yr._____ 2 yr._____ 3 yr._____ 4 yr._____

Annual_____ Termination_____ Other_____
(Specify)

APPRAISAL DATE_____ **SHIFT**_____ **DATE HIRED**_____

INSTRUCTIONS:
1. Indicate your judgment by circling the figure which best describes the employee's attribute. Give your rating with utmost care and thought.
2. Use your own judgment. Disregard general impressions. Concentrate on one factor at a time.
3. Remember instances that are typical of the individual's work and way of acting.

1. Job knowledge—skill Desire to keep abreast	Outstandingly good; thorough, systematic 10 9	Above average; needs minimal guidance 8 7	Adequate for Classifications: Routine guidance 6 5	Needs more than average guidance 4 3	Inadequate; requires excessive guidance 2 1
2. Quality of work accuracy, thoroughness	Excellent, regardless of circumstances 10 9	High quality, little checking required 8 7	Good, consistent with standards. Routine checking required 6 5	Variable; needs careful checking 4 3	Below standard for Classification 2 1
3. Quantity of work	Energetic, highly productive 10 9	Usually does more than required 8 7	Good, average output 6 5	Does only required minimum 4 3	Insufficient, needs prodding 2 1
4. Initiative	Actively seeks more responsibility, resourceful 10 9	Constructive thinker. Suggests improvements 8 7	Usually able to go ahead. Occasional new ideas 6 5	Merely conforms 4 3	Resists change or new ideas 2 1
5. Ability to work with others	Pleasant, willing, excellent rapport 10 9	Courteous, helpful to team members 8 7	Usually works well with others 6 5	Tends to be uncooperative 4 3	Unsatisfactory, frequent clashes 2 1
6. Mental alertness	Outstanding. Grasps new ideas and duties immediately 10 9	Learns quickly; needs little instruction 8 7	Normal ability in learning new methods 6 5	Needs repeated detailed instructions 4 3	Comprehension questionable. Often seems confused 2 1
7. Dependability in response to direction	Easily directed, profits from constructive comments 10 9	Accepts direction readily. Seldom needs reminders 8 7	Usually follows instructions, needs some repetition 6 5	Resentful, makes excuses 4 3	Disregards directions; does not admit mistakes; blames others 2 1
8. Neatness, work appearance	Fastidious in appearance and work 10 9	Neat, well-groomed, work area tidy 8 7	Appearance and work satisfactory 6 5	Often careless about grooming and work area 4 3	Untidy about person and work area 2 1
9. Attendance punctuality	Exemplary record 10 9	Rarely absent or tardy 8 7	Usually present and on time 6 5	Frequently late, often absent 4 3	Unreliable 2 1

Capacity for advancement (Check one) ☐ Very promising ☐ Able to handle more than present job ☐ Appropriately classified. Gaining experience ☐ Limited to present job ☐ Negative

SUPERVISOR'S COMMENTS:_____   **EMPLOYEE'S COMMENTS:**_____

SUPERVISOR'S SIGNATURE_____   **EMPLOYEE'S SIGNATURE**_____
DATE_____   **DEPARTMENT HEAD**_____

Figure 9-6 Performance Appraisal Report. (Source: Mount Carmel Mercy Hospital and Medical Center, Detroit, Michigan. Used by permission.)

The key elements of management development are
1. An analysis of the managerial requirements of the organization.
2. An evaluation of the present management skills and capabilities.
3. Planning a development program based on differences in steps 1 and 2.
4. Carrying out the program.
5. Evaluating the results of the program on a continuing basis and relating it back to the first four steps.

There are a number of approaches to management development; they may be either internal or external to the organization. Internally, job rotation has been used to some extent to develop assistant level administrative personnel. Periodic seminars or "management clubs" for exchanging ideas and viewpoints can be helpful. Other approaches, including the coaching of lower level managers by top managers, inclusion on important committees, and such simple things as required reading lists, have all been used with some degree of success.

Externally, university and association development programs, if well conceived, well developed, and well taught may be the most effective management development programs available. There are a few universities which offer such programs specifically for health administrators. There are many seminars and conferences which managers can attend in order to develop themselves further. The American College of Hospital Administrators uses this approach in their extensive program for developing health administrators. [11]

WAGE AND SALARY ADMINISTRATION

One of the most important aspects of maintaining a suitable work force is the administration of wages and salaries (employee income), which make up 60 to 70 per cent of the hospital's total operating costs. It affects not only the ability of the organization to attract suitable employees but also employee attitude and morale.

The commonly accepted definition of *wage and salary administration* includes those activities concerned with the establishment and implementation of suitable policies and practices dealing with employee compensation (activities such as development and maintenance of wage structures and job evaluations).

Basic Concepts. There are a number of basic concepts of wage and salary administration which are important to the manager. The reader should keep in mind that the wage and salary program is administered by the Personnel Department in most organizations, but the individual manager is responsible for the application of the program in his or her department. Dale S. Beach has provided these generally accepted guidelines for a wage and salary program:[12]

---

[11]The reader who is interested in training and development should see Donald L. Kirkpatrick, *A Practical Guide for Supervisory Training and Development.* Reading, Mass.: Addison-Wesley Publishing Co., 1971; and Robert A. Desatnick, *A Concise Guide to Management Development.* New York: The American Management Association, 1970.

[12]Beach, op. cit. p. 652. Adapted by permission of the publisher. Copyright 1975.

A. There should be a definite plan in which differences in pay for jobs are based upon variation in job requirements, such as skill, effort, responsibility, and job conditions.

B. The general level of wages and salaries should be reasonable, in line with that prevailing in other health care organizations and industries in the area.

C. The plan should carefully distinguish between jobs and employees. A job carries a certain wage rate, and a person is assigned to fill it at that rate.

D. Equal pay for equal work is particularly relevant at this time in that the Sixth U.S. Circuit Court of Appeals has reversed a lower court decision and has ordered a retrial in the case involving back wages for nurses aides. Previously, the hospital had paid a differential to orderlies because of the "extra duties" imposed upon them. The Sixth Circuit cited the Fourth Circuit's opinion in Brennan versus Prince William Hospitals 503 F.2d 282 (1974), and the court reiterated the principles of that case: "Higher pay is not related to extra duties when one or more of the following circumstances exist: (1) Some male employees receive higher pay without doing the extra work. (2) Female employees also perform extra duties of equal skilled effort and responsibility. (3) Qualified female employees are not given the opportunity to do the extra work. (4) The supposed extra duties do not in fact exist. (5) The extra task assumes a minimal amount of time and is of peripheral importance. (6) Third persons who do the extra task as their primary job are paid less than the male employees in question."

The Federal Equal Pay Act of June 10, 1963 specifically outlines its aim as that of eliminating differentials in pay based solely on sex. It makes it unlawful for an employer to pay wages at a rate less than the rate at which he pays wages to employees of the opposite sex in established jobs which require equal skill, effort, and responsibility, and which are performed under similar working conditions. Thus skill, effort, responsibility, and working conditions are tests of equality of the rates.

In regard to equal pay, the standards have been set so that the target is only wage differentials based upon sex. Differentials based upon any other factor are not affected. Discrimination unrelated to wages is also not affected; in this respect, the coverage is so much more restricted than the general ban on sex discrimination in Title VII of the Civil Rights Act.

E. An equitable means should be adopted for recognizing individual differences in ability and contribution.

F. There should be a clearly established procedure for hearing and adjusting wage complaints. This may be integrated with the regular grievance procedure, if one exists.

G. The employees, and the union if there is one, should be adequately informed about the procedures used to establish wage rates. Every employee should be informed of his own position in the wage and salary structure. Secrecy in wage matters should not be used as a cover-up for a haphazard and unreasonable wage program.

There are a number of advantages for both employees and managers in a well-structured and well administered wage and salary program. For example,

1. Employees are paid according to the requirements of their jobs. Skilled employees receive more compensation than unskilled employees; thus inequities tend to be reduced.

2. The chance for favoritism to creep into the assigning of wage rates is greatly minimized.

3. Job sequences and lines of promotion are established where applicable.

4. Employee morale and motivation are increased because the wage program is explainable and based upon facts. Employees know where they stand.
5. The manager can systematically plan for and control his labor costs.
6. It aids in attracting qualified employees by paying adequately for all jobs.
7. In dealing with a union, the manager can explain the basis for his wage program because it is based upon systematic analysis of job and wage facts.

   Job Evaluation. Job evaluation, a formalized system for determining the relative value of all jobs within an organization, is the heart of a wage and salary administration program. All jobs are analyzed and a written job description, which includes the specifications for that job, is prepared. At this point, the jobs are rated through the use of a job evaluation plan with the objective of establishing either specific rates of pay for each job or a specific wage range for each job. A complete discussion of the various approaches to job evaluation is beyond the scope of this text; however, most of the personnel administration textbooks available have a comprehensive treatment of this important subject.

   There are four major methods of job evaluation commonly used. Figure 9–7 summarizes these methods. The two least complex of these four methods, the ranking and the job classification method, are the dominant ones used in the health care field. The other two systems, the point system and the factor comparison system, are quite complex, and although they are used occasionally in certain hospitals, they are more commonly used in the larger corporate organizations in American business.

   The system utilized in the health care field that possesses the greatest advantages is the job classification method. We will briefly describe how this method works. It is important to note that one of the major objectives of any job evaluation system is to establish a relationship of internal and external consistency. All jobs within an organization should relate to one another in such a way that persons with the more responsible jobs are paid more. Responsibility is one of the major factors used in determining the relative value of one job as compared to another. Some of the other factors are the skill that is necessary on a job, the degree of physical effort necessary, and the working conditions. If jobs within a health care organization are evaluated properly, and if it is found that certain jobs which have a higher valuation than others receive significantly lower pay, then internal inconsistency exists. This can be corrected with a consistent pay system wherein persons with jobs that are rated higher are paid more than those with jobs that have a lower rating. While this may appear to be oversimplified, its importance cannot be overstressed. External consistency refers to the comparison of the jobs within a health care organization with similar jobs in other health care organizations or in other industries.

   In the job classification method of job evaluation, various jobs that share a similar amount of responsibility, skill, effort, and working conditions are grouped together. After the jobs are grouped into clusters, each cluster is ranked one with another. As a result, job clusters are ranked in such a way that the more difficult jobs are rated higher than the less difficult jobs. A typical large hospital, for example, may have as many as 200 or 300 different jobs. It would be quite a task to rank 300 jobs in terms of value to the organization. However, if these 200 or 300 jobs were examined and those jobs that were similar were placed in various clusters, one might come up with 15, 20, or even 25

NONQUANTITATIVE MEASURES		QUANTITATIVE EVALUATION MEASURES	
Ranking Method	Job Classification Method	Factor-Comparison Method	Point Method
The job analysis. A narrative description of the job with the duties, responsibilities, degree of difficulty, and required qualifications clearly brought out.		The job analysis. A narrative statement of duties and qualifications. In addition, the job is broken down into the important compensable factors, such as required experience and training, mental effort, and physical effort. The amount to which each factor is present in the job is indicated by a short narrative statement.	
Method of Relating Jobs	Method of Relating Jobs	Method of Relating Jobs	Method of Relating Jobs
Jobs are ranked in their order of relative difficulty or value to the hospital, and grade levels are sometimes defined after the jobs have been ranked.	Jobs are allocated to grade levels which are defined arbitrarily prior to evaluating jobs.	Jobs are related by factorial comparison. The factors used are assumed to be fundamental to all jobs and of universal application. The point values are set after analysis of jobs from existing rates of key jobs, and degrees of each factor are expressed by sample jobs.	Jobs are related by factorial analysis. A restricted number of fairly specific factors is selected for application to a limited number of types of work. The point values are predetermined before analysis of jobs and are decided arbitrarily, and the degree of each factor is expressed by a definition.

Figure 9-7 Comparison of the four basic methods of job evaluation. (Source: Job Evaluation Systems, United States Department of Labor.)

different clusters. Within each cluster, the jobs would be considered of approximately equal value to the organization. Then, the task would be to rank each cluster, which constitutes the essence of the job classification method of job evaluation. After the job clusters have been ranked, a wage rate or range is established for each.[13]

For example, salary pay grade 1 may be composed of similar unskilled jobs that are utilitarian in nature. There may be as few as one or two jobs, or as many as 50 in a given pay grade. The important point is that they must be relatively similar in nature and in value to the organization. Where a particular job is classified is not affected by the quality of the individual employee's performance within the organization; nor is such a placement affected by the quantity of work being performed. The important point is that *jobs* are slotted, not individual employees. It is also important that in each salary grade the slotted jobs are similar enough to warrant common treatment; the same class description would apply and identical salary ranges would be applied to all.

Not everyone within any particular salary grade will receive the same wage or salary. Persons who have been with the organization for a short period of time may be at the lower part of the pay range, while others, through merit and seniority, may be near the top of the pay range. Generally, new employees will start at the beginning salary of their pay grade. In some instances, if a particular employee has a good deal of experience, he may be started toward the middle of the pay range. Specific policies for each health care organization should be established as a basis for slotting new employees and for determining a method of progression of existing employees within each salary grade.

The health care organization should make it very clear to all supervisors and department heads that employees do not receive pay beyond the salary range established for any particular job classification. The only way that employees can receive additional money would be through (a) an across-the-board pay increase to all employees, (b) promotion to a higher salary grade, or (c) if a particular job was reclassified into a higher pay grade because of increased importance of the job to the health care facility.

Any job classification plan must be flexible. Future jobs will have to be evaluated and appropriately classified. In all cases, department heads should be up to date on what is going on and be involved in the steps along the way. There will be a strong tendency for department heads to evaluate people rather than jobs. The Personnel Department occupies a key role in the coordination of all these activities.

There will be many pressures to create exceptions to the program. Strong department heads in radiology and pathology may expect their medical secretaries to be paid more than medical secretaries in other departments. If a hospital has one morgue attendant who would be difficult to replace, they may not want to lose him. If he receives a good offer from another hospital, they may pressure the Personnel Department to rank the job higher. Pleas may be made

---

[13]For a complete listing of all the specific steps to be taken in establishing a job classification method of job evaluation for any health care facility, see: Thomas R. O'Donovan, "Establishing a wage and salary program, Part I and Part II. *Hospital Management, 19*:49, May, 1964, and :54, June, 1964.

to add to the importance of the job of the diener because of the degree of adverseness in working conditions, in order to move the job up one or two pay grades.

All job evaluation systems are subject to this kind of pressure, because jobs have to be filled. The Personnel Department cannot maintain equity and consistency alone; it is also the responsibility of the manager. A sound wage and salary administration program is extremely important. The role of area practice and competitive forces must be reckoned with. The pay range that the hospital presents must be high enough to attract capable candidates for positions. In the determination of the relative value of certain jobs, the political issues sometimes play a more important role than the objective factors involved in careful evaluation.

The handling of the mechanics for establishing a sound wage and salary program offers numerous opportunities to achieve high morale. The Personnel Department will conduct many interviews throughout the total process. This presents a continuing opportunity to aid the organization in building a cohesive work force. Establishing the job evaluation program is rarely as difficult as administering it over the years. Problems that arise in organization dynamics must be turned into opportunities for ongoing progress in employee-employer relationships. If the health care organization delays in achieving the advantages of a sound wage and salary program, they may find the employees seeking to unionize as a vehicle to force the development of an equitable and consistent (in their eyes) compensation system.

It is also important for the manager to have a basic understanding of the laws affecting compensation. The most important legislation in this regard is the Fair Labor Standards Act (FLSA) of 1938, amended in 1967 to include many health care facilities.[14]

Under the provisions of the FLSA, hospitals have the option of paying overtime to employees for hours worked in excess of 40 in a seven day period or 80 in a 14 day period, assuming the work day is eight hours. No employer whose workers are protected by the minimum wage requirements may discriminate on the basis of sex in the payment of wages for equal work performed. The act also sets a minimum age of 16 years for general employment and 18 years for work declared hazardous by the Secretary of Labor. Minors who are 14 and 15 years of age may be employed outside school hours in certain occupations and under specified conditions. The evaluations, judgments, determinations, and decisions relating to wage and salary administration are subject to review by the Wage and Hour Division of the Department of Labor to determine actual compliance with the law. Official inquiries and follow up investigations can be made arbitrarily or as the result of an employee complaint. Through either or both of these approaches, conformity with FLSA requirements is objectively measured to protect the rights of both employees and employers.

---

[14]Complete copies of the Fair Labor Standards Act are available in the government documents section of most university and public libraries. Individual copies may be obtained from the Superintendent of Documents, Government Printing Office, Washington, D.C. 20402, or at the nearest office of the United States Labor Department's Wage and Hour and Public Contracts Division.

DISCIPLINE

Perhaps no other aspect of the health care organization's relationship with its employees is less understood than that of discipline. Most people immediately associate discipline with the negative concept of punishment. In a broader sense, it also has a positive meaning which managers should strive to develop. This involves "the creation of an attitude among employees and a climate which causes employees to willingly conform to established rules and regulations because they realize that they are in their best interest as well as the best interest of the organization."[15]

An effective disciplinary program should be based on due process. The due process concept as applied to personnel management is based upon four assumptions which are usually upheld by arbitrators: (1) the rules must be reasonable, (2) the employee must have a clear understanding of what is expected of him, (3) the employer has a right to have a well-disciplined, cooperative work force, and (4) the employer has the authority to administer discipline when rules are violated.[16]

To effectively carry out the concept of due process, a formal disciplinary procedure must be established. There is no best way to set up the procedure. However, it should contain certain provisions:[17]

1. Penalties should be based on specific charges. The charges and their underlying reasons should be clear and provable (for example incompetence, negligence, and misconduct).
2. All employees must be treated consistently under the disciplinary program; however, the background and circumstances of each case should be considered separately.
3. Penalties should be progressive and related to the offense. Typical penalties in progressive order of severity are
   a. Simple oral warning.
   b. Oral warning that is noted in the person's employment record.
   c. Written warning noted in employment record.
   d. Suspension from the job, usually varying from one day to two weeks.
   e. Discharge.
4. Rules and regulations must be reasonable.
5. There must be a provision for appeal.

The inclusion of these provisions does not guarantee that a disciplinary program will meet its objectives; however these provisions can go a long way toward ensuring a positive approach to discipline in the health care facility.

HEALTH AND SAFETY

A final aspect of maintaining a work force is ensuring on the job health and safety. Health care facilities, like other types of organizations, have long been concerned with the health and safety of their employees in the work set-

---

[15] Beach, op. cit. p. 600.
[16] Joseph B. Wallenberger, "Acceptable work rules and penalties, a company guide." *Personnel*, 50:27, July, 1963.
[17] This procedure is adapted from Beach, op. cit. pp. 606–609.

ting, although the real impetus for formal health and safety programs came with the enactment of Workmen's Compensation laws in the various states, mostly between 1910 and 1925. These laws hold employers financially responsible for work injuries without regard to who is at fault.

More recently, the enactment of the Occupational Safety and Health Act of 1970 (OSHA) promises to have far-reaching implications for all types of organizations. The law has the objective of ensuring a safe and healthy place for people to work in. It invests the Secretary of Labor with the authority and obligation to promulgate mandatory federal safety and health standards.

Section 5(a) of the Act provides that every employer must furnish each employee with a place to work which is free from recognized hazards causing or likely to cause death or serious physical harm.

Section 5(b) provides that each employee must comply with occupational safety and health standards and all rules and orders issued under the Act.

No one can argue with the objectives of this Act. However, there is much skepticism among managers as to whether or not the objectives are realistically attainable. The Act is in its early stages but the staff required to operate this arm of the Federal government has already grown considerably. Not only has the staff increased in size but also its budget requirements are expanding at record rates. In 1976, the President asked Congress for 263.4 million dollars to fund the Federal Occupational Safety and Health efforts in three executive departments and one independent agency during fiscal year 1977. The Department of Labor's Occupational Safety and Health Administration is slated to receive 128 million dollars, an increase of nearly 12 million dollars over funds approved by Congress in 1975. Within the Department of Health, Education, and Welfare, the National Institute for Occupational Safety and Health would receive 37.1 million dollars; the Interior Department's Mining Enforcement and Safety Administration has requested 90.1 million. The budget provides 6.2 million dollars for funding the Occupational Safety and Health Review Commission during fiscal year 1977. A total of 135 new positions have been requested for fiscal year 1977, which will bring the total OSHA employment to 2306 by the end of the year. It is clear at this point, that a major new impetus for employers to be conerned about health and safety of their workers is contained in OSHA.

PENSION PROGRAMS

Although pension programs are only one of a variety of employee benefit programs provided for most health care employees, they have particular significance, since they demonstrate the progressive involvement of the Federal government in hospital employer-employee relations.

The Employee Retirement Income Security Act (ERISA) was enacted by the Congress in 1974. This piece of social legislation has caused a basic philosophical change regarding pension plans to take place over the last several years. The basic change in the pension commitment is from the old theory of pension as a reward for long and faithful service or as a device to hold personnel, to the new theory that pensions are not a gratuity but a contractual right, a form of deferred wages, and a right of employment such as workmen's compensation and unemployment compensation. We now have this legislation because people had lost benefits that they thought they were entitled to when pension plans were terminated for reasons such as plant closings, bankruptcies, sale or merger of business, or voluntary termination.

Given the fact that ERISA is a fact of life and is now having and will in the future have far reaching effects upon the management of employee benefit programs, effective management of the legal requirements of the act will provide new opportunities for employee communications that will help health care organizations maintain their employees.

The stated policy of the ERISA is to protect the interests of the participants in employee benefit plans (both pension and welfare) and their beneficiaries. To carry out this policy, Congress has set up specific requirements for the preparation and filing of reports, for making available planned documents, and for making statements of individual employees' benefits available. In terms of day-to-day work and expense these requirements may be quite troublesome at first, but properly applied they can open doors to improve employer-employee relations.

After taking a good look at all of the new requirements for the communication of benefits to employees, it becomes evident that pension laws shift the burden from the employees (who had to ask for information prior to the law) to the employers (who now must provide this information as a matter of course).

Seen in this light, the best approach (and the most practical) may be to view the new requirements as an investment toward attracting and retaining good employees.

SUMMARY

Staffing serves the important purpose of bringing the health care organization to life by manning it with competent people through selection and development of personnel. The responsibility for staffing rests with the line manager, although he is usually assisted in this by the Personnel Department. This activity has been broken down into two parts in this chapter: obtaining employees and maintaining employees.

The beginning point in obtaining employees is manpower planning—the determination of manpower requirements for the present and the future and the means of meeting those requirements.

The basic component in maintaining employees is a complete understanding of their performance in the organization. This understanding comes from employee appraisal, and can lead to rational training and development of employees, in addition to equitable compensation.

DISCUSSION QUESTIONS

1. Describe in general terms the activities that are characteristic of manpower acquisition and maintenance.

2. What are the responsibilities of the Personnel Department in the health care organization?

3. What are the responsibilities of the individual managers throughout the health care organization in regard to manpower acquisition and maintenance?

4. Describe the five steps necessary to sound manpower planning.

5. What are the relationships between job analysis, job description, and job specification?

6. What information is usually obtained in the selection of new employees? How?

7. What role does employee appraisal play in maintaining the personnel of a health care organization? How is this appraisal carried out?

8. What is a wage and salary program? Why is it important in the modern health care organization?

9. What is job evaluation? What is its relationship to a wage and salary program?

10. Describe how legislation since 1964 has affected the staffing process.

11. What is the relationship between staffing and the organizing process discussed in the two previous chapters?

INCIDENTS

1. PERSONAL DAYS

The King General Hospital is located in a large urban area and has 415 beds. One of the personnel policies of this hospital is that employees are given two weeks vacation per year and are allowed one day per month of sick day accumulation. For those employees who need some personal time off, such as to close on a mortgage on a new home, or any other reasonable purpose for needing a personal day off, four days per year are allowed for personal business, provided that staffing conditions permit it, and also provided that the employee gives at least three working days' notice to his supervisor in making the request.

One day a nurse makes an appointment to see the administrator because she feels she has been mistreated. She had called early one morning last week to notify her department that she would be an hour late because her car wouldn't start. Approximately an hour later, she found that her car was not going to be repaired until later in the day, and she called again, asking that a personal day be charged against her because there was no way for her to get to the hospital. She was informed that no disciplinary action would be taken for her being absent (because this certainly was a valid reason), but because she did not give the three days' personal leave notice she would be docked a day's pay. The employee had 18 days of accumulated vacation, had four personal days in her "bank," had not taken a sick day for the past year, and had a good work record during the 10 years she had worked for the hospital.

The administrator referred the problem to the Department of Nursing Service and notified the Personnel Director. Nursing Service upheld the docking of the day's pay because this is the policy that they apply around-the-clock to all members of the Department of Nursing Service. After an investigation by the Personnel Director, it was found that in some of the other departments, especially the smaller ones, a great deal of leniency in matters such as this was extended by certain department heads. In fact, investigation found many examples where employees who called in unable to attend work because of car problems and similar reasons were instead granted a sick or vacation day in order to circumvent the three-day notice for personal days as stated in the Personnel Policies Manual of the hospital.

A. As administrator of the hospital, what would you do about this inconsistency in the application of personnel policies? Should the personal day policy be changed?

B. What would you do about the specific request of the nurse?

C. Comment on the following statement: "An organization should have sound and fair personnel policies because employees have a right to them, and we should treat all employees in as dignified and fair a way as possible."

2. FALSIFIED APPLICATION

Frieda Schumacher has been employed by Green Valley Hospital (450 beds) as an R.N. for five years. She first came to the hospital seven years ago, when she was 20, and was enrolled in the hospital's diploma program. After her graduation at the top of her class two years later, she began working on the afternoon shift. During that period her performance was excellent. She is a very likeable, warm, compassionate, and respected individual who is willing to go out of her way to assist employees and patients. Frieda is married, has a two year old child, is a dedicated mother, and is active in church and community affairs. When she took a three month maternity leave for the birth of her child, her supervisor found out how valuable she really was.

Last week, she was one of three nurses being considered for promotion to supervisor. In comparison with the others, she was by far the most qualified. As a matter of policy, all individuals being considered for promotion to positions of major responsibility (Frieda would be responsible for controlling narcotics kept at the nursing station), are subject to a routine background investigation by an outside agency.

Much to the Director's dismay, the investigation revealed that when Frieda was 17 years old she was arrested for and convicted on drunken driving, a felony charge. When Frieda applied for admission to the diploma program and completed the employment application, she did not reveal this fact. In fact, on the employment form a specific question asked if the applicant had ever been convicted of a felony. Frieda had responded "No." Furthermore, in bold print on the application blank is the statement that "intentional falsification of information on this application will result in immediate discharge."

When the Director of Nursing Service confronted Frieda with this particular fact, she stated, "I was a young girl at the time and was in the company of several other teenagers. We were foolish and didn't think; I certainly would never do anything like that again."

A. What action should be taken against Frieda? Should she be discharged? Should she be promoted?

B. Is the policy that "falsification of information on an application form will result in immediate discharge" valid?

C. If Frieda was not discharged, what impact would it have? Would it establish an unwanted precedent?

This Chapter Contains:

Chapter 10

LABOR RELATIONS

"The problems and challenges of labor relations in the health services industry have only recently gained widespread attention among those engaged in the delivery of health care. Health administrators, faced with demands for more and higher quality health services and, simultaneously, with closer examination of medical costs by consumers and government, have become particularly concerned about the threat of union organization and collective bargaining."

(Metzger and Pointer)[1]

INTRODUCTION

In the preceding statement, Norman Metzger and Dennis Pointer make a very important observation—labor relations has only recently been given widespread attention by health care organizations and those who manage them. This leads to obvious questions of why labor relations is important and why attention is now being given to the area by health care administrators.

IMPORTANCE OF LABOR RELATIONS

In the previous chapter we discussed the fact that manpower is one of the most important of all input resources for health care organizations. They are labor intensive—a substantial portion of their expenditures is in the form of payroll. With the increasing ratio of employees to patients, attention should be given to staffing patterns, compensation rates, and employee utilization, since they eventually affect the efficiency of health care organizations. Furthermore, attention should be given to the subject of unionization and the impact that unions can have on these areas.

"Labor relations" is a generic term used to describe the employer-employee relationship, yet it is often used to convey the relationship between the employer and union. The nature of that relationship is important because unions representing health care organization employees negotiate with the administration concerning such matters of employment as wages, promotional policies, discipline procedures, work assignments, and seniority provisions. Consequently, the nature of the employer-union relationship and specific agreements between the two can ultimately affect the organization's costs and its utilization of employees, as well as influence the decision-making, planning, executing, and controlling processes.

---

[1] Norman Metzger and Dennis D. Pointer, *Labor-Management Relations in the Health Services Industry.* Washington, D.C.: The Science and Health Publications, Inc., 1972, p. xix.

Whatever term is used by those involved — unionization, collective bargaining, professional association representation — dealing with an employees' organization is one of the many emotionally involved issues facing the health care industry and its organizations in the 1970's. "All unions are bad." Are they? "All unions are good." Are they? Some will contend that there is nothing worse than a union. Others argue that unions are the only reason for employers being semi-humane and responsible in dealing with their employees. Granted, unionization is an explosive issue, perhaps more so than any other, but that does not mean it should be ignored. In fact, it is because hostility can occur, damage can be done, and destructiveness can result from confrontation that it is important to examine the subject of labor relations, specifically unionization.

RECENT ATTENTION

The primary factor that has caused health care organizations to direct their attention to the area of labor relations is the recent rise of unionization in the health care industry. In comparison with the industrial sector, unionization efforts in health care organizations are fairly recent phenomena. Although scattered instances are reported by Metzger and Pointer as early as 1919,[2] it has only been during the past decade that the unionization of health care organizations increased substantially. Among the various unions and associations representing employees are the 1199 locals of the National Hospital and Nursing Home Employees' Union, the Teamsters, the American Federation of State, County and Municipal Employees Union, The American Nurses' Association, and various state Nurses' Associations.

There are three main reasons why health care organizations were relatively non-union. First, they attracted little attention on the part of national labor organizations, which were directing most of their time and effort toward industry. Second, professionalism and the humanitarian nature of health care organizations led many employees to conclude that it was not appropriate to join a union. Third, the unique reimbursement methods for most health care facilities, based largely on costs, do not incorporate the "profit concept" nor the corollary concept of earnings being available for distribution to employees.

The acceleration of the unionization movement in health care organizations can be attributed to several factors. First, the civil rights movement of the late 1960's focused in part on the conditions of unskilled and semi-skilled minority workers who frequently are employed in lower level positions in health care facilities. As a result, the anti-discrimination and employee recognition groups found reasons for joining forces. Second, because of the changing values and viewpoints in our society, professional employees, such as nurses, are no longer averse to joining a union. Third, hospitalization coverage through federal programs such as Medicare and Medicaid pay for the care of many who were formerly indigent patients. The notion of health care facilities absorbing the cost of charity care is now largely limited as a rationale for paying low wages. Fourth, health care employees no longer accept "psychic" income

---

[2] *Ibid.* p. 22.

derived from working for a humanitarian organization in lieu of adequate wages. Finally, poor personnel practices and poor first line supervision in health care facilities have caused employees to seek a vehicle for rectification.

Consequently, union activity has grown in the health care industry. For example, in 1973 almost 1200 (17 per cent) of the nation's hospitals had at least one collective bargaining agreement.[3] The number of unionized facilities doubled between 1967 and 1973, and it has been predicted that the number will still increase substantially during the next few years. Therefore, several conclusions can be drawn. First, unions are here to stay. Second, organizing efforts are increasing in intensity. Third, unions often improve employment conditions for their members and function as an environmental force with which health care organizations, and their managers, must cope. Finally, inept management can cause employees to seek representation or it can create a post-union entry atmosphere of hostility. For these reasons, health care organizations have begun to give serious attention to the area of labor relations.

Because of the importance of labor relations, we will focus on five specific subject areas in this chapter: (1) the history of the labor movement, (2) federal labor legislation as it applies to health care organizations, (3) reasons why employees join unions, (4) the role of the administration in labor relations, and (5) collective bargaining.

HISTORY OF UNIONIZATION

The history of unionization in the United States can be divided into two eras—before 1930 and after 1930.

PRE-1930 ERA

Union activity in the United States can be traced back to 1792. In that year, a local union was formed by the journeymen cordwainers (shoemakers) of Philadelphia.[4] There was, however, relatively little union activity until the late 1800's. Even though the Knights of Labor were organized by a group of tailors in Philadelphia in 1869, 11 years later there were only 9000 craft members.[5] In 1886 the American Federation of Labor (AFL) was formed by Samuel Gompers; by 1898 it had 278,000 members, and shortly after the turn of the century it absorbed the Knights of Labor.[6] Other examples are the formation of the Industry Workers of the World in 1905 and the establishment of the United States Department of Labor in 1913.[7]

From the 1800's until the 1930's union membership rose gradually. It

---

[3] Donald F. Phillips, "Taft-Hartley: What to expect." *Hospitals, 48*:18b, July 1, 1974.

[4] Lloyd G. Reynolds, *Labor Economics and Labor Relations.* Englewood Cliffs, New Jersey: Prentice-Hall, 1970, p. 323.

[5] Arthur A. Sloane and Fred Witney, *Labor Relations.* Englewood Cliffs, New Jersey: Prentice-Hall, 1972, p. 57.

[6] *Ibid.* p. 61.

[7] Wendell French, *The Personnel Management Process.* Boston: Houghton Mifflin, 1974, pp. 729–730.

increased in prosperity and decreased in depression. Membership was generally confined to the skilled crafts and it was not until 1930 to 1947 that the basic manufacturing industries were organized.

There were a number of reasons for the lack of organizational success during the pre-1930 era: the government's pro-business attitude, employee fear, and the attitude of employers. It is the latter which gave rise to the bloody Carnegie Steel (1892) and Pullman (1894) strikes. Sloane and Witney describe the prevailing management attitude of the time:

> . . . organized labor still had a severe problem to contend with in the 1890's: the deep desire of the nation's industrialists, now themselves strongly centralized in this era of trusts and other forms of consolidations, to regain unilateral control of employee affairs. Not since the 1870's had the forces of management been as determined, as formidable, or as successful in opposing unionism.[8]

Viewing Figure 10–1, it is possible to note that there were less than a million union members at the turn of the century. By 1910, membership had risen to 2 million and peaked at 5.1 million in 1920.

---

[8] Sloane and Witney, op. cit. p. 61.

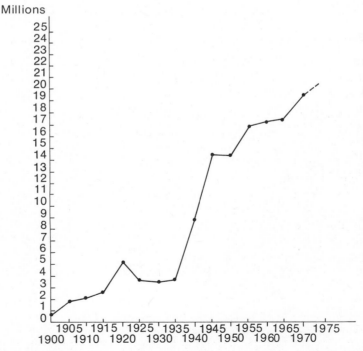

Figure 10–1 Total United States union membership. (Source: Data for 1900–1925, includes Canadian union membership, which approximates 6 per cent of the total; *Handbook of Labor Statistics*, Bureau of Labor Statistics, United States Department of Labor, 1950. Data for 1930–1970 excludes Canadian union membership. *Handbook of Labor Statistics*, Bureau of Labor Statistics, U. S. Department of Labor, 1973.

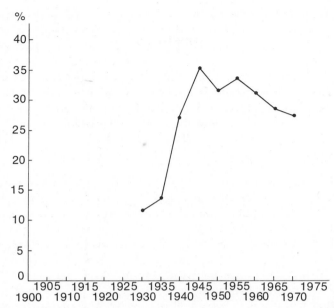

Figure 10-2 United States union membership as a percentage of the nonagricultural work force. (Source: *Handbook of Labor Statistics*, Bureau of Labor Statistics, U. S. Department of Labor, 1973.)

POST-1930 ERA

Beginning with the early 1930's, union membership in the United States increased substantially. The sharp increase in the total number of union members and this membership as a percentage of the non-agricultural work force can be noted by viewing Figures 10-1 and 10-2 respectively. The primary impetus giving rise to the unionization movement was the federal legislation passed during the 1930's.

During the early portion of this period basic industries such as steel, autos, and rubber were unionized. Starting in the 1950's, union membership as a percentage of the non-agricultural work force began to decline. This was due to the fact that most union organizing occurred in the manufacturing industries and focused on blue collar workers. Since 1950, the percentage of blue collar workers in the total labor force has declined and that of service employees has grown. As a result, many unions began to organize service employees, and in the late 1960's organization efforts began to be directed toward health care employees.

FEDERAL LABOR LEGISLATION

Generally, it can be said that prior to the 1930's the federal government had an anti-union attitude. However, during the depression an attitude shift occurred. The Protestant Ethic, factory systems, and common law employer property rights philosophies were being influenced by the Social Ethic. The depression contributed to an emerging awareness on the part of Congress that it had responsibilities to the working class that needed to be fulfilled. That change of attitude was expressed in 1932 by passage of the Norris-LaGuardia Act. The Wagner Act was enacted in 1935, and was amended by the Taft-Hartley Act in 1947.

Although there had been other federal labor legislation before this time (Railway Labor Act of 1926) and after (Landrum-Griffin Act of 1959), our attention will focus on The Norris-LaGuardia, Wagner, and Taft-Hartley Acts, along with the 1974 hospital amendment to the Taft-Hartley Act.

NORRIS-LAGUARDIA ACT (1932)

The Norris-LaGuardia Act of 1932, officially called The Anti-Injunction Act,[9] was a landmark piece of legislation. It represented a major change in Congress' attitude toward labor-management relations. The basic philosophy of the Act was that the individual employee was at a disadvantage when bargaining with his employer. Consequently, to enable the individual employee ". . . to protect his freedom of labor . . ." the Act prohibited two employer practices: the first was the "Yellow Dog" contract; the second was a restriction of the use of court injunctions in labor disputes.

Yellow Dog Contracts.   Section 3 of the Norris-LaGuardia Act specified that an employer could not require a contract to state that the employee would not join a union when doing so would be a breach of the contract and cause for termination of employment. The Act stated that such contracts are ". . . hereby declared to be contrary to the public policy of The United States (and) shall not be enforceable in any court. . . ."[10]

Injunctions.   The Norris-LaGuardia Act also focused on the use of federal court injunctions in labor disputes. Prior to 1932, preliminary court injunctions were frequently issued to forestall union activity (such as a strike) that could cause "irreparable" harm while the court examined the merits of the situation. Employers had often been able to seek and obtain court injunctions enjoining union activity from courts sympathetic to employers. Though activities such as strikes or picketing were not illegal, failure to comply with court injunctions was. The Norris-LaGuardia Act did not require employers to recognize or bargain with unions. They could take action to prevent unionization; however, they were stripped of unmeritorious legal protection (injunction).

THE WAGNER ACT OF 1935

The second major piece of legislation dealing with labor-management relations to be enacted in the 1930's was the Wagner Act.[11] Officially it is called the National Labor Relations Act of 1935. Many have charged that the Wagner Act

---

[9] For a copy of the Norris-LaGuardia Act see *The Statutes at Large of The United States of America* from December 1931 to March 1933. Washington, D.C.: U.S. Government Printing Office, *48*:70, Part I.

[10] *Ibid.* p. 70.

[11] For a copy of the Wagner Act see *The Statutes of the United States of America* from January 1935 to June 1936. Washington, D.C.: U.S. Government Printing Office, *49*:449, Part I.

Table 10–1 Employer Unfair Labor Practices (and Examples)[13]

1. *To interfere with, restrain, or coerce employees in the exercise of their rights to organize*
   (threaten employees with loss of job if they vote for a union)

   (grant wage increases deliberately timed to discourage employees from joining a union)

2. *To dominate or interfere with the affairs of a union*
   (take an active part in the affairs of a union, such as a nurse supervisor actively participating in a nurses' association representing R.N.'s)

   (show favoritism to one union over another in an organization attempt)

3. *To discriminate in regard to hiring, tenure, or any employment condition for the purpose of encouraging or discouraging membership in any union organization*
   (discharge an employee if he urges others to join a union)

   (demote an employee for union activity)

4. *To discriminate against or discharge an employee because he has filed charges or given testimony under this Act.*
   (discriminate against, fire, or demote an employee because he gave testimony to NLRB officials or filed charges against the employer with the NLRB)

5. *To refuse to bargain collectively with representatives of the employees; that is, "bargain in good faith"*
   (refuse to provide financial data, if requested by the union, when the health care organization pleads losses)

   (refuse to bargain about a "mandatory" subject such as hours and wages)

   (refuse to meet with union representatives duly appointed by a certified bargaining unit)

   (take unilateral action in current conditions of employment without notifying the union, such as subcontracting x-ray or food service activities if those employees are currently unionized)

was one-sided in favor of unions. Their point is substantiated by noting that the philosophy or intent of the Wagner Act was to
1. rectify the existing employer-employee power imbalance by creating conditions which would enable unions to grow in strength,
2. restrain certain forms of employer coercion, and
3. enable unionism to spread throughout all sectors of the economy.[12]

The principle of the Wagner Act was that employees had the right to organize and to bargain collectively, free from employer influence or coercion. To implement this, employer unfair labor practices were itemized and the National Labor Relations Board (NLRB) was established to oversee issues involving union recognition and collective bargaining.

Employer Unfair Labor Practices. Section 8 of the Wagner Act itemizes five employer unfair labor practices which are covered by current labor law. These practices are presented in summary form in Table 10–1, with examples. Basically, they indicate how an employer *cannot* behave toward employees who want to unionize and, in addition, specify how the employer should deal with

---

[12] Reynolds, op. cit. pp. 462–463.
[13] The following are drawn from National Labor Relations Board, *A Layman's Guide to Basic Law Under the National Labor Relations Act.* Washington, D.C.: U.S. Government Printing Office, 1971, pp. 19–29.

the certified representative (union) of the employees. In other words, bargain in good faith.

National Labor Relations Board. The second major provision of the Wagner Act dealt with the establishment of the National Labor Relations Board (NLRB). The Board was responsible for overseeing two specific areas: (1) union recognition and (2) the means for settling unfair labor practices. Concerning the first function the position of the Wagner Act was that the representative of a majority of the employees for an appropriate bargaining unit shall be the exclusive agent for the purpose of collective bargaining. Basically, if a majority of the employees wished to have a union representative they could impose their will upon the minority. The NLRB was to conduct elections for representatives and certify the exclusive agent for a particular bargaining unit.

Prior to the Wagner Act, unions often had to strike to force employers to recognize them as the employee's bargaining agent. With the Wagner Act, that situation changed. At the request of the employees, the board would hold an election and if a majority wanted a particular union to represent them, that union became their exclusive bargaining agent. Furthermore, the employer had to bargain in good faith with that agent.

The second function of the NLRB concerned unfair labor practices by employers. If it was found that an employer unfair labor practice had occurred, the NLRB could seek remedy through the courts. Although the Act did not make an unfair labor practice a crime or permit penalties or fines for violation, "the teeth in the Wagner Act became apparent only when the courts began to uphold NLRB orders instructing employers to reinstate with back pay, employees who had been discharged in violation of the Act."[14]

As can be noted by the employer unfair labor practices listed in Table 10–1, as of 1935 constraints never before imposed had to be followed by employers. Restrictions on labor's behavior were minimal. In terms of the Act, its purposes were accomplished. In fact, the balance of power had swung so far in favor of labor that Congress passed the Taft-Hartley Act in 1947 to rectify the situation.

TAFT-HARTLEY ACT OF 1947

In passing the Wagner Act in 1935, Congress' intent was to provide a legal environment which would enable unions to grow in size and strength and to remedy the one-sided power balance favoring the employer. This was accomplished during the following decade. In fact, unions lost some of their public favor in the years immediately after World War II. With the changeover to peacetime production, rising prices, and pent up consumer demand, unions struck as never before.[15] Many people felt that the pendulum of power had swung all the way from employer to union and that a balance of power was necessary.

---

[14] Edwin F. Beal, Edward D. Wickersham, and Philip Kienast, *The Practice of Collective Bargaining*. Homewood, Illinois: Richard D. Irwin, 1972, p. 163.
[15] Sloane and Witney, op. cit. pp. 76–77.

In 1947, the Taft-Hartley Act, officially titled The Labor Management Relations Act of 1947,[16] amended the Wagner Act of 1935. Its purpose was

> ... to define and protect the rights of employees and employer, to encourage collective bargaining, and to eliminate certain practices on the part of labor and management that are harmful to the general welfare.[17]

The major provisions of the Taft-Hartley Act concerned changes in the structure of the NLRB, protection of employee rights, enumeration of *union* unfair labor practices, legislative prescriptions for certain bargaining procedures, and procedures for handling national emergencies.[18] We will examine each of these provisions next.

National Labor Relations Board.   The National Labor Relations Board was split into two segments. The first was the general counsel, which had responsibility for investigating and prosecuting. The second segment was the five man board, which was responsible for hearing cases. The purpose of this structural change was to separate the prosecuting of cases from the judging of them.

Employee Protection.   Another major change was that the Taft-Hartley Act afforded protection not only to workers who wished to organize but also to workers who did not. When a "substantial" number of employees wish to have a recognition election (30 per cent of the unit), the NLRB will conduct one. If a majority of the employees do not want the union to represent them, section 9,c,3 prohibits any union from petitioning for another representative election for one year. Therefore, employees and employers will not be harassed. Similarly, with a majority vote, employees can exercise their right to decertify a union that is currently representing them (section 9e).

Union Unfair Labor Practices.   The major provision of the 1947 Taft-Hartley Act was the enumeration of union unfair labor practices. Just as the employer unfair labor practices specified in the 1935 Wagner Act restrained an employer's actions, the union unfair labor practices restrained the actions of labor organizations, thus bringing about a closer balance of power. The union unfair labor practices contained in section 8b of the Act are presented in summarized form in Table 10–2 along with examples.

Bargaining Procedures.   Other provisions of the 1947 Act specified that (1) handbilling, unless threatening, was not an unfair labor practice; (2) a 60 day notice of contract termination or modification must be given to the other party; (3) supervisors could not be part of a bargaining unit; (4) guards and professional employees could not be mixed with other employees in a bargaining unit unless the professional employees concurred.

The Taft-Hartley Act contained other provisions such as the 80 day cooling off period in national emergency disputes during which there could be no strike. It was further amended by the 1959 Landrum-Griffin Act, formally

---

[16] For a copy of the Taft-Hartley Act see *United States Statutes at Large* 1947, Washington, D.C.: U.S. Government Printing Office, 1948, *61*:136, Part I.

[17] National Labor Relations Board, op. cit. p. 1.

[18] Beal, Wickersham, and Kienast, op. cit. pp. 163–169.

Table 10-2   Union Unfair Labor Practices (and Examples)[19]

---

1. *To restrain or coerce employees in the exercise of their right to join or not to join a union except when an agreement is made by the employer and union that a condition of employment will be joining the union (called a union security clause authorizing a "union shop")*
   (picket as a mass and physically bar other employees from entering a health care facility)

   (act violently toward non-union employees)

   (threaten employees for not supporting union activities)

2. *To cause an employer to discriminate against an employee other than for non-payment of dues or initiation fees*
   (cause an employer to discriminate against an employee for anti-union activity)

   (force the employer to hire only workers "satisfactory" to the union)

3. *To refuse to bargain with an employer in "good faith"*
   (insist on negotiating illegal provisions such as the administration's prerogative to appoint supervisors)

   (refuse to meet with the employer's representative)

   (terminate an existing contract or strike without the appropriate notice)

4. *To engage, induce, encourage, threaten, or coerce any individual to engage in strikes, refusal to work, or boycott where the objective is to*
   (a) force or require any employer or self-employed person to recognize or join any labor organization or employer organization
   (b) force or require an employer or self-employed person to cease using the products of or doing business with another person, or force any other employer to recognize or bargain with the union unless it has been certified by the NLRB
   (c) force an employer to apply pressure to another employer to recognize a union. Examples are: picketing a hospital so that it will apply pressure on a subcontractor (Food Service, Maintenance, Emergency Department) to recognize a union, or forcing an employer to only do business with others, such as suppliers, who have a union, or picketing by another union for recognition when a different one is already certified

5. *To charge excessive or discriminatory membership fees*
   (charge a higher initiation fee to employees who did not join the union until after a union-security agreement [union shop] is in force)

6. *To cause an employer to give payment for services not performed (featherbedding)*
   (force an employer to add people to the payroll when they are not needed)

   (force payment to employees who provide no services)

---

known as The Labor-Management Reporting and Disclosure Act of 1959. While the Landrum-Griffin Act primarily addressed itself to internal union affairs, such as elections of officers, and provided safeguards for union members, Title VII added a seventh unfair union practice dealing with the picketing of an employer for recognition of a second union when one union has been certified by the NLRB.

The impact of the Taft-Hartley Act was substantial. Unlike the Wagner Act, it specified that the NLRB could issue cease and desist orders and could go to court to enjoin activities relative to a complaint (section 10e). Although the

---

[19] The following are drawn from National Labor Relations Board, op. cit. pp. 29–44.

Act was essentially remedial, it did provide for fines and imprisonment for specific acts such as interfering with the performance of an NLRB board member's duties.[20]

1974 NONPROFIT HOSPITAL AMENDMENTS TO THE TAFT-HARTLEY ACT[21]

The Taft-Hartley Act of 1947 specifically excluded from its definition of an employer ". . . any corporation or association operating a hospital, if no part of the net earnings inures to the benefit of any private sharholder or individual. . ." (section 2,2). Since any governmental organization (federal, state, or local) including hospitals was also excluded, only those health care institutions run for profit fell under the provisions of the Act. Furthermore, it is important to note that the NLRB was granted authority to specify standards for determining if an organization (employer) affected interstate commerce. The standard applied to long-term-care facilities run for profit was $100,000 in revenue per year, and a $250,000 revenue per year standard was applied to hospitals run for profit.[22] Before the 1974 amendment, nonprofit hospitals did not fall within the coverage of the Taft-Hartley Act and the NLRB did not have jurisdiction. State laws, however, did apply.

On August 25, 1974, Public Law 93–360, the Nonprofit Hospital Amendments to the Taft-Hartley Act became effective.[23] The amendments delete the "nonprofit hospital exclusion" of the 1947 Act and as a result, nonprofit health care organizations now fall within the scope of the National Labor Relations Act. Health care organizations, as well as unions, must comply with the recognition, election, and unfair labor practice provisions of the Act. In terms of the Act, health care organizations

> . . . shall include any hospital, convalesce hospital, health maintenance organization, health clinic, nursing home, extended care facility, or any other institution devoted to the care of sick, infirm or aged persons [2(2) (b) (14)].

The General Counsel of the NLRB, in his memorandum of interpretation,[24] which considers the Act and legislative history, has concluded, in the absence of a court decision to the contrary, that the definition of health service delivery concerns both inpatient or outpatient care. Spas, diet clinics, and muscle-building organizations do not fall within the definition of health care organizations. The 1974 amendment did make special unique provisions for health care organizations in the areas of (1) contract notices, (2) notification

---

[20] Ibid. p. 5.

[21] The material in this section is adapted from: Jonathon S. Rakich, "The impact of the 1974 Taft-Hartley Amendment on health care facilities," Business Law Review, 7:4, December, 1974. Used by permission of the publisher.

[22] National Labor Relations Board, op. cit. p. 46.

[23] For a copy of the "Nonprofit Hospital Amendments to the Taft-Hartley Act" see P L 93–360, 94th Congress, S. 3203, July 26, 1974.

[24] For a copy of the guidelines issued by the General Counsel of the National Labor Relations Board for use by Board Regional Offices in unfair labor practice cases arising under the 1974 Nonprofit Hospital Amendments to the Taft-Hartley Act see Labor Relations Reporter, 86:371, August 26, 1974.

preceding a strike, (3) conciliation of labor disputes, and (4) individuals with religious convictions.[25]

Contract Notices.   Since health care organizations provide unique and essential services for patients, the amendment requires a 90 day, versus a 60 day, notification to the other party to modify an existing contract and a 60 day notice to the Federal Mediation and Conciliation Service (FMCS) and the applicable state agency. If a breakdown occurs when bargaining for an initial contract following certification and recognition, a 30 day notice must be given to the FMCS and the appropriate state agency before a strike can be called. The purpose of these provisions is to provide a longer period of time for the parties to reach an agreement, plan for a work stoppage, and enable the FMCS to provide assistance.

Strike Notice.   Another exception for health care organizations is the strike notice. Specifically, the union must give at least ten days' notice to the employer and the FMCS preceding a work stoppage, which cannot occur before the end of the 90 day notice of a desire to change an existing contract. In the case of bargaining for an initial contract after recognition, the notice cannot be given until the end of the 30 day notice of an impasse. The purpose of the strike notice is to allow the health care organizations to discharge or transfer their patients, or otherwise plan for the continuity of their care. However, it was not intended that the organization would use this period to stockpile supplies or bring in large numbers of supervisory employees.

Conciliation of Labor Disputes.   Section 213 provides that if, in the opinion of the Director of FMCS, ". . . a threatened strike or lockout affecting a health care institution will . . . substantially interrupt the delivery of health care in the locality concerned . . ." he can appoint an impartial board of inquiry to help resolve the issue. The Act specifies various time constraints for the appointment of the board, the investigation, and the reporting during which the employer and union must maintain the status quo unless they both agree to a change. This enables the FMCS to enter into the discussions and help resolve issues involving health care organizations before they break down totally.

Individuals with Religious Convictions.   PL 93–360 added to Title 1 section 19. It exempts health care organization employees from paying dues to a union, even if there is a union shop agreement, when the individual ". . . is a member of and adheres to established and traditional tenets or teachings of a bona fide religion, body, or sect which has historically held religious conscientious objections to joining or financially supporting labor organizations. . . ." The individual must, however, donate an equivalent amount to a charitable fund approved by the institution and the labor organization. The purpose of this provision was to recognize the unique position of the employees in many of the nation's religiously affiliated hospitals and long-term-care facilities.

Impact of Taft-Hartley on Health Care Organizations.   Some writers, along with Phillips,[26] have argued that the net effect of the 1974 Hospital Amendments to the Taft-Hartley Act will be a significant increase in union ac-

---

[25] For further discussion of these provisions see Dennis D. Pointer and Norman Metzger, *The National Labor Relations Act.* New York: Spectrum Publications, 1975, Chapters 4 and 8.

[26] Phillips, op. cit. p. 18b.

tivity. Schwartz states that strikes and work stoppages not perceived as being legitimate by the public will boomerang.[27] Others, including Metzger,[28] contend that consistency of law will now occur because the former exemption of nonprofit hospitals caused inconsistent and sometimes disadvantageous decisions by states. Finally, Pointer contends that coverage will lead to an explosion of union activity in the health care industry similar to those of the auto and steel industries during the 1930's as well as the possible erosion of the administration's managerial flexibility.[29] Regardless of the various predictions, some of the minimum effects of the amendment will be

1. the requirement that nonprofit, nongovernmental health care facilities and union organizations will have to function within the new constraint of existing statutory and administrative laws with which the former party has had little experience;
2. specific recognitional, renewal, and strike notices will be required;
3. the costs incurred by facilities in connection with recognition elections will increase since recognition efforts now have the benefit of law;
4. consistency, for better or worse, will result, since the federal coverage of nonprofit, nongovernmental hospitals will pre-empt previous state coverage;
5. finally, confusion will be present for an undetermined period of time until the NLRB and the courts settle questions raised by the general counsel of the NLRB as to what constitutes a strike notice, what constitutes a bona fide religion, and the definition of common bargaining units.

Probably that which has the most important impact on both health care organizations and unions is the fact that both must be cautious of their actions so that unfair labor practices do not occur. For instance, two relatively innocent examples can be used to demonstrate how easily an employer unfair labor practice can occur. The first is organizational support in terms of release time, tuition, or registration fees for nurse supervisors attending a nurse association meeting (conference) when that association also acts as a bargaining agent for the facility's R.N.'s.[30] The second involves an organization's general no solicitation/distribution policy that would also infringe on the employee's right to unionize.[31]

REASONS WHY EMPLOYEES JOIN UNIONS

With an acquaintance of the union movement and federal laws, we will next examine the reasons employees join unions (there are a number of them). Most of the reasons can be related to the desire for need fulfillment. Representative of employees' needs are such items as compensation, job security,

---

[27] Harry Schwartz, "Public will not tolerate disruptive strikes." *Hospitals, 49*:46, November 16, 1975.

[28] Norman Metzger, "Labor relations." *Hospitals, 44*:80, March 16, 1970.

[29] Dennis Dale Pointer, "How the 1974 Taft-Hartley Amendments will affect health care facilities." *Hospital Progress, 55*:68, Part 1, October, 1974.

[30] William J. Emanuel, "Hospital policy: Professional associations as unions," *Hospital Progress, 57*:53, January, 1976.

[31] Richard L. Epstein, "Guide to NLRB rules on solicitation and distribution." *Hospitals, 49*:44, August 16, 1975.

Table 10-3 Summary of Various Reasons Why Employees Join Unions

CONDITIONS OF EMPLOYMENT
Concern for matters such as
1. Pay and consistency among pay grades
2. Fringe benefits—such as hospitalization insurance, holidays, vacation time, bereavement time
3. Physical and nonphysical working conditions, such as work breaks, clean-up time, safety conditions, parking, and security
4. Hours of employment
5. The scheduling of employees and the assignment of specific work activities

DEMOCRACY IN THE WORK SETTING
Concern with unfair, unwarranted, or inconsistent administrative actions often restrained by the establishment of procedures for
1. Layoffs, typically based on a seniority basis
2. Promotions, typically based on a combination of seniority and qualifications
3. Dismissal of employees
4. Disciplining of employees

CONTENT OF EMPLOYMENT
Concern for the atmosphere of employment such as
1. Desire to be treated as a human being
2. The ability to have some control over one's job and the factors that affect it
3. Being kept informed and listened to through the establishment of communication channels often accomplished with a grievance procedure
4. Desire to apply pressure to force supervision to be humanistic toward employees

affiliation with co-workers, plus the feeling that one's abilities are being used and the individual's point of view is being heard by the administration. These causal factors can be grouped into three major categories. The first category concerns the conditions of employment; the second relates to democracy in the work setting where unwarranted or inconsistent administrative actions can be restrained; the third involves the content of employment.

Table 10-3 provides a list summarizing these various factors. An understanding of them is important, since administrative inattention to these factors can lead to dissatisfaction on the part of employees. *When that occurs, a union is often perceived as a vehicle to bring dissatisfactions to the attention of the administrator and to rectify them.*

CONDITIONS OF EMPLOYMENT

Metzger and Pointer indicate that wages, fringe benefits, and inconsistency among job classifications are major factors encouraging employees to unionize.[32] Although low in the past, wages in health care organizations today are fairly competitive with many industrial organizations. Fringe benefits such as holidays, hospitalization insurance, and life insurance are a related concern of employees. Furthermore, physical and nonphysical working conditions such as coffee breaks, clean-up time, the hours of employment, and scheduling are conditions of employment which are important to employees.

---

[32] Metzger and Pointer, op. cit. p. 120.

DEMOCRACY OF THE WORK SETTING

Democracy in the work setting deals with another group of factors that can cause employees to organize. This refers specifically to the establishment of procedures that would restrain unfair, unwarranted, or inconsistent administrative action. Matters of concern would be the determination of which employees are to be "laid off," procedures for promotion, discipline, employee appraisal, compensation increases, and so forth. Elkin, for example, indicates that a union contract generally establishes the criteria and procedures that lead to this democracy in the work setting.[33] Administrative abuses in promotion, discipline, and so on will influence employees to seek a means of protecting themselves, or at least force the administration to establish procedures and criteria which will be consistently applied.

CONTENT OF EMPLOYMENT

The content of employment refers to the total atmosphere of employment. Most people want to be treated as individuals rather than just as another resource and want to know that supervisors have a sincere concern for their welfare. Furthermore, the ability to expand one's job responsibility, engage in valid participation in decision-making about one's job, and assume additional responsibilities are things most employees seek from their job.

The desire to be kept informed and also to be heard is very important to employees. Lack of information creates a vacuum leading to uncertainty and can be perceived as threatening. By the same token, the inability to be heard can be very frustrating. One of the functions of a union is to provide a grievance procedure that is basically an upward channel of communication. Imberman states that the administration's ignorance of what is troubling the employees is a major oversight. Attention should be given to listening and trying to "understand the hourly employee who, after all, makes the decision about unions."[34] We can include the desire to have our abilities utilized, the sense of accomplishment resulting from our job, and the ability to have some control over the parameters of one's job as other factors that may induce employees to join unions.[35]

The health care organization manager should be aware of the many factors that cause employee dissatisfaction. We have discussed some of them, but there are others. The perceptive manager will be cognizant of the factors of concern inherent in the conditions of work, democracy of the work setting, and content of the employment categories. Early rectification of deficiencies will do much to strengthen the employer-employee relationship. If they are not rectified, employees may seek a union in order to eliminate the dissatisfactions they have. As a result, the role of the administration is to promote a positive and constructive employer-employee relationship.

---

[33] Randyl D. Elkin, "Negotiating and administering a union contract." *Hospital Progress*, 56:41, January, 1975.

[34] A. A. Imberman, "Communication an effective weapon against unionization." *Hospital Progress*, 54:56, December, 1973.

[35] Donald F. Phillips, "New demands of nurses—Part 1." *Hospitals*, 48:31, August 16, 1974.

ROLE OF THE ADMINISTRATION IN LABOR RELATIONS

The administration of the health care organization is responsible for the delivery of high quality patient care at a reasonable cost, in addition to being responsive to the needs and concerns of its personnel and the community. The American Hospital Association (AHA) in its "Statement on Employee Relations for Health Care Institutions" indicates that for these responsibilities to be discharged, requisite activities are (1) the establishment of a progressive employee relations program, and (2) the establishment of personnel policies that contribute positively to the welfare of the employed and the employer. In Table 10–4, seven specific principles to be used as guides for the development of personnel policies and practices by health care organizations are presented. Table 10–5 presents 14 personnel policies and practices suggested by the AHA.

CONCERNS

Traditionally, the areas of concern for health care organizations vis-a-vis unions have been the following: (1) that costs would increase owing to higher wages, (2) that strikes could occur, and (3) that administrative flexibility relative to employee utilization could be lost. Although these concerns are real, blind obedience to a strategy of "fighting" unionization can cause more harm than good. The spirit of the AHA statement can be summarized in the word "positive." Another word could be "constructive." Careful examination of the statement's principles would indicate that its basic message is to be sensitive to the needs of employees. Administrative sensitivity along with constructive policies and procedures can do much to decrease the number of reasons why employees might wish to unionize. This does not, however, imply that the man-

---

Table 10–4   American Hospital Association Principles of Employee Relations

The employee relations policies and practices of the health care institution should be guided by principles that are fair and equitable in uniform application to all individuals and that will contribute positively to the welfare of both the employing institution and the employee. These principles include the provision of

Job security and job satisfaction

Opportunities for self-expression

Potential for growth in knowledge and skills, with defined means for career mobility and promotion

Promotion and implementation of affirmative action programs and practices and the use of appropriate techniques for nondiscriminatory selection and placement

Recognition for accomplishment

An awareness that it is people, at all levels of the organization, that make it work

Compensation programs covering wages, salaries, and supplemental benefits guided by and commensurate with community standards

---

(Source: Reprinted by permission. From "Statement on employee relations for health care institutions," developed by the American Hospital Association, 1975.)

Table 10–5 American Hospital Association Employee Relations
Policies and Practices

Establishment of a centrally administered and professionally managed personnel program

Publication and uniform administration of personnel policies and practices

Evaluation of job applicants on the basis of their potential and qualifications consistent with job requirements

Programs to enable the full use of the individual's potentialities through orientation, training, upgrading, and other personnel development techniques

Training and continuing development of all levels of management

Fair and equitable compensation that is competitive with community standards for wages and benefits

Maintenance of equitable compensation levels among all employees, with compensation based on skill, ability, and job requirements

Maintenance of a sound performance evaluation system to assist in employee development, with equitable standards uniformly applied to all employees

Provisions for channels of communication within the institution to involve individuals in the development of policies and procedures affecting them and to facilitate and encourage constructive responses and suggestions concerning work to be performed.

Establishment of a standard procedure of due process whereby employee complaints or grievances can be heard promptly and effectively resolved

Maintenance of reasonable working schedules compatible with patient care requirements

Working conditions that are conducive to efficient work habits and that provide safety and comfort

An employee health program

Periodic review and updating of personnel policies and practices, which may include use of professional consultation in evaluation of the total program

Where collective bargaining agreements are in effect, every effort should be made to ensure that the agreements do not interfere with good employee relations policies and practices as described above.

(Source: Reprinted by permission. From "Statement on employee relations for health care institutions," developed by the American Hospital Association, 1975.)

ager's responsibility to the patients and the community can be ignored. There must be a balance between responsibilities and concerns.

Concerning the increased costs that could result from unionization, it can be argued that the cost issue is really neutral. If the organization truly seeks to be responsible to its personnel, remuneration in the form of wages, salaries, and fringe benefits will be commensurate with community standards. It should be pointed out that if compensation is perceived by the employees as being appropriate, they probably will not view the formation of a union as a vehicle to rectify low compensation.

Similarly, the concern about strikes or work stoppages carries economic as well as patient welfare costs. Work stoppages in particular are unacceptable to the traditional constituents of the health care organizations: patients, governing authorities, and society. Therefore, the benefits derived from thwarting the use of this union leverage device by resisting unions may be too costly in terms of patient care responsibilities.

The final concern to which costs can be assigned is administrative flexibility. Typically, the most lasting effect of a union is to lessen the administration's prerogative to manage. Since the health care industry is characterized by rapid growth in size and employment, due to the increasing demand for service, the need for its organizations to effectively and efficiently utilize their personnel is of paramount importance. Health care organizations are labor intensive. Any influence that constrains the utilization of employees could have a serious impact on the area of costs and efficiency. Therefore, the issue of administrative control over personnel should provide an adequate rationale, from a cost-benefit analysis of all issues, for implementing a "positive" employee relations program.

THE ISSUE

The American Hospital Association cites poor first line supervision, poorly developed personnel policies and practices, and the breakdown of some facets of employer-employee relations, such as communication and consistency, as some of the major reasons that induce health care employees to unionize. Furthermore, the Association states that it is both easier and wiser to take affirmative and constructive steps in advance of a union organization campaign.

The issue relative to labor relations is that positive and constructive policies and practices should be implemented regardless of whether or not the organization is unionized. If a union is not present, these practices will fulfill the organization's responsibility toward its personnel as well as create an atmosphere in which employees will find no useful value in unionizing. If the facility is about to be or already is unionized, these same policies and practices would not only be required but also greatly diminish the built-in hostility between the two negotiating parties. A positive and constructive attitude toward employee relations makes good management sense in and of itself. The implementation of that attitude requires that certain steps be taken. They will be presented next.

CONSTRUCTIVE STEPS[36]

The development of the personnel functional area is a must and should involve all aspects covering employment and working conditions. Appropriate job descriptions and job specifications should be developed so that the employees are aware of what is expected of them. The wage and benefit levels should be updated in order to provide internal consistency between job classifications as well as to be externally competitive. The appraisal method should be as objective as possible and based on criteria deemed important with respect to job performance. Policies that affect the employees should be communicated to them, particularly those related to promotion, discipline, and job tenure.

---

[36] The material in this section is adapted from Jonathon S. Rakich, "Hospital unionization: Causes and effects." Used by permission from the quarterly journal of the American College of Hospital Administrators. *Hospital Administration, 18*:14, Winter, 1973.

Attention should be given to the activities characteristic of manpower acquisition and maintenance that were presented in the previous chapter.

The establishment of an upward communication channel through which employee grievances can be examined and acted upon without jeopardy is important. The ability to feel that the administration is interested in legitimate complaints serves to decrease employee dissatisfaction. The upward communication channel serves two functions. First, it can make the administration aware of the many irritants related to the job which may seem insignificant but are, nevertheless, important to employees. Second, it can serve as a vehicle for releasing employee frustration. A positive administrative response would be to institute a formal grievance procedure through the Personnel Office. The right of appeal would eliminate arbitrary decisions by supervisors. The procedure must be perceived by the employees as being legitimate. Employee participation in instituting the grievance procedure would serve to promote legitimacy and to instill in them a sense of commitment to making it work. When possible, rectifying issues such as job conditions, parking, and work schedules helps to minimize employee dissatisfaction.

The establishment and use of a downward communication channel serves to keep the employees informed. The dissemination of information dealing with policies and procedures reduces the possibility of grapevine distortion. Often a simple ignorance of the facts or the reasons behind management's actions can lead to employee counteractions. Full communication with employees is a good management practice. The communication method may be informal or formalized through the use of internal media such as a house organ, employee handbook, or administrative announcements.

If a sense of importance to the successful operation of the organization can be fostered in the employees, their identification with their jobs (and therefore, the organization) can be enhanced. Involved employees are committed employees. Reminders to the employee indicating his importance to the total team effort can be constructive. They are particularly helpful to those who occupy the lower occupational or status positions. An employee newsletter, for example, honoring outstanding or long service employees instills a sense of pride.

Procedures designed to give the individual some control over his or her job environment, when possible, are a secondary step toward fostering commitment to the organization. Promotion based on merit, but with seniority consideration, enables the individual to exercise some control over his destiny. Furthermore, progressive policies directed toward upgrading employees' skill levels are a good investment. In-service training programs, professional conference support, or leaves of absence for education may enable employees to upgrade their occupational status and circumvent blocked promotional paths.

Finally, the supervisor's role is important in setting the total employee relations tone. A people-oriented supervisor is often much more effective than one who is primarily task oriented. The supervisor's awareness of employee feelings, the treatment of subordinates as individuals, and a sincere concern for their job-related problems will remove many intangible causal factors related to unionization. It is recognized that many of the health care organization's operational areas, such as the nursing service, may require close and detailed supervision. The employee's ability to participate, or at least to express an opinion, in job-related decisions is important. Very possibly, the assignment of some work activities may be left to the work group's discretion, provided it does not interfere with the effective operation of the unit.

COLLECTIVE BARGAINING

Up to this point, we have described the impact a union can have on a health care organization, the federal labor laws that define the manner in which the employer and union must interact, some of the reasons why employees may desire to join a union, and various positive labor relations steps the organization may consider. However, even if a sound labor relations program is developed, there remains the likelihood that employees may unionize. Should that be the case, the administration of the organization and representatives of the union will engage in collective bargaining.

The activities of union recognition, negotiation, and contract administration are characteristic of collective bargaining. The mutually agreed upon provisions of an employer-union contract establish the parameters, and both the administration of the health care organization and the employees' representative (union) must conduct themselves in accordance with the responsibilities each must fulfill. As a result, the contract obtained through collective bargaining becomes the *"private law"* for both parties. Federal and state laws do not prescribe specific contract provisions, but they do set limits on how recognition can be accomplished, indicate the range of behavior and bargaining issues that are legal, and mandate that both parties bargain fairly and in good faith.

RECOGNITION

Collective bargaining begins when a union has been recognized. Recognition can be accomplished in several ways. First, the employees may simply ask the administration to recognize a union as their representative. Since most employers do not voluntarily recognize a union, the second method—recognition with governmental intervention—is generally followed.

Since nongovernmental health care organizations, both profit and nonprofit, fall within the scope of federal labor legislation, both the employer and the employees must follow certain recognition procedures prescribed by the Taft-Hartley Act and subsequent amendments. If requested, a certification election will be held by the NLRB, provided a substantial number of employees (generally 30 per cent) wish to have a recognition election. If a majority of the employees vote for the union, the NLRB will certify the representative (union), and the organization must bargain with it. If a majority of the employees do not vote for the union, then another election cannot be held by any union for one year.

Furthermore, in addition to defining the recognition procedure, federal law specifies that the employer and union may not interfere with the employees' rights to organize by actively taking steps to influence the outcome of the election. (See the employer and union unfair labor practices presented in Tables 10–1 and 10–2.) The law also specifies certain requirements for the establishment of bargaining units. For example, guards and professional employees such as RN's cannot be mixed with nurse's aides and ward assistants, nor can supervisors be part of the union.

NEGOTIATION

Once a union has been certified as the representative of a group of employees, initial negotiations can begin. Generally, much preparation time will be spent by both parties; warm-up meetings may be held; proposals and counter proposals will be made. In the negotiations, the following issues may be discussed:[37] (1) conditions of employment, (2) employee and union security, (3) management rights, (4) discipline and grievance procedure, and (5) contract duration.

Conditions of employment generally concern wages, fringe benefits, health and safety, vacation time, holidays, leaves of absence, and so on. Employee security would relate to the manner in which layoffs, promotions, transfers, bumping, and the like would occur. Generally, seniority is the major criterion.

Union security relates to the union's desire to secure and strengthen its position. The employer may agree to a contract provision stating that all new employees within a class that is represented must join the union after a brief period (generally 30 days). This is known as a union shop. At the minimum, the union may seek to write an agency shop provision into the contract requiring an employee who does not join the union to pay the equivalent of union dues to it. Finally, there may be contract agreement for a check-off provision allowing the employer to deduct union dues from each member's pay for remittance to the union, making the latter's collection much easier.

Management rights may be specified during the negotiation, written into the contract, and be binding until it is mutually agreed to alter those provisions. Examples might cover management's stated prerogative in areas such as requiring that employees work overtime, scheduling, determination of job content, transferring employees, the right to determine who will be hired, and so on.

Generally, the establishment of a grievance procedure will be negotiated and become part of the contract. This procedure consists of a formalized series of steps for resolving contract disputes while the contract is in force. A contract dispute results when either the employer or employees feel that the other party has not lived up to the terms of the contract. Disputes or grievances can range from the transferring of workers to changing the content of the job (if that is part of the contract) to discipline. For example, the contract may specify a series of disciplinary steps which must be followed for certain infractions of behavior. Absenteeism, insubordination, theft, and violence could be some of the many categories of behavior covered. Part of the contract may be a sequence of disciplinary steps such as an oral warning for the first occurrence of the infraction, followed by a written warning for the second infraction, then disciplinary layoff (perhaps one week without pay), and finally, termination. Furthermore, it may be specified that certain categories of infraction may not

---

[37] William F. Glueck, *Personnel: A Diagnostic Approach.* Dallas: Business Publications, Inc., 1974, pp. 582–584.

require the first several disciplinary steps. Physically striking a supervisor may carry a penalty of "up to and including discharge" without the other steps having to be met. If, in this case, an employee feels the procedure has not been followed, he can file a grievance.

The specified procedure for handling the grievance may involve first the supervisor and union steward, then the personnel manager, and finally the administrator meeting with a union official. Should a consensus not be reached on the resolution of the grievance, an arbitrator (a neutral third party) may hear the facts and render a decision, either advisory or binding depending upon the agreement between the employer and union.[38]

Whatever the agreements are between the health care organization and the union, once ratified, they become binding. This contract becomes the "private law" between the two parties. In reaching their agreement, federal legislation places restrictions on how the parties must act toward each other and what can and cannot be part of the contract. For example, once a union has been recognized, the employer must bargain in good faith, as must the union. They must meet with each other's representatives, cannot interfere with the rights of the other, and so on. In addition, the union can request and the employer must bargain about "mandatory" issues. These include issues which would relate to such conditions of employment as pay and working hours. Federal law further stipulates that a union can seek to bargain, although not necessarily reach agreement, about "nonmandatory" issues such as establishing grievance procedure, seniority, discipline, and union security. The employer does not have to bargain about nonmandatory issues and a refusal would not be an employer unfair labor practice. Finally, neither party can negotiate binding "unlawful" terms, such as a union shop wherein the newly hired employee must be a union member before he can be hired, that supervisors be included in a bargaining unit, that the health care organization pressure a sub-contractor to recognize a union, and so on.

IMPASSES

During negotiation, whether it be for an initial contract or the revision of an existing one, an impasse may occur if the parties do not agree. There are several options available to the employer and the union at this time. The union may call a strike, after appropriate notification, and have its employees refuse to work. The purpose of a strike is to place an economic burden on the employer so that he will be encouraged to modify his position. For health care organizations, a strike can be very costly in terms of money and also patient welfare. Picture a situation in which a strike causes a facility to curtail admissions and the occupancy rate falls from 94 per cent to 50 per cent. Since revenues would be sharply curtailed, generally more so than costs can be reduced, financial losses will result.

If a health organization is struck by a union, it has the option of hiring other workers. However, given the large numbers of professionals and the critical interdependence of work effort among the members of the health team in

---

[38] For an example of contract negotiation and the resulting provisions, see Barry W. Singleton, "Negotiating a collective bargaining agreement." *Hospital Progress,* 56:57, 80, October, 1975.

health care organizations, those employees on strike may not be replaceable or the facility may not be able to function without them. If, for example, the nurses walk out, they will not be replaced easily. Or, if the maintenance employees strike, the facility may have difficulty in keeping operations going for an extended period of time. Furthermore, if the employees are legitimately striking because the employer is committing an unfair labor practice, such as refusing to negotiate about a "mandatory" issue like wages or meet with the union representative, the employer must reinstate those striking workers even if it means discharging the replacements. However, if the strike is not one called because the employer is committing an unfair labor practice or if the union is striking illegally and committing an unfair labor practice, the employer is not required to reinstate the striking employees.

Another option available to the employer and the union when an impasse is reached is mediation and conciliation; in such a situation assistance is requested from the state or the Federal Mediation and Conciliation Service. Basically, the mediator (a neutral third party) meets with both parties, attempts to stimulate negotiation, and tries to persuade them to agree on a solution. However, the mediator has no authority other than that of persuasion. Consequently, the impasse could remain. A subsequent option would be arbitration; here both parties agree to abide by the arbitrator's recommendations. However, during contract negotiations the employer and the union generally do not want to give up their authority to a third party. As a result, arbitration is usually used to settle grievances during the life of an existing contract rather than as a method to resolve impasses during contract negotiations.[39]

Regardless of the method, at some point in time an agreement will be reached. That contract will then become the "private law" between the two parties and both must abide by its provisions.

SUMMARY

In recent years, health care organizations have begun to focus attention on the area of labor relations, specifically on unionization. In this chapter we offered reasons why that attention is important, along with some reasons for the increasing trend of unionization in health care organizations. Because of cost and other implications, the administration was encouraged to give attention to the relationship which exists between itself and its employees, since whether or not a health care organization becomes unionized has much to do with the nature of that relationship. Unionization is an emotionally charged and explosive issue. Severe hostility can be enormously destructive. The theme offered by the AHA is summarized as "positive," meaning that the organization should take a positive labor relations posture.

The labor movement during the pre- and post-1930 eras was briefly described in this chapter. It was during the latter period that federal legislation sympathetic to labor was passed. The Wagner Act (1935) and the Taft-Hartley Act (1947), respectively, set forth unfair labor practices for employers and unions. In 1974, the Taft-Hartley Act was amended to include within its

---

[39] Edwin B. Flippo, *Principles of Personnel Management.* New York: McGraw-Hill, 1976, p. 498.

provisions nonprofit health care organizations. The importance of this law lies in the fact that health care organizations and unions must now comply with federal labor law relative to recognition, negotiation, and general conduct. New restrictions are now imposed on both parties. Various reasons why employees join unions were presented, along with a discussion of the administration's role in labor relations. Finally, a brief overview of steps in collective bargaining was presented.

DISCUSSION QUESTIONS

1. Discuss the reasons why health care organizations have begun to focus attention on labor relations, particularly unionization.

2. Discuss why a sound employer-employee relationship is important for health care organizations. Presuming that an unsound relationship leads to unionization, what impact would be expected?

3. a) From the point of view of the employee, what are the pros and cons of joining a union?
   b) What are the pros and cons from the employer's point of view? Can a union be beneficial to the health care organization?
   c) Should health care professionals unionize? Discuss and support your position.

4. Discuss the meaning and give examples of the employer and union unfair labor practices. How do they restrain behavior for both parties?

5. A number of reasons were given as to why employees join unions. Identify and discuss others.

6. It was stated in this chapter that "the issue relative to labor relations is that positive and constructive policies and practices should be implemented regardless of whether a facility is unionized." Do you agree? Why?

INCIDENTS

1. HANDOUTS

Four months ago one of the five hospitals in the urban area in which your hospital is located was unionized. Yesterday, the same union that won recognition at the other hospital and negotiated a contract was passing out literature to the hourly employees of your hospital as they were leaving their jobs at the end of the day. The personnel director became aware of the activity and informed the administrator. They held an immediate impromptu meeting to discuss the various actions that they could take to thwart the unionization effort. Given the information that the recently unionized hospital agreed to a 9 per cent hourly pay increase for its employees (your last pay increase five months ago was 3 per cent), the administrator and personnel director wondered what they should do. The personnel director suggested that he hold meetings with the employees on their various shifts as soon as possible in order to get a "better feel" of the employees' morale and their attitudes. Their thinking had not gone past that.

A. If you were the personnel director, what would you suggest to the administrator?

B. Is there anything that the administration should have done previously?

C. Is it too late?

D. Can they urge their employees not to join the union?

2. MISMANAGEMENT AND UNIONIZATION

Two administrators are discussing collective bargaining in hospitals. The first administrator says that in the city where he comes from there are over 30 hospitals, and three of them are unionized. It is his opinion that since 90 per cent of the hospitals of this particular city are not unionized, the administrations of the three unionized hospitals must have been guilty of gross mismanagement in order to have the employees vote in favor of a union. The second administrator counters this argument by saying that there are many issues that lead to the situation wherein employees will vote for a union without the administration of that hospital being guilty of mismanagement or not having a good relationship with employees.

A. Which view do you hold, and why?

3. THE FIRING OF SAM

On Friday afternoon the manager of the Food Service Department in a large metropolitan hospital, Mrs. Lincoln, was asked to confer with the personnel director. On the preceding Wednesday, she had fired Sam Smith, who was 25 and had worked for the hospital for one year. He was fired for "insubordination, threatening and causing bodily harm" to his supervisor, who reported to Mrs. Lincoln. The incident occurred after the supervisor asked Sam to scrape the food from some excessively burnt pots and pans. His regular job was that of washing pots and pans but they had never been this badly burnt before. Sam refused, saying that he did not have a scraper, only soap pads, and he wasn't going to clean any pots and pans without a scraper. The supervisor again directed Sam to scrape the pots and pans. Immediately after the second order, Sam turned angrily toward the supervisor—nose to nose—and said, "If you say one more word about those pots and pans, I'll break your arm." As he walked away to leave the building, he brushed the supervisor aside, knocking her down. The supervisor reported the incident to Mrs. Lincoln, who immediately filled out a dismissal form which was sent to the personnel director. He notified Sam at home that he had been fired.

On Friday morning, Sam filed a grievance through his union steward, contending that his discharge did not follow the specified disciplinary steps in the union contract and that he should be reinstated with back pay. The union steward met with the personnel director in order to resolve the issue. He pointed out that the contract called for the following sequential disciplinary steps for insubordination: (1) oral warning, (2) written warning, (3) disciplinary layoff, and finally, (4) termination. Contending that Sam was not even given a written warning and that it was his first offense, the union steward stated that Sam's discharge was in violation of the contract and he *must* be reinstated. The personnel director, on the other hand, argued that the contract specified that physically striking or harming others carried disciplinary action "up to and including discharge," and that neither a written warning nor disciplinary layoff was necessary. In addition, the personnel manager said that "by reason of walking off his job as he did, he in fact quit."

The personnel director wanted to meet with Mrs. Lincoln in order to make sure that his facts were correct, and they were. Since the contract requires binding arbitration if a dispute is not resolved, the personnel manager was considering the alternatives of reinstating Sam or submitting the dispute to arbitration which would eventually cost the hospital at least $1000.

A. What are the implications of the alternative "reinstate" that the personnel director should consider?

B. Should Mrs. Lincoln or the supervisor have anything to say about the decision reached? What repercussions could there be for them if Sam is reinstated?

C. If you were the arbitrator, what would your decision be? Why?

Part IV

ORGANIZATIONAL DYNAMICS

In Part III, *ORGANIZATIONAL DESIGN AND STRUCTURE,* we focused on the organizing process. In this part, *ORGANIZATIONAL DYNAMICS,* we will focus on the executing process. As indicated in Chapter 2, the executing process is social in nature and is concerned with initiating action within the organization. Those activities characteristic of the executing process are (a) motivating, (b) leading and supervising, and (c) communicating with employees so that planned work within the organization setting will occur.

This part contains three intertwining chapters. In the first chapter, Motivation of Employees, we focus on the theories of motivation; that is, what causes people to behave and act as they do. An understanding of human needs and how they cause behavior is mandatory for any manager, who must know how and in what way he can induce people to act (behave) and perform their duties.

In the second chapter, Leadership and Supervision, we describe a key aspect of managing people — leading and supervising them. Various styles will be presented along with a leadership contingency model. In the final chapter, Communication, we present the flows, importance, and some of the barriers to effective communication.

Motivation, leadership and supervision, and communication are the three interrelated activities which characterize the executing process. Without communication, what and how things are to be done cannot be conveyed. Without leadership, focused direction of the efforts of personnel will not occur. Without motivation, it is difficult to induce subordinates to perform. Since the executing process deals with getting things done *through* people, it represents the *dynamics* of organization.

This Chapter Contains:

- The Concept of Motivation
    Definition and Model
- Motivation Theories
    Classical Theory
    Hierarchy of Needs Theory
    Two-factor Theory
    Expectancy Theory
- Application of Motivational Theory
    Theory X
    Theory Y
- Summary
- Discussion Questions
- Incidents

Chapter 11

MOTIVATION OF EMPLOYEES

"The job of administrators is a most difficult one because, instead of performing the technical operations themselves, they must induce others to carry them out according to previously determined plans. The work of administrators will be fruitless unless the various members of their organizations are willing to contribute their efforts to the achievement of common objectives. Therefore, the primary function of administrators is to induce voluntary cooperation on the part of their subordinates and associates. It follows from this that the most important qualifications of administrators are (1) an understanding of why persons are willing to contribute their efforts and (2) skill in obtaining cooperation from the members of an organization in working toward planned objectives."

(Ted R. Brannen)[1]

INTRODUCTION

The manager in a health care organization may be adept at planning for and organizing the human and physical resources at his command but, as the preceding quote indicates, unless the manager can get the people in the organization to do what must be done, he or she will not succeed. This and the two chapters that follow deal with the topic of getting organizational participants to do what must be done. This is the executing process of management, and unless it is done effectively, the planning, organizing, and controlling efforts will be largely wasted. Motivation will be dealt with in this chapter; leadership will be covered in Chapter 12; and communication will be discussed in Chapter 13. These three topics are intertwined and, in the end, explain how the manager gets other people to do the necessary work of the health care organization.

---

[1]Ted R. Brannen, "The organization as a social system." *Hospital Administration, 4*:19, Spring, 1959.

THE CONCEPT OF MOTIVATION

Why do people behave the way they do? How do you obtain the cooperation of others? A major ingredient in the answer to this is motivation. The concept of motivation is both simple and complex. It is simple because the behavior of individuals is goal-directed and either externally or internally induced. It is complex because the mechanism which induces behavior consists of the individual's needs, wants, and desires, and these are shaped, affected, and satisfied in many different ways.

MOTIVATION DEFINED AND MODELED

Why does one person work harder than another? Why is one more cooperative than another? The answers to these questions can be traced to the fact that people have needs to satisfy and will behave in certain ways in order to achieve satisfaction. In other words, people's needs cause them to undertake a pattern of behavior. For example, a hungry person *needs* food, is *driven* by hunger, and is *motivated* by the desire for food in order to satisfy the need. Using just this information, it is possible to design a simple model of motivation (see Fig. 11–1). We may thus define *motivation as self or externally induced behavior which occurs in order to bring about or maintain need fulfillment.* All people have needs that they seek to fulfill. We could ask, why do you work? It could be to earn an income in order to house, feed, and clothe yourself and your family—to satisfy your physiological needs. Or, do you work for a health care organization in order to satisfy a desire (need) to serve humanity. Why do people train themselves to become registered nurses, doctors, or pharmacists? The point is, people have needs which they attempt to satisfy. These needs become goals, and people behave in a way they feel will satisfy them.

When we discern behavioral patterns that will enable us to satisfy our needs, we repeat those patterns until they no longer contribute to goal (need) fulfillment. If we have a need for praise and recognition from our immediate supervisor, the likely behavior pattern will be exceptional job performance. If praise and recognition occur, we can assume that continued performance will result in more praise. This learned behavior pattern is presented as the lower loop in Figure 11–1.

Thus, the motivational model presented in Figure 11–1 explains the behavior of individuals conceptually. However, what happens when we are blocked from fulfilling our needs? What happens if you work extremely hard—above and way beyond the call of duty—and there are no rewards, so that your needs are not fulfilled?

A phenomenon of behavior is that there are times when it cannot be explained rationally. When a behavioral pattern we perceive as leading to need fulfillment is blocked, we often react and behave in an irrational manner.

The manager should know what kinds of behavior this frustration gener-

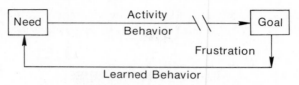

Figure 11-1   Motivation model.

ates. In general, frustration occurs when one is blocked from fulfilling needs (see the motivation model in Fig. 11-1). It is important for the manager to recognize and understand frustration as it affects subordinates' behavior. Frustration may occur when an employee has a strong need for esteem but his or her job cannot fulfill this need. One form of behavior may be frequent absenteeism, a questioning of one's own abilities, negativism ("I don't care if you fire me"), or actual self-termination (quitting).

Defense Mechanisms.   The individual's reaction to frustration may not be chosen consciously but may be the product of unconscious learning. Many of these unconscious reactions to the tension created by frustration are called *defense mechanisms.*

The following are some of the most common defense mechanisms:[2]

Withdrawal.   One way to avoid frustration is to withdraw or avoid frustrating situations. This may result in physically leaving the scene but more likely will result in apathy.

Displacement.   Often it is not possible to be aggressive toward the person who is causing the frustration (a superior for example) so the aggression is directed toward another person—a wife or a child or a peer—or some object.

Compensation.   Sometimes a person goes overboard in one area of activity to make up for deficiencies in another area.

Repression.   Sometimes a person can repress a frustrating situation by losing awareness of the situation that would cause frustration if allowed to remain at the conscious level of the mind.

Regression.   Some people revert to childlike behavior in their attempt to avoid an unpleasant reality. This often exhibits itself as horseplay in the work setting.

Rationalization.   People are often able to convince themselves that a reason for not being able to satisfy a need lies outside themselves. This is often less ego-deflating than the real reason. For example, a medical technologist may explain poor lab work by blaming obsolete equipment rather than some deficiency of his or her own.

---

[2]Wendell French, *The Personnel Management Process.* Boston: Houghton-Mifflin Company, 1974, pp. 95–97.

In order to fully understand the needs-behavior-frustration components of the motivation model, we will next present various motivation theories.

MOTIVATION THEORIES

The complexity of motivating human behavior can be further illustrated by examining the diversity of theoretical underpinnings developed to explain it. This diversity, which often presents a problem for the student, can be explained by pointing out that motivation is not fully understood. Authorities disagree on how motivation occurs and on what causes it. Research is underway which may eventually lead to a complete understanding, but until that time we will have to realize that our knowledge of motivation is not complete.

Several of the most important motivation theories are described in this section. These theories can be divided into two broad categories: *content theories* and *process theories.*

Content theories attempt to identify specifically *what* it is within the individual, or the environment, that initiates, sustains, and eventually terminates behavior. In contrast, process theories attempt to explain *how* behavior is initiated, sustained, and terminated. These theories define the variables that explain motivated behavior and then try to show how the variables interact and influence each other to produce certain behavioral patterns within people.[3] Examples of the theoretical development of motivation in both areas are cited below.

CLASSICAL THEORY

The most basic example of a content theory can be traced back to the work of Frederick W. Taylor in the early 1900's.[4] Taylor, one of the founders of what is called Scientific Management, observed management from a shop level point of view. He felt that work could be arranged and jobs designed to maximize efficiency. Pursuant to his approach was the premise that man is primarily economically motivated. As a result, he developed a differential price rate (incentive) system of compensation as a motivational device to induce workers to produce more.

The straight-forward power of money as a motivator is not so great today. In fact, it never fully explained motivation for all people. To believe it did, or does, would mean ignoring all those who have forsaken financial security for the betterment of their fellow man. Money can motivate *some* people to *some* extent but it is not the whole answer to motivation — it is not the only need men work to satisfy.

---

[3]John P. Campbell, Marvin D. Dunnette, Edward E. Lawler III, and Karl E. Weick, Jr., *Managerial Behavior, Performance, and Effectiveness.* New York: McGraw-Hill Book Company, 1970, p. 341.
[4]Frederick W. Taylor, *Scientific Management.* New York: Harper and Brothers, Publishers, 1919.

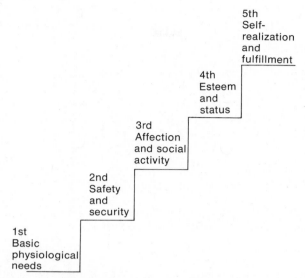

Figure 11–2 Hierarchy of human needs. (From Maslow, Abraham, *Psychological Review*, 50:4, July, 1943. Copyright © by The American Psychological Association. "Reprinted by permission.")

HIERARCHY OF NEEDS

Abraham H. Maslow, a psychologist, formulated one of the most widely known content theories of motivation. In his theory, he stressed two fundamental premises. The first is that man is a wanting animal whose needs depend on what he already has. Only needs not yet satisfied can influence behavior; an adequately fulfilled need is not a motivator. The second premise is that man's needs are arranged in a hierarchy of importance. Once a particular need is fulfilled, another emerges and demands fulfillment.

Need Hierarchy. Maslow's need theory, first publicized in the early 1940's, stressed a hierarchy with certain "higher" needs becoming dominant after other "lower" needs were satisfied.[5] Figure 11–2 illustrates the hierarchy. Each of Maslow's need categories is briefly described below.

1. *Physiological needs.* This category consists of the basic survival needs for food, water, and so on.
2. *Safety and security needs.* Once the survival needs are met, attention can be turned to ensuring continued survival by protecting oneself against physical harm and deprivation.
3. *Affection and social activity needs.* This third level is related to the social and gregarious nature of man. This is something of a breaking point in the hierarchy in that it begins to get away from the physical or quasiphysical needs of the first two levels. These needs exhibit themselves in man's need for as-

[5]Abraham H. Maslow, "A theory of human motivation." *Psychological Review*, July, 1943, pp. 370–396. Copyright © 1943 by the American Psychological Association. Used by permission.

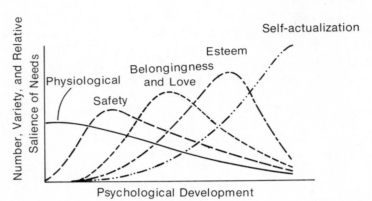

Figure 11-3 Relative importance of needs as motivators. (From David Krech, Richard S. Crutchfield, and Egerton L. Ballachey, page 77: *Individual In Society.* Copyright © 1962 by McGraw-Hill Inc. Used by permission of the McGraw-Hill Book Company.)

sociation or companionship with others, for belonging to groups, and for giving and receiving friendship and affection.

4. *Esteem and status needs.* These are the needs for self-respect or self-esteem that come from an awareness of one's importance to others. One's status or level of importance relative to others is an important need in this category.

5. *Self-realization needs.* This highest level of human needs includes the need to achieve the fullest development of one's potential. It exhibits itself in the need to be creative and to have the opportunity for self-expression.

For purposes of analysis or discussion these categories can be separated, but in truth they are interacting within the individual. Lower level needs are never completely satisfied; they recur from time to time. The need for esteem and self-realization is such that once they become important to a person he seeks indefinitely for more satisfaction of them. The need hierarchy model essentially points out that satisfied needs are no longer strong motivating forces. People are motivated by what they are *seeking* much more than by what they already have.

Needs Change. It can be further pointed out that people's needs change over time. Figure 11-3 shows the relative mix of needs for an individual as he develops and as circumstances change.[6] Our needs also change among generations. The needs (wants, desires) of our parents are quite different from ours. They were content with one car; we want two. Figure 11-3 also illustrates progressive changes and the relative importance, number, and variety of needs during one's development. Finally, the diagram shows that the peak of a "lower" level need must be passed before a "higher" level need becomes a dominant motivating force.

Because this theory is applied in the work setting, it is necessary to realize that all health care employees have a variety of needs motivating them. The

---

[6]Orlando Behling and Mitchell B. Shapiro, "Motivation theory: Source of solution or part of problem?" *Business Horizons, 17*:61, February, 1974.

manager's task is to develop situations which will permit employees to satisfy their needs. Within the health care field there is much built-in satisfaction in comparison with manufacturing and other industries. Nevertheless, the astute health care manager will recognize what needs are important to motivate each subordinate. When possible, the manager will alter approach, rewards, job assignments, and so on, to maximize need fulfillment for as many subordinates as possible. For example, some people have a continuous need to be reassured that they are doing well; others do not like to be bothered while working. If the manager gave more attention to the former individual, it would help to fulfill the employee's need; however, close attention would be perceived as meddling and would detract from the latter employee's need fulfillment. Different people have different needs and should be managed in different ways.

TWO-FACTOR THEORY

In 1959, Herzberg, Mausner, and Snyderman reported research findings which suggested that people have two sets of needs: their need as animals to avoid pain, and their need as humans to grow psychologically. These findings led them to advance a "dual-factor" theory of motivation.[7]

Whereas previous theories of motivation (Taylor and Maslow) were based on causal inferences of the theorists, and deduction from their own insights and experience, the dual-factor theory of motivation was inferred from a study of need satisfactions and the reported motivational effects of these satisfactions on a sample of 200 engineers and accountants. The subjects were first requested to recall a time when they had felt exceptionally good about their jobs. By further questioning, the investigators sought to determine the reasons for their subjects' feelings of satisfaction, and whether these feelings had affected their performance, personal relationships, and well-being. Finally, the sequence of events that served to return the workers' attitudes to "normal" was elicited.

In a second set of interviews, the same subjects were asked to describe incidents in which their feelings about their job were exceptionally negative—instances where their negative feelings were related to some event on the job. Herzberg and his associates came to the conclusion that job satisfaction consisted of two separate and independent dimensions.[8]

---

[7]Frederick Herzberg, Bernard Mausner, and Barbara Snyderman, *The Motivation to Work*, 2nd ed. New York: John Wiley and Sons, Inc., 1959.

[8]For some interesting studies of the Herzberg dual-factor theory in health care organizations see

(a) Beaufort B. Longest, Jr., "Job satisfaction for registered nurses in the hospital setting." *Journal of Nursing Administration, 4*:46, May-June, 1974.

(b) Glennadee A. Nichols, "Important satisfying and dissatisfying aspects of nurses." *Supervisor Nurse, 5*:10, January, 1974.

(c) David E. Schrieber and Stanley Sloan, "An occupational analysis of job satisfaction in a public hospital," *Hospital Management, 108*:26, 30, 32, August, 1969.

(d) John W. Slocum, Jr., Gerald A. Susman, and John E. Sheridan, "An analysis of need satisfaction and job performance among professional and paraprofessional hospital personnel." *Nursing Research, 21*:338, July-August, 1972.

(e) Catherine Harman White and Maureen Claire Maguire, "Job satisfaction and dissatisfaction among hospital nursing supervisors." *Nursing Research, 22*:25, January-February, 1973.

Maintenance Dimension (Dissatisfiers). There are some conditions of the job which dissatisfy employees when they are absent. However, the presence of these conditions does not necessarily lead to a high degree of motivation. Herzberg called them *maintenance* factors, since they are necessary in order to maintain a reasonable level of satisfaction. He also noted that many of these factors have been perceived by managers as motivators, but that they are actually more potent as dissatisfiers (demotivators) when they are absent. He concluded that there were ten maintenance factors:

1. Organizational policy and administration
2. Technical supervision
3. Interpersonal relations with supervisor
4. Interpersonal relations with peers
5. Interpersonal relations with subordinates
6. Salary
7. Job security
8. Personal life
9. Work conditions
10. Status

Motivational Dimension (Satisfiers). There are other job conditions that, if present, tend to build high levels of motivation and job satisfaction. However,

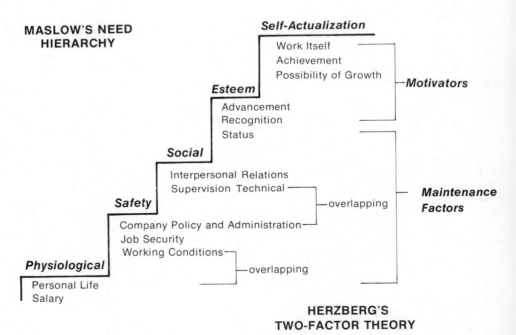

Figure 11–4 Comparison of the Maslow and Herzberg models. (Source: Richard M. Hodgetts, *Management Theory Process and Practice*. Philadelphia: W. B. Saunders Co., 1975, p. 326. Used by permission of the publisher. Also see Keith Davis, *Human Behavior at Work*. New York: McGraw-Hill Book Company, 1972, p. 59.)

if these conditions are not present, it does not prove to be highly dissatisfying. Herzberg described six of these factors as *motivational* factors or satisfiers:

1. Achievement
2. Recognition
3. Advancement
4. The work itself
5. The possibility of growth
6. Responsibility

When the Herzberg and Maslow models are compared, it can be seen that they both emphasize the same set of relationships. Both are content theories; they look at *what* motivates human behavior. Maslow looked at the human needs of the individual, while Herzberg focused on how the job conditions affect the individual's basic needs. Figure 11–4 illustrates this point.

The basic advance of Herzberg's theory of motivation over the Maslow model of need-priority is that Herzberg's theory shows the distinction between maintenance and motivational factors and, most importantly for the application of motivation theory in the work place, Herzberg shows that motivation tends to be derived from the work itself. This, however, is not to say that the Herzberg motivating factors are equally important for all people. For example, House and Wigdor have ranked the ten factors which Herzberg used in terms of their satisfaction of workers' needs as follows:[9]

1. Achievement
2. Recognition
3. Work itself
4. Responsibility
5. Advancement
6. Policy and administration
7. Supervision, technical
8. Working conditions
9. Interpersonal relations
10. Salary

In contrast, Longest has developed the following ranking of the motivational factors for registered nurses in a hospital setting:[10]

1. Achievement
2. Interpersonal relations
3. Work itself
4. Policy and administration
5. Responsibility
6. Supervision—technical
7. Salary
8. Working conditions
9. Recognition
10. Advancement

---

[9]R. J. House and L. A. Wigdor, "Herzberg's dual-factor theory of job satisfaction and motivation: A review of the evidence and a criticism." *Personnel Psychology, 20*:20, 1967.
[10]Beaufort B. Longest, Jr., op. cit. p. 51.

The difference between these two rankings occurs with three factors: interpersonal relations, recognition, and advancement. This illustrates that needs vary with workers and organizational settings. As with any general theory, the motivation theories must be applied with great care. Longest suggests that the most important implication of his study for hospital managers is

> . . . the very high ranking given to *interpersonal relations* between the registered nurse and her superiors in the organization as a factor influencing her job satisfaction. The fact that R.N.'s rank this factor so high may very well stem from their feeling that this is an area where they have been treated badly. Clearly, the registered nurses are concerned about this factor.[11]

Herzberg's two-factor theory has extended Maslow's need hierarchy to motivation in the work place but it has its flaws — and its critics. Schwab, DeVitt, and Cummings, in a study involving both managerial and professional workers, found that the maintenance factors were as useful in motivating employees as the motivational factors were.[12]

Where does this leave us? It must be concluded that the Maslow and Herzberg theories of motivation are generalizations and, on the surface, oversimplify the nature of motivation. This is not to say that they are not useful. On the contrary, both theories provide a frame of reference, manner of thinking, and conceptual foundation that can be useful to managers who must motivate their employees. However, to make the link between individual need satisfaction and the achievement of organization objectives, we will review the process theories of motivation.[13]

EXPECTANCY THEORY

The process theories of motivation attempt to explain how behavior is initiated. We shall examine two that are based on the theory of expectancy, which proposes that a person will generally be a high performer if he or she feels (expects) that there is a good chance that high performance will result in certain preferred outcome (usually more positive outcomes, such as rewards, than negative outcomes, such as discipline).[14]

Preference–Expectancy.   Victor H. Vroom has developed a preference–expectancy theory which suggests that motivation is a product of expectancy (what one thinks will result from certain actions) and preference (what one would like to have result from certain actions or behavior).[15] The preference–expectancy theory is more an explanation of the motivation phenomenon than

---

[11]*Ibid.* p. 51.

[12] Donald P. Schwab, H. William DeVitt, and Larry L. Cummings. "A test of the adequacy of the two-factor theory as a predictor of self-report performance effects," *Personnel Psychology,* 24:293, Summer, 1971.

[13]Richard M. Hodgetts, *Management: Theory, Process and Practice.* Philadelphia: W. B. Saunders Company, 1975, p. 326.

[14]Larry L. Cummings and Donald P. Schwab, *Performance in Organizations: Determinants and Appraisal.* Glenview, Ill.: Scott, Foresman and Co., 1973, p. 31.

[15]Victor H. Vroom, *Work and Motivation.* New York: John Wiley and Sons, Inc., 1964 (especially Chapter 2).

a description of what motivates (as in the content theories we have looked at). Vroom's theory explains how two variables (preference and expectation) work to determine motivation.

Preference. In Vroom's model, preference refers to the possible outcomes an individual might experience as the result of certain behavior. If, for example, a clerk in the Business Office files more documents than other clerks, he or she may receive higher pay, get a promotion, impress the supervisor, or make co-workers jealous. Many other outcomes are possible, including the possibility that nothing will happen. However, the clerk clearly has a preference.

Expectancy. Expectancy, the other part of the Vroom model, is the individual's expectation that from behavior a desired outcome will happen. An individual with a preference for an outcome must also feel that he can achieve it by doing certain things. The importance of the Vroom model lies in its emphasis of the fact that motivation is individualistic and in its dependency upon the individual's having a specific, preferred outcome that is coupled with a belief or expectation that certain activities or behavior will bring about this outcome.

PORTER AND LAWLER'S MODEL

A second modern process theory based on expectancy theory is that proposed by Porter and Lawler.[16] According to their theory, people are motivated by future expectations that are based on previously learned experiences. Figure 11–5 illustrates the Porter-Lawler theory. This model is more comprehensive than Vroom's because it includes the relationship between rewards and performance.

Although the model is very straightforward, the reader should be aware of the fact that the wavy line between performance and extrinsic rewards denotes that the two are not always directly related and the semi-wavy line between performance and intrinsic rewards indicates that a direct relationship exists *only if* the job has been designed to allow a person who performs well to actually feel a sense of accomplishment.

Furthermore, the model suggests that performance causes satisfaction. This is in contrast to the view held by many authorities who believe that satisfaction causes performance. No one really knows, at this point, which comes first. Obviously, the complexity of human motivation is not fully understood even yet. In addition, in this model, whether or not the cost of high job satisfaction (higher pay, better working conditions, sense of accomplishment from one's job, and so on) is offset by higher levels of job performance is not considered. There are jobs (such as on an assembly line) where it may not be applicable. However, as a rule, health care organizations rely heavily upon the cooperation, performance, and high quality of work effort among their many professional and semi-professional employees. In this setting, the concept of job satisfaction and its linkage to performance appears to be worthy of careful consideration by health care organization managers.

---

[16]Lyman W. Porter and Edward E. Lawler III, *Managerial Attitudes and Performance.* Homewood, Ill.: Richard D. Irwin, Inc., and The Dorsey Press, 1968.

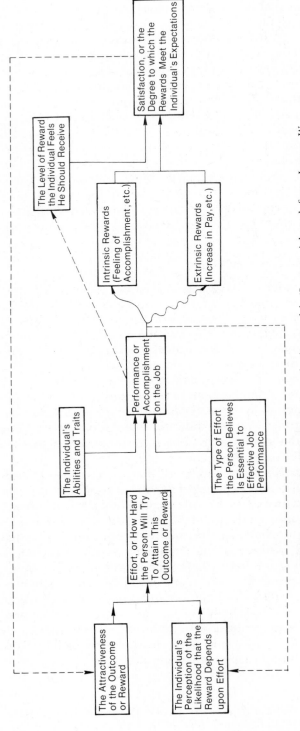

Figure 11-5 Porter and Lawler's motivation model. (Source: Adapted from Lyman W. Porter and Edward E. Lawler III, *Managerial Attitudes and Performance.* Homewood, Ill.: Richard D. Irwin Co. 1968, p. 165, by Richard M. Hodgetts, *Management Theory, Process, and Practice.* Philadelphia: W. B. Saunders, 1975, p. 331. Used by permission of both publishers.)

We have looked at five motivation theories. All are different, yet all are related; the common thread between these theories is that motivation is goal-directed behavior. For Taylor, the goal was simple: money. Maslow suggested a range of needs which are shared by all human beings and which exist in a hierarchy. Herzberg's two-factor theory develops a distinction between maintenance factors (necessary to avoid dissatisfaction) and motivational factors (necessary to motivate workers). Vroom and Porter and Lawler suggest ways to understand the motivational process: individual preference as to outcome of activities and behavior coupled with expectation that the desired outcome can be achieved.

THE APPLICATION OF MOTIVATION THEORY

The present state of motivation theory does not permit us to say with unassailable conviction *what* motivates people or *how* the phenomenon takes place. The theories are constantly challenged, expanded, and sometimes discarded. Yet, the health care manager is faced with the day-to-day operational necessity of motivating employees. An important factor contributing to the manager's success will be his or her *attitude* about people. When all the theorizing about motivation is done, the manager must, at some point, apply theory to real situations.

In the field of health care delivery, this is quite a challenge since so much of motivation is beyond the direct control of managers. A great deal of the motivation for performance comes from the individual employee and is due to his or her professional training and background. Many administrators and assistant administrators have attempted to motivate physicians who head up departments and have been quite unsuccessful. What works with the Laundry Manager does not always work with the Chief of Surgery, although certainly there are exceptions to this general statement of motivational dynamics. Part of the reason for this is that professional training tends to develop a strong sense of independence in people, and a manager's attempts to control or influence a professional person often do not meet with success.

If one analyzes what has been discovered about human nature, a number of important facts present themselves:

No One Is An Average Person. People differ in terms of basic mental abilities, personality, interests, level of aspiration, energy, education, experience, and so on. From the day of birth, each person is unique. For the rest of our lives the people, things, and events we contact make us even more different, because they constitute a part of our experience. Attempts to take some kind of arithmetical average of people will fail, as will attempts to deal with individuals as if they represented some hypothetical average. Many health care managers are unsuccessful because they take a standard, across-the-board way of relating to other people in almost every situation. This tendency is exhibited by many managers because, at least as they view it, it greatly simplifies their job.

People Work to Satisfy Their Own Needs. All normal human behavior is caused by a need structure. Workers have a perception of their needs that often differs from what management thinks they have. Furthermore, not all workers perceive their needs in the same way. The medical technologist values "independence" more so than maids or dietary aides. An even more complex factor is that as individuals grow older, their perception of their needs changes. These facts make it very difficult for a manager, especially one who supervises a large number of people, to create an environment in which all workers can satisfy their needs. After all, the manager only *thinks* he or she knows what the workers' needs are. This is made even more complex because needs differ from one worker to another, and the needs of an individual are constantly changing. Yet, the manager must keep in mind that getting a worker to carry out a directive is "caused behavior." Since this behavior is caused in part by the employee's attempt to satisfy a personal need, the manager has only two ways to get the employee to carry out the directive. *The manager can get the employee to understand that a desired action will increase the employee's need fulfillment, or the manager can convince the employee that to carry out the directive is to avoid a decreased need fulfillment.*

What this means is that management's ability to motivate successfully depends almost entirely on the fact that, from the employees' point of view, management controls the means by which the employees can meet many of their needs. This is why it is much more difficult to motivate professionally trained employees as compared to nonprofessional employees.

People Respond to Leadership.   There is a great deal of evidence that people respond to leadership. Yet, the reasons for this are not well understood. It is clear that a leader who can help others meet their needs as they perceive them will be followed. It is important for the manager to take advantage of this characteristic of human nature in the work setting. Leadership is not something that can be entirely taught. However, there are certain techniques (styles) that have been formulated which can be useful to the manager in the role of leader. We will examine these techniques in the next chapter.

The manager should keep these facts about human behavior in mind when trying to motivate subordinates. The manner in which motivation is approached will depend largely on the manager's attitude about the basic nature of man.

THEORIES X AND Y

One of the most prevalent styles of management is centralized direction and control. This strong pattern has deep roots in the long and successful experience of religious and military organizations. The line of authority, or command, goes directly from the top down through the various layers of the organization with delegation of authority; but full and detailed accountability goes up the line.

What is commonly called the autocratic or authoritarian style of management has arisen, in part, as an outgrowth of strong centralization of control. In its extreme form, such a management style begins to relate closely to the classic "Theory X" of Douglas McGregor.

The assumptions behind this view of management have been carefully formulated by McGregor, who has developed the following foundation for his "Theory X":

1. The average human being has an inherent dislike of work and will avoid it if he can.
2. Because of this human characteristic of dislike of work, most people must be coerced, controlled, directed, threatened with punishment to get them to put forth adequate effort toward the achievement of organizational objectives.
3. The average human being prefers to be closely directed, wishes to avoid responsibility, has relatively little ambition, wants security above all.[17]

Behavioral science research has clearly demonstrated that management based on the Theory X point of view is definitely not effective over a long period of time, especially in the health care field. Workers subjected to management based upon these assumptions take little initiative, make few innovations, and enjoy no sense of achievement or job satisfaction. Most health care employees will not function under the stringent, centralized direction and control implicit in the Theory X approach to management.

Fortunately, a contrasting concept of management has evolved and is highly applicable to health care organizations. It is based on the belief that the most effective way to get results is to *work with* people rather than to *use* them. The quality of the relationships within the organization is what Mary Parker Follett, an early writer on management, called "co-action," as contrasted with coercion.[18]

Douglas McGregor calls this alternative to the traditional view of management "Theory Y":

Above all, the assumptions of Theory Y point up the fact that the limits on human collaboration in the organizational setting are not limits of human nature but of management's ingenuity in discovering how to realize the potential represented by its human resources. Theory X offers management an easy rationalization for ineffective organizational performance. It is due to the nature of the human resources with which we must work. Theory Y, on the other hand, places the problems squarely in the lap of management. If employees are lazy, indifferent, unwilling to take responsibility, intransigent, uncreative, uncooperative, Theory Y implies that the causes lie in management's methods of organization and control.[19]

In what McGregor calls "Theory Y," the assumptions about human behavior in organizations are as follows:

1. The expenditure of physical and mental effort in work is as natural as play or rest. The average human being does not inherently dislike work. Depending upon controllable conditions, work may be a source of satisfaction (and will be voluntarily performed) or a source of punishment (and will be avoided if possible).

---

[17]Douglas McGregor, *The Human Side of Enterprise*. New York: McGraw-Hill Book Company, 1960, pp. 33–34. Used by permission of the publisher.
[18]Mary Parker Follett, *Creative Experience*. New York: Longmans Green and Company, Inc., 1924, p. XIII.
[19]Douglas McGregor. op. cit., p. 48. Used by permission of the publisher.

2. External control and the threat of punishment are not the only mean~ f
   ing about effort toward organizational objectives. Man will e
   and self-control in the service of objectives to which he is
3. Commitment to objectives is a function of the rewards
   achievement. The most significant of such rewards, e.g., the
   ego and self-actualization needs, can be direct products
   toward organizational objectives.
4. The average human being learns under proper conditio:
   but to seek responsibility. Avoidance of responsibility, lack
   phasis on security are generally consequences of expe
   human characteristics.
5. The capacity to exercise a relatively high degree of imagi:
   creativity in the solution of organizational problems is wid
   tributed in the population.
6. Under conditions of modern industrial life, the intellectu:
   average human being are only partly utilized.[20]

Theory X and Theory Y concern the attitudes t
toward employees. They are important concepts and are
because they represent a dichotomy in how the manager n
of motivating others. The manager who operates under T
will see his or her task to be the creation of an organizati(
the health care worker can find satisfaction and, therefor
performing on the job.

SUMMARY

Motivation was defined as either externally or self-indu
occurs in order to satisfy or maintain need satisfaction. The
motivation (classical, hierarchy of needs, and two-factor thec
theory of motivation (represented by Vroom's preference-
and the Porter-Lawler model) were also presented. Since
portant factor in the application of motivation theory to the
zation is the *attitude* of the manager about those he or she
McGregor Theory X and Theory Y dichotomy was describe
manager to understand his or her attitudes about people.

---

[20]*Ibid.* pp. 47–48. Used by permission of the publisher.

DISCUSSION QUESTIONS

tional model in Figure 11–1, think of an example of unusual be-
d in at work. Identify the need you were attempting to fulfill, how
ed, and what defense mechanism resulted. Do the same for one

nilarity and difference between the Maslow need hierarchy and the
notivational theories.

was made that as people develop, become older, and mature,
Explain why and give examples.

4. Ide...   al situations (jobs) in a health care organization where you think
a manager should be more of a Theory X person than a Theory Y person. Discuss the factors characteristic of those situations which are similar. Identify several situations
(jobs) when you feel a manager should take on the Theory Y style. Discuss the factors
characteristic of those situations which are similar.

5. Basically, people are motivated (behave) to satisfy needs. As a manager, how
do you motivate a person who just doesn't care about anything? Discuss. Is there a point
in time when that type of person should be terminated? Why?

INCIDENTS

1. TIME CLOCK

At the present time, your organization requires that all employees except department heads punch a time card. This means that nurses and head nurses, and so on, receive pay only for time clocked in on the time card. In other words, if the employee is
late an hour, he or she is docked an hour. Certain of your professional employees,
including registered dietitians, social workers with Master's degrees, and medical technologists, have requested that they be removed from the "rigorous controls" of the time
clock.
  A. What factors prompted the professional employees to make their request?
  B. What might happen if the request is not granted?
  C. If the request were granted to the professional employees, how would you
     predict the other "non-professional" employees would react?

2. JOB RECLASSIFICATION

The secretary reporting to the full-time salaried Chief of Medicine is in Pay Grade 7.
Betty, the employee occupying this position, is doing an outstanding job, and the
department head would like to promote her one or possibly two pay grades in order to
give her a good raise. The level of her current job responsibility is similar to other positions in Pay Grade 7. With the exception of her outstanding merit, attitude, initiative, and
willingness to work hard, there is no other basis for reclassifying the position to a higher

pay grade, since the responsibilities do not justify it. Because of the great amo
pressure that is being exerted by the Chief of Medicine, this is becoming qu
problem for the Administrator.

A. How might Betty react if her job classification is not changed so a
increase could be given? Why?

B. How might the Chief of Medicine react if the Administrator does not gra
request? Why?

C. If the job classification is changed and higher pay given without a change
sponsibilities, how would other Pay Grade 7 employees react? Why?

D. If you were the Administrator and decided to grant the doctor's wish, what
you do to minimize the likelihood that other employees would react adverse
you decided not to grant the request, how would you approach him and e
your decision?

3. BILL'S PROMOTION?

At the DEF Community Hospital there was an opening for a dietary supervisor.
Harris applied, and her background was judged by the Personnel Department ar
Director of the Dietary Department to be well suited for this position.

A few days after Kathy had started to work, she ran into some problems. The
ous dietary supervisor had been fired for stealing, and most of the dietary aide
that Bill Warner would be promoted to the supervisory position. The Director o
Dietary Department told Kathy that Bill had been considered, but was thought to b
young for that much responsibility.

It soon became evident that while Bill was co-operative, many of the empl
were not. When one of the dietary employees was unhappy with an assignment he
would tell Kathy that if Bill had been appointed supervisor such problems woul
have occurred. Many comments were made as Kathy continued her supervisory a
ties. Some of these comments were very embarrassing for her, because it
suggested that she had friends in the Administration who gave her the job c
friendship, rather than because she was competent.

Then Kathy got an idea. Since Bill was so close to the employees, she delega
him the authority for coordinating the daily job assignments. Bill was delighted
this assignment and did an excellent job. As a result, Kathy had less contact with t
dividual dietary employees, and she began to depend upon Bill in these relations
Bill was apparently happy, and the employees were quite satisfied. One day
suggested to Kathy that he be given a raise to reflect his new responsibilities. Sin
was doing such an effective job, she requested that his job description be reviewe
the Personnel Department and that he should be given a promotion and a pay rai
recognize the fine job he was doing. The Personnel Department turned the request
because Kathy had had no approval for the action she took in the first place.

A. If you were Kathy, what would you do now?

B. In her dealings with Bill, was Kathy using Theory X or Y? Discuss.

C. How does the health care organization's promotion policy affect the motivati
employees?

D. What problems now exist in motivating Bill?

E. What should the Director of the Dietary Department do now?

F. What other issues do you feel are important in this case?

4. SUSAN'S FAMILY

For the past four years, Susan has been a medical record clerk at the XYZ Hos
and her work has nearly always been perfect. After her return from vacation, it bec
evident that her accuracy had begun to slip. Occasionally, key information on the r
cal chart was not followed up properly. Certain charts that were deficient were not
ted by Susan and these omissions could have been serious during, for exampl
inspection by the Joint Commission on Accreditation of Hospitals. Today, the Direc

Medical Records noticed a major error that could have had a very strong effect on patient care in a specific situation. When confronted, Susan mentioned that she had a serious illness in the family, spent her vacation caring for this relative, and the worry caused her loss of attention.

    A. What should the Director of Medical Records do regarding Susan?

    B. Are the usual tools and principles of motivation going to readily apply to correcting this situation?

This Chapter Contains:

- Introduction

- Definition of Leadership

- Who Is a Leader

- Dimensions of Leader Behavior
- Degree of Decision-Making Authority
  Overseeing Work Activity

- Contingency Leadership Model

- Summary

- Discussion Questions

- Incidents

Chapter 12

LEADERSHIP

"The endurance of organizations depends upon the
quality of leadership...."

(Chester I. Barnard)[1]

INTRODUCTION

For the organization to endure and for quality patient care to be provided, leadership is required. The simple reason for this is that an important part of management consists of dealing with and working through people. Furthermore, someone must determine, initiate, coordinate, influence, and oversee the work activities of other individuals. In our examination of the subject of leadership, we will begin by asking the following questions: Who are leaders? What are the dimensions of leader behavior? How do leaders know what behavior is most effective? These are some of the questions we propose to answer in this chapter.

DEFINITION OF LEADERSHIP

Leadership is a very complex subject and has been defined in a number of different ways. Cartwright and Zander, in their review of the literature, propose that leadership consists of the acts and activities of one person that contribute to performance by others (the group).[2] Kron refers to leadership as making people want to do something.[3] It has also been viewed as "influencing others at a particular time in a particular situation to strive willingly to attain organizational objectives."[4] Fiedler and Chemers describe leadership as an unequal influence and power relationship with the followers accepting the leader's legitimate right to make decisions.[5] According to Hodgetts, "...leadership is the process of influencing people to direct their efforts toward the achievement

[1]Chester Barnard, *Functions of the Executive.* Cambridge: Harvard University Press, 1958, p. 282.
[2]Dorwin Cartwright and Alvin Zander, *Group Dynamics: Research and Theory.* New York: Harper and Row Publishers, 1968, pp. 304–305.
[3]Thora Kron, *The Management of Patient Care: Putting Leadership Skills to Work.* Philadelphia: W. B. Saunders Co., 1971, p. 44.
[4]Robert T. Golembiewski, "Three styles of leadership and their uses." *Personnel, 38*:35, July, 1961.
[5]Fred E. Fiedler and Martin E. Chemers, *Leadership and Effective Management.* Glenview, Illinois: Scott, Foresman and Company, 1974, p. 4.

of particular goals."[6] The elements that these definitions have in common are *group, goals, influence,* and *acceptance.* In other words, a leader leads those in the organization who are subordinates reporting to him or her (and, in some instances, other employees who do not report). This individual influences, instructs, and commands the work effort of others in order to accomplish a purpose, such as attaining objectives (organizational or personal) that, as a rule, have been translated into specific work activities. This implies that the leader's role consists of determining what is to be accomplished, influencing others, and directing their efforts toward that purpose. It further implies that those being led, those whom we call the "followers," accept the leader's role and influence over them. We can combine these elements and define leadership as the process by which one person designates "what is to be done" and influences (instructs, commands) the efforts of others in order to accomplish specific purposes (objectives and work tasks).

WHO IS A LEADER?

Viewed in an organizational context there are two types of leaders: formal and informal. The formal leaders are those appointed to positions of authority by the organization who are responsible for making sure that specific work is performed by those who report to them. Informal leaders can also be present within the organization. Specifically, in work groups there may be an individual who, by reason of respect, age, knowledge of the job, and other characteristics, is looked upon by the group as their leader or spokesman. Although this individual is not a formal leader appointed by the organization, he or she is the group's informal leader and does influence them.

In some situations the leadership (influence) of the formal and informal leaders may create conflict if the objectives of the two differ and they both influence the same group or set of employees. Occasionally, the group will be influenced to a greater degree by the informal leader than by the formal leader. In these instances, the formal leader may have to alter his or her manner of influence, perhaps through the use of negative sanctions.

Although the dynamics of organizational conflict and role clashes between formal and informal leaders are important subjects, their treatment is beyond the scope of this book. Our attention will be directed toward an examination of leadership as it relates to the managing of health care organizations, by inspecting the leader behavior of those formally appointed by the organization. *Therefore, we will basically treat the manager–subordinate situation.* This is not to say that all managers are leaders, nor that all leaders are as effective as they might be. However, in most instances, managers do lead others. They generally have subordinates reporting to them (those to be led), and they seek to obtain cooperation from others and to influence them in order to direct work effort toward the accomplishment of specific purposes.

---

[6]Richard M. Hodgetts, *Management Theory, Process and Practice.* Philadelphia: W. B. Saunders Company, 1975, p. 342.

DIMENSIONS OF LEADER BEHAVIOR

The accepted manner for studying leadership is through the examination of "Leader Behavior." This is done by examining how a leader (in our case, the formally appointed manager) behaves while attempting to lead others. There are two dimensions to leader behavior which we will examine. The first is behavior in relation to the degree of decision-making authority held by the leader or relinquished to the group. The second dimension is the manner in which the leader interacts with others and the way in which he or she oversees (supervises) the accomplishment of specific work activities.

DEGREE OF DECISION-MAKING AUTHORITY HELD BY THE MANAGER

Fiedler and Chemers have indicated that leadership includes the concept of decision-making authority. In the relationship between the leader and those being led, the latter have accepted the former's legitimate right to have influence or power — to make decisions and be responsible for them.[7] Obviously, in any organization activity involving two or more people, someone must be responsible for the determination of what is to be accomplished, how, by whom, and when. Thus, the decision-making authority dimension of leader behavior sets the overall leader–follower (manager–subordinate) relationship in terms of determining direction and scope of work activities along with how and when they will be performed.

MANNER OF OVERSEEING THE ACCOMPLISHMENT OF WORK ACTIVITY

The second dimension of leader behavior concerns the manner in which the leader oversees the predetermined work activity of others. Overseeing implies not only monitoring work but also specifically assigning tasks as well as directing, instructing, and influencing others (typically, subordinates). It also carries the connotation of a relationship that is the result of the leader's concern for workers or output or both, the way in which rules are enforced, the closeness between the leader and the subordinates, and the degree to which they are represented to others in the organization by the leader. Generally, this dimension of leader behavior is called "supervision." For the sake of convention, we will use this term when referring to the leader behavior dimension of overseeing the accomplishment of work activity.

STYLES OF LEADER AUTHORITY AND SUPERVISION

Various terms such as "autocratic"–"democratic" have been attached to the decision-making authority dimension of leader behavior vis-a-vis the manager and the subordinates.[8] These labels are traditionally called "styles of leader decision authority" and can be displayed on a continuum. In addition, terms

---

[7] Fiedler and Chemers, op. cit. p. 4.

[8] For a classic development of these styles see Ralph White and Ronald Lippit, "Leader behavior and member reaction in three social climates." in *Group Dynamics*, Dorwin Cartwright and Alvin Zander eds., Evanston: Row Peterson and Company, 1960, pp. 527–553.

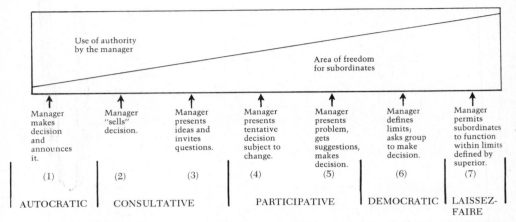

Figure 12-1 Continuum of leader decision-making authority. (Adapted from Robert Tannenbaum and Warren H. Schmidt, "How to choose a leadership pattern," *Harvard Business Review*, 36:96, March–April, 1958. Used by permission of the publisher.)

such as "employee centered" and "work centered" have been used to describe various supervisory styles used by the manager in overseeing work activity. Rather than being a continuum, they represent opposites characterizing the way in which the manager interacts with subordinates.[9]

In 1958, Robert Tannenbaum and Warren H. Schmidt formulated a continuum basically describing the decision-making authority dimension of leader behavior.[10] The continuum presented in Figure 12-1 has two polar ends with changing degrees of manager–subordinate decision-making authority. Tannenbaum and Schmidt have provided descriptions indicating the degree of decision-making authority held by the manager. At the bottom of the continuum, we have added commonly used labels ranging from "autocratic" to "laissez-faire." These labels are general descriptions of whoever determines the what, when, and how for work activities to be accomplished.

Autocratic.   In the continuum of leader authority presented in Figure 12-1 the "autocratic" end represents the manager who makes decisions and announces them to the group (see description 1).[11] The use of the autocratic style of leader decision authority means that the manager has made a decision pertaining to what the purpose of the group activity is, how the group activity is to be structured, and who is to be assigned to what specific tasks. The total interacting relationship and the work setting have been decided by the manager. The role of subordinates is to carry out orders without having any opportunity to materially alter the decisions that have been made. The manager provides little opportunity for a subordinate to participate in making decisions.

In health care settings, we seldom see the pure form of the autocratic leader decision authority style exercised by administrative personnel. It is often

---

[9]*Ibid.* pp. 554–570. Also see Rensis Likert, *New Patterns of Management.* New York: McGraw-Hill, 1961, Chapter 1.

[10]Robert Tannenbaum and Warren H. Schmidt, "How to choose a leadership pattern." *Harvard Business Review*, 36:95, March–April, 1958. (A revised and somewhat altered version of this may be found in *Harvard Business Review*, May–June, 1973, pp. 162–175, 178–180.)

[11]*Ibid.* p. 97.

the physician who adopts this style as the individual responsible for the activities required for patient care. Out of necessity, the physician must make decisions that no one else can. Consequently, he or she will make decisions and announce them to other personnel, such as nurses and technicians, who will be expected to carry out the activities without deviation. In fact, the physician in health care occupies the unique position of having responsibility via medical staff bylaws and an enormous amount of authority in patient care coordination, without having any formal hospital management-delegated authority (see Chapter 8, The Structure of Health Care Organizations). The authority–responsibility of physicians is, therefore, far different from that of salaried health care managers.

Consultative. The "consultative" style of leader decision authority appears to the right of "autocratic" and is characterized by descriptions 2 and 3. In this situation, the manager "sells" the decision or presents ideas and invites questions from subordinates, or both.[12] Specifically, the manager makes decisions concerning the work activity to be carried out, its purpose, how it is to be done, when, and by whom, and attempts to sell the subordinates on the decisions. Tannenbaum and Schmidt indicate that the manager may recognize the possibility of some resistance and invite questions; however, unless overwhelming reasons cause a change in the decisions made, they stand.[13]

Participative. Descriptions 4 and 5 of the continuum indicate that the manager presents a tentative decision which is subject to change or presents the problem to the subordinates, gets suggestions, and then makes the decision.[14] This represents the "participative" style of leader decision authority. The manager identifies the purposes, the problems, and the means by which the activities should be carried out; presents a tentative decision already made or seeks subordinate opinion; then, makes the decision. In this instance the "area of decision freedom for subordinates" is much greater and the "use of authority by the manager" is much smaller than with the autocratic and consultative styles.

Participative management, as we will see in a subsequent section, is a very powerful motivator in enabling employees to have some measure of influence and control over work-related activities. The work group can influence the decisions made concerning work activities and their purpose.

Democratic. Description 6 of the continuum represents the "democratic" style of leader decision authority. In this case, the manager defines the limits of the situation and the problem to be solved and asks the group to make decisions. The subordinates have a relatively large "area of decision freedom," as indicated in Figure 12–1. The boundaries of activity are set by the manager, who permits the group to make decisions within those restrictions.[15] For example, a nurse supervisor allows only RN's to give medication, but permits them to decide among themselves who will give the medication and who will perform other tasks that must be done.

Laissez-faire. The term "laissez-faire" was originally coined for the doc-

---

[12]*Ibid.* p. 97.
[13]*Ibid.* p. 97.
[14]*Ibid.* p. 97.
[15]*Ibid.* p. 97.

trine that government should not interfere with commerce. It is sometimes called "free rein."

Viewing description 7 in Figure 12–1, we see that subordinates are permitted to function within the limits set by the manager's own superior. There is no interference within the group by the manager, who, although participating in the decision-making, attempts to do so with no more influence than any other member of the group. Since the subordinates basically have complete freedom in making decisions, with minimum participation by the manager, this style falls on the far right end of the Tannenbaum–Schmidt leader authority continuum. The manager is merely a figurehead.[16] This style of leader decision authority is rarely found in health care organizations.

DETERMINANTS OF LEADER AUTHORITY STYLE: AUTOCRATIC TO DEMOCRATIC—WHICH IS CORRECT?

It was previously mentioned that no single leader decision authority style is correct all of the time. The manager must adapt and change the style to fit the situation. The autocratic style must be used by the physician in the operating room. By the same token, the democratic approach may not be appropriate when dealing with clerical or unskilled employees, but may be quite appropriate when dealing with groups of professional employees in the Laboratory or Radiology Department.

Factors Affecting Style.   The leader decision authority style adopted by the manager depends a great deal on factors such as (1) the importance of the results, (2) the nature of the work, (3) the characteristics of the workers, and (4) the personal characteristics of the manager.[17] If work activity must be performed immediately, perhaps under disaster or crisis conditions, the health care manager may have to adopt a style from the autocratic end of the continuum. At other times, when work need not be done immediately, another style, perhaps consultative or participative, may be used.

The type of work being performed by subordinates can influence which style is most appropriate. If it is routine, clerical, and must have a specific sequence flow, the manager may be more consultative than democratic in determining what, how, and when work activity will be performed. However, if the work is creative, flexible, and other departments do not rely on its timely completion, the manager may be able to adopt a participative or democratic style. Certainly, the manager of the billing or accounts receivable department will adopt a different leader authority style than the manager of a medical research department will.

The subordinates' characteristics—their training, education, motivation,

---

[16]*Ibid.* p. 97.
[17]For various discussions see
  (a) *Ibid.* pp. 98–101.
  (b) Golembiewski, op. cit. p. 36.
  (c) J. C. Wofford, "Managerial behavior, situational factors, and productivity and morale." *Administrative Science Quarterly, 16*:12, March, 1971.
  (d) Gordon E. O'Brien "Leadership in organizational settings." *Journal of Applied Behavioral Science, 5*:45, January–March, 1969.

and experience—can influence the leader authority style adopted by the manager. This factor is closely related to the type of work, since personnel skills tend to correspond closely with the work required. If the subordinates are skilled professionals, as opposed to unskilled, the manager may seek their opinions more readily (consultative or participative style) in connection with the determination of the work to be performed. If they are unskilled, not necessarily dependable, or inexperienced employees, the manager may have to make most of the decisions. Furthermore, there are some employees who, because of their value systems or previous experiences, will not accept decision responsibility if it is offered.

Finally, the personal characteristics of the manager can affect the leader authority style adopted. Some individuals, by reason of their personality traits, previous experiences, values, and cultural background, function better under one style or another and may find it difficult to change with the situation. The physician who becomes a health care organization administrator may find it difficult to readjust his or her style because of previous training and experience. In the doctor–patient relationship, the doctor has always been the primary decision-maker. As an administrator, a participative approach is often more appropriate, particularly when supervising professionals.

No One Style Is Always Appropriate. No one style is appropriate at all times. Which style is correct can only be answered after an evaluation of the situation including the work environment, what is to be done, the nature of the employees, the personality of the manager, and the organizational climate. This is not to say that a leader authority approach cannot be suggested. We will next describe more fully the participative style, its merits, and benefits that can be derived if used successfully.

PARTICIPATIVE LEADERSHIP

There is a great deal of evidence supporting the contention that a participative leader decision authority style can have a favorable effect on organizational productivity and efficiency.[18] Other advantages of employee participation in decisions that affect the work setting are the following:[19]

1. There is a tendency for the employees to identify with the organization more closely and, as a result, their motivation is enhanced. If people have some say about their job situation they tend to be more enthusiastic in carrying out the plans that have been developed. Since a large percentage of health care employees are professionally trained, this style may be particularly applicable in health care organizations.
2. Participation can be a means to overcome resistance to change. Those who

---

[18]See
  (a) Likert, op. cit. pp. 92–93;
  (b) Larry E. Greiner, "What managers think of participative leadership." *Harvard Business Review, 51*:111, March–April, 1973.
  (c) David J. Cherrington and J. Owen Cherrington, "Participation, performance, and appraisal," *Business Horizons, 17*:40, December, 1974.
[19]Thomas R. O'Donovan, "Can the 'participative' approach to management help the decision-makers?" *Hospital Management, 112*:16, July, 1971.

participate in decisions that cause change will understand it and be less likely to resist it.

3. Participation can enhance the personal growth and development of organization members. By participating in decisions, employees gain from experience.

4. Participation enables a wider range of ideas and experiences to be brought to bear on a problem. Often employees who are close to the situation can solve it more easily, and sometimes better, than the manager because of their familiarity with it.

5. Participation can increase organizational flexibility by reason of the wider experiences employees will have about the job situation.

Although efficiency and productivity can result under both participative and autocratic styles, sometimes a question of short-term versus long-term benefits arises. A rigid work setting with very little participation in the decision-making by employees can achieve high output. However, it may only be for a short time. We cannot conclude that the participative approach always does or does not increase productivity. It depends on the individual situation.

In order to make full use of a participative approach, certain guidelines are suggested.[20]

1. The urgency of the results should be such that there is adequate time to seek the opinions of the employees.

2. The personnel should have expertise and skill in the matters under consideration. It makes little sense to ask nurse aides to participate in the formulation of major overall hospital policies.

3. The cost of possible error should be considered. When you ask others to participate, there is a risk that mistakes will be made. Obviously, areas of direct patient care may not lend themselves to employee participation because of the high cost of error.

4. A quick shift in style should be cautioned against. Employees should be prepared for the change in order to reduce skepticism and to build their confidence.

5. The employees must be willing to participate. Some people do not want the responsibility that participation entails. Furthermore, the climate of respect between the manager and the group should be such that the employees are not afraid to make their opinions known.

6. Finally, the participative style must be used with sincerity and must be legitimate. Specifically, the manager who frequently asks subordinates to participate, yet has no intention of following their recommendations will soon lose the support and acceptance of the group. Once that mistrust arises, they may never view the participative style as being legitimate. This does not mean that the manager cannot reject their recommendations; however, if they are rejected, it is the manager's responsibility to justify his decision.

It is our view that for health care organizations there cannot be long-term maximization of patient care without a reasonable level of participate decision-making from the health care team. A large part of the health care field is made up of professionals and they simply do not tolerate being left out of the

---

[20]*Ibid.* p. 17.

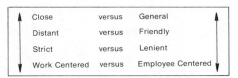

Figure 12–2 Supervisory styles.

decision-making process. The point is, managers should examine themselves, the costs, and the benefits of the leader authority style they use.

SUPERVISORY STYLES

In our previous discussion we stated that the second dimension of leader behavior, labeled "supervision," depicts the manner in which the leader (manager) interacts with the followers (subordinates) in the actual carrying out of the work activities. In other words, the way the accomplishment of specific work activity is overseen. Various styles of supervision can be used to denote that manner of interaction and are presented in Figure 12–2.[21] The first style discussed depicts how closely the manager oversees employees in the performance of their duties. The second describes the social distance the manager maintains. The third deals with how strict the supervision is in terms of rules and regulations. The fourth style discussed is whether the manager's orientation toward employees is employee or work centered. In the discussion of each style, observations will be made concerning variables that might cause the use of one or the other style contrasts.

Close Versus General Supervision.[22] "Close" versus "general" supervision refers to the degree to which the manager oversees the actual work activities of subordinates. Characteristics to be considered are the degree of delegation and how closely the subordinate's performance is monitored. Whether or not the manager should supervise subordinates closely or generally depends on a large number of factors related to the job setting—the people, the nature of their work, and so on. People holding unskilled or clerical health care jobs tend to require closer supervision than those in professional or managerial jobs; for example, maids and ward assistants generally need closer supervision than skilled technicians and nurses. The supervision of unskilled or clerical employees is generally related to the specifics of job performance; supervision of professional or managerial employees is more often concerned with checking results.

New employees tend to require closer supervision than experienced employees who have been on the job for a long period of time. Close supervision is not only necessary for inexperienced and unskilled employees, but also for emergency situations. In such instances, it may be necessary to give very specific instructions and follow every detail very closely. The surgeon–nurse relationship in the operating room is one example.

[21] See: Katz and Kahn "Leadership practices." in *Group Dynamics,* pp. 554–570.
[22] Thomas R. O'Donovan, "Effective supervision requires leadership." *Hospital Progress, 46*:65, February, 1965.

Generally, managers who have confidence in the ability of their subordinates will tend to supervise in a general way, while those who do not have this confidence, for reasons such as lack of subordinate motivation, skill, or training, will tend to oversee activities in closer detail. Obviously, if supervision is *too* general, control over results can be reduced and serious error could occur.

Distant Versus Friendly Supervision.[23]   The appropriateness of either the "distant" or the "friendly" supervisory style cannot be easily answered. The manager should be distant enough to retain the respect of subordinates, yet friendly enough to work effectively with them. If the manager is too friendly, socializes excessively, and is considered "one of the gang" it may hamper discipline, when it is necessary, or prevent effective supervision of the work activity. On the other hand, a too distant, "aloof" attitude may be interpreted by the employees as a lack of interest in them as individuals, and may result in lower employee motivation.

Strict Versus Lenient Supervision.[24]   The concept of the "strict" versus "lenient" supervisory style concerns the manner in which the manager enforces rules, policies, and overall employee conduct while overseeing the accomplishment of work activity. Although behavior and performance compliance will require firmness, the manager should also be fair. If performance standards are not imposed, both performance and respect can degenerate. It is important that strictness be reasonable. If the manager has unreasonable expectations and adheres strictly to policies and rules, then the voluntary cooperation of the group may be lost.

Employee Centered Versus Work Centered Supervision.[25]   The categorization of "employee" versus "work" centered supervision defines the tone of relations between the manager and the group in carrying out work activities. The employee centered health care manager views subordinates as being the center of the productivity wheel, the key ingredient to getting things done. This type of manager is interested in the subordinate's well-being, morale, and aspirations, and in whether his or her abilities are being utilized. Here, the manner of carrying out work activities is interpreted as being the positive motivation of subordinates rather than motivation through the use of negative sanctions. This is not a "slap on the back," superficial concern for employees but a recognition of their importance.

In contrast, managers adopting the work centered style when overseeing work activity tend to ignore the human factor in the job setting and concentrate on the production and technical aspects of the job. He or she is more concerned with immediate output than with developing strong interpersonal relationships based on respect with the employees. Typically, this manager is not concerned with the employees as individuals who have needs and aspirations, but views them as just another resource.

SUPERVISORY STYLE—WHICH IS CORRECT?

We have addressed the question "Autocratic to democratic—which is correct?" We will respond in a similar manner to the question "Supervisory

---

[23]*Ibid.* p. 66.
[24]*Ibid.* p. 66.
[25]*Ibid.* pp. 66–67.

style—which is correct?" It depends. No one supervisory style used by the manager for the accomplishment of work activities will be proper in all situations. The nature of the work, the urgency of the results, the characteristics of the workers, and the personality of the manager, among other things, are all factors in the work situation. The correct prescription will depend on these factors.

Cluster of Styles. There is another point that should be made regarding supervisory style. In Figure 12–2, it can be noted that there is a vertical arrow beside each column. This means that the four descriptive supervisory style contrasts we have examined tend to cluster along the two separate columns. In other words, the manager who can be described as "employee centered" tends to be lenient and friendly, and oversees activities in a general manner. In contrast, the manager who can be characterized as "work centered" tends to be strict and distant, and oversees activities in a close manner.

Linkage to Leader Authority Style. By the same token, the manager who can be characterized by the "employee centered" supervisory style would tend to fall toward the right side of the leader authority style continuum presented in Figure 12–2. He would more likely be "participative" or "democratic." In a similar manner, the manager characterized as being "work centered" would tend to have a leader authority style more toward the "consultative" or "autocratic" end of the continuum.

We have attempted to provide some linkage between the contrast of supervisory styles such as employee centered, and work centered, and the general polar ends of the leader authority style continuum. Supervisory style characterizes the leader behavior dimension and involves the manner in which the manager oversees the accomplishment of work activity—how it is done—and the relationship between manager and those being led. The leader authority style continuum portrays the leader behavior dimension and involves the amount of decision-making authority the manager holds or relinquishes to the group. Although the broad characterization of these two dimensions of leader behavior that we gave previously is not a truism, the generalization might prove worth considering.

Linkage to Managerial Approach. In addition, we would like to make several other observations for the reader to consider. In the previous chapter, Motivation of Employees, we discussed the Maslow need hierarchy, presented a model of human behavior, and dealt with Douglas McGregor's Theory X and Theory Y. Although the linkage is not precise, there are some generalizations that can be made. Typically, the manager with (1) an "employee centered" supervisory style and (2) a leader authority style more toward the "participative"–"democratic" end of the continuum could be regarded as being a Theory Y type of individual. This could correspond with the assumptions that McGregor makes concerning that managerial approach. In addition, we could also make a broad generalization that the manager classified as having (1) a "work centered," supervisory style and (2) a leader authority style toward the "consultative"–"autocratic" end of the continuum, would be a Theory X type of individual.

An important point should be interjected at this time. A labeling in terms of "good–bad" and "black–white" in regard to Theory X and Theory Y, leader authority styles, and supervisory styles might be construed here. *Beware!* It is not inconsistent for some of these descriptors to be mixed. It is also not inconsistent for the manager to vary to some degree between styles in different situations. For example, in her normal setting the head nurse may adopt an employee centered supervisory style with perhaps a consultative or participative leader authority style to deal with those who report to her. However, in a crisis, for whatever period of time, her style must adapt to the situation.

The perceptive manager can determine when and how to change leader behavior styles. No one style is correct for all situations. The point is, when you motivate and lead people, it is necessary to mix rewards, balance job satisfaction, and modify the leader authority and supervisory style ingredients to fit the followers, the time, and the place.

CONTINGENCY LEADERSHIP MODEL

Initially, we made the point that leadership is complex. We have also presented two dimensions of leader behavior. The first dimension dealt with the degree of decision-making authority held or relinquished to the group by the manager (leader decision authority style); the second dealt with the manner in which the manager oversees the accomplishment of specific work activity (supervisory style). We have alluded to the fact that the two sets of styles can be linked with each other. In addition, we emphasized the fact that no one style is necessarily correct but that the nature of the work, the urgency of the results, the characteristics of the workers, and the personality of the manager, (i.e., the sum of the situation) influence what is most appropriate. In other words, the appropriate pattern of leadership is *contingent* upon the situation.

In this section, we will present a leadership model—the "Contingency Model of Leadership"—developed by Fred Fiedler after extensive research over many years. Professor Fiedler examined various situational conditions with the purpose of identifying which style of leader behavior would be most appropriate given those conditions. While his model is by no means all-encompassing, and does not examine all possible variables, it does represent a major step toward the understanding of the complex subject of leadership.

On first glance, the leadership contingency model appears to be complicated. It is. We will attempt to condense its basic elements. To summarize, the model attempts to predict under what conditions (situations) the two broad leadership styles would be most effective in terms of group job performance. Those two styles are labeled by Fiedler as (1) "relations-motivated" and (2) "task-motivated." Fiedler's leader style labels differ from those we previously presented. His style labels can be construed as close approximations of "employee centered" and "work centered." As will be pointed out, he focuses primarily on the second dimension of leader behavior—the accomplishment of work activity—as opposed to the decision authority dimension.

Leadership Style Measurement. The two leadership styles labeled "relations-motivated" and "task-motivated" are measured by the Least Preferred Co-worker (LPC) questionnaire. The manager is asked to think of a present or past co-worker with whom he liked to work the *least*. The questionnaire contains attribute sets such as "Pleasant–Unpleasant" with eight response points between the two.[26]

Fiedler and Chemers conclude from their research that the manager with a high LPC score tends to seek strong emotional ties with others and is primarily motivated to seek close interpersonal relations. The reason for this is that if the manager thinks fairly positively of his *least* preferred coworker, he will tend to be more *people oriented*. On the other hand, a manager who has a low LPC score tends to be *task-motivated*, with interpersonal relationships having lower priority.[27]

SITUATIONAL CONDITIONS

The second aspect of the leadership contingency model incorporates the situational conditions of (a) leader–member relations, (b) task structure, and (c) position power.

Leader–Member Relations

One way of measuring the leader–member relations condition is by asking the group to respond to ten sets of attributes such as "Friendly–Unfriendly" which will indicate whether or not they accept and endorse their manager. A high score indicates good leader–member relations, while a low score indicates the opposite. Good leader–member relations implies that the manager is able to obtain compliance with minimum effort whereas poor leader–member relations implies compliance but given with reservation and reluctance.[28]

Task Structure

The task structure condition characterizes whether the tasks to be performed are unstructured or structured. Fiedler and Chemers point out that in an unstructured task situation the manager's expertise will not necessarily be greater than that of the group. As a result, an unstructured task implies correspondingly lower control and influence by the manager.

A structured task is a job situation that has specific instructions, general guidelines, and standard procedures provided for its completion. On the other hand, an unstructured task has only a vague and inexplicit procedure without step-by-step guidelines.[29]

Position Power

The position power condition reveals the degree of power vested in the manager by reason of his or her position. Position power refers to the legitimate authority that the manager has to reward or punish, hire or fire, promote or demote, and so on.[30]

Figure 12–3 presents the "Situational Favorableness Dimension" of the Fiedler model. It includes the combination of conditions that can exist relative to the three conditions of leader–member relations (good–poor), the task structure (high–low), and the manager's position power (strong–weak).

There are multiple combinations of conditions which result in eight spe-

---

[26]Fiedler and Chemers, op. cit. pp. 74–77.
[27]*Ibid.* pp. 76–77.
[28]*Ibid.* pp. 64–66.
[29]*Ibid.* pp. 66–68.
[30]*Ibid.* pp. 68–69.

THE SITUATIONAL FAVORABLENESS DIMENSION.

	I	II	III	IV	V	VI	VII	VIII
Leader–member Relations	Good				Poor			
Task Structure	High		Low		High		Low	
Position Power	Strong	Weak	Strong	Weak	Strong	Weak	Strong	Weak
Most Appropriate leadership style	T	T	T	R	R	R	R	T

T = Task-motivated

R = Relations motivated

Figure 12–3 Situational favorableness dimension of the contingency model of leadership. (Source: Adapted from Fred E. Fiedler, *Leadership.* Copyright © 1971 General Learning Corporation. Reprinted by permission of Silver Burdett Company).

cific possible situations. For example, in situation I there are good leader–member relations, high task structure, and strong position power. The question is, which type of leadership style, "relations-motivated" or "task-motivated" is best in this situation? The same question can be asked for each of the other seven situations.

In their research, Fiedler and his associates correlated group job performance with leadership style (relations-motivated and task-motivated) for each of the eight situational conditions (I–VIII). Their findings, presented in Figure 12–3, indicated that job performance tended to be higher in situations IV, V, VI, and VII when the manager was relations-motivated and higher in situations I, II, III, VIII when the manager was task-motivated.[31]

Although this model does not include all of the variables which affect the situation, it does include some, and is somewhat predictive. For example, Fiedler's research would indicate that in a situation of good leader–member relations, low task structure, and weak position power, the relations-motivated manager would tend to be more effective.

The contingency model is presented to reiterate our original statement that the most effective leader behavior is contingent upon the situation. Fiedler's model develops a theory based on three situational elements. This by no means ends the leadership theories. Nor can we restrict ourselves to these three conditions. However, the contingency theory, as presented, does offer some predictability between style and job performance.

[31]*Ibid.* pp. 77–81.

SUMMARY

This chapter is the second of three presenting integral parts of the executing process. We previously examined motivation; in this chapter we focused on leadership; and in the next chapter we will present the subject of communication. The heart of management is dealing with people. As a result, to be effective, all managers must motivate, lead, and communicate with others.

Leadership is a very complex subject. We presented its characteristic elements — group, goals, influence, and acceptance. Leadership was defined as that process by which one person designates "what is to be done" and influences others in order to accomplish specific purposes. Our attention was directed to the leader behavior of those formally appointed by the organization (manager–subordinate context). We also presented two dimensions of leader behavior: (1) the degree of decision-making authority held by the leader or relinquished to the group, and (2) the manner in which the leader interacts with others when overseeing the accomplishment of specific work activity.

Various styles of the two dimensions of leader behavior were presented. The leader decision authority styles ranged on a continuum from autocratic to laissez-faire. The supervisory styles were sets ranging from close–general to work centered–employee centered. Furthermore, factors such as the importance of the results, the type of work performed, the characteristics of the subordinates, and the personal characteristics of the managers were described as influencing the appropriateness of these leader behavior styles. Finally, a contingency leadership model was presented.

DISCUSSION QUESTIONS

1. How are the terms "group," "goals," "influence," and "acceptance" related to leadership? Can any of them be excluded?

2. Discuss the distinction between the various leader decision authority styles as well as the various supervisory styles.

3. Some have argued that leaders are born not made, and that all great leaders have certain common traits. Discuss.

4. Think of a health care manager you have worked for or have known and describe his or her leader decision authority style and supervisory style. Are the styles linked?

5. Identify and discuss the factors that influence an individual's leader decision authority and supervisory styles. Are there others?

INCIDENTS

1. GROUP DECISION

John Stevens, a hospital department head, recently attended a management seminar on decision-making. Professor Smith, who conducted the seminar, particularly impressed Mr. Stevens with his thoughts on group decision-making.

On the basis of research and experience, Professor Smith was convinced that employees, if given the opportunity, could meet together, intelligently consider, and then formulate quality decisions that would be enthusiastically accepted. In other words, the manager should follow the participative style.

Returning to his department at the conclusion of the seminar, Mr. Stevens decided to practice some of the principles he had learned. He called together the 25 employees of his department and told them that the production standards established several years previously were now too low in view of the recent installation of some automated equipment. He gave the employees the opportunity to discuss the mitigating circumstances and to decide among themselves, as a group, what their standards should be. Mr. Stevens, on leaving the room, believed that the employees would doubtlessly establish much higher standards than he himself would have dared propose.

After an hour of discussion the group summoned Mr. Stevens and notified him that, contrary to his opinion, their group decision was that the standards were already too high, and since they had been given the authority to establish their own standards, they were making a reduction of 10 per cent.

These standards are far too low to permit the department to do its work with the present number of employees. Yet, it is clear to Mr. Stevens that his refusal to accept the group decision could have serious implications. Stevens is in a mess.

A. How did he get there?

B. How could he have avoided it?

C. What should he do now?

(Source: Beaufort B. Longest, Jr., *Business Management of Health Care Providers*. Chicago: Hospital Financial Management Association, 1975. Used by permission of the publisher.)

2. CHARLOTTE COOK

Charlotte Cook is an RN who has three LPN's (Sally, Mary, and Betty) reporting to her during the day shift at Longview Nursing Home. She is 48 years old and has worked for Stanley George, the Administrator, for the past ten years.

Charlotte has been confronted with a leadership problem. Sally, who has worked for Charlotte for five years is 40 years old, cooperative, dependable, skilled, and an excellent performer. In fact, Charlotte has such confidence in Sally that she often leaves her in charge when she leaves the floor. Mary, who is 28, transferred from the evening shift two months ago after having worked there for one year. The administrator told Charlotte that he was transferring Mary because she could not get along with the new RN supervisor on that shift. The new RN is two years younger than Mary and they had a personality clash. In fact, rumors circulated that Mary resented the new RN because she was not satisfied with either Mary's performance or attitude. Furthermore, the previous supervisor and Mary were very close socially, she was not demanding of Mary, and she often made exceptions for her. The other second shift LPN's resented this and would have nothing to do with Mary.

Betty is 30 years old and has worked for Charlotte for the year she has been at Longview. Her performance is acceptable, she requires some direct supervision, and she and Charlotte have a good relationship.

Four weeks ago Mary began complaining to Sally and Betty. She criticized Mr. George and Mrs. Cook, and was generally "anti-everything" about Longview and its staff, particularly the new second shift RN and Charlotte. She was uncooperative, often did her job wrong, and gossiped with the patients.

Charlotte has noticed that Mary seems to always be with Betty during their free time and that Betty tends to side with Mary. Charlotte feels that if the situation is ignored, matters could get worse. Presume that LPN's are hard to get and that Charlotte doesn't want to discharge Mary, at least for the present.

A. How should Charlotte change the supervisory style she uses with Sally, when she interacts with Mary?

B. How should Charlotte approach and interact with Sally?

C. What should Charlotte do if Mary does not change?

D. Did Mr. George do the correct thing in transferring Mary?

E. What could Mr. George have done to remedy the situation at the time he transferred Mary?

3. PROMOTION DENIED

The Assistant Director of the Department of Housekeeping was very lax in keeping the time records of the employees. He had an informal system of allowing them 15 or 20 minutes tardiness leeway without docking them, against hospital policy. He is now retired, and a new assistant director has been appointed. The new man docks everybody, according to hospital policy. One of the employees who was up for promotion to housekeeping supervisor suddenly had three tardiness offenses charged against him, and Personnel has denied his promotion. As Director of the Housekeeping Department you have just found out all of this for the first time, and you are now trying very hard to have the Personnel Department excuse these tardiness offenses because they were allowed by the previous Assistant Director of the Housekeeping Department, and because you feel that the employee is very competent and deserves a promotion.

A. Should the housekeeping employee be promoted to supervisor?

B. What problems do you now face in having a new Assistant Director for the Housekeeping Department?

This Chapter Contains:

- Introduction
- Communication Defined
- Organizational Communication
- Communication Flows
    Downward
    Upward
    Horizontal
- Barriers to Communication
    Environmental Barriers
    Personal Barriers
- Informal Communication
- Summary
- Discussion Questions
- Incidents

Chapter 13

COMMUNICATION

"Communication is a means, not an end. It serves as the lubricant fostering the smooth operation of the management process(es)."

(George Terry)[1]

INTRODUCTION

The management processes of decision-making, planning, organizing, executing, and controlling depend on effective communication. Without it, plans and objectives would go no further than the person who originated them; the organization would exist only as a conglomeration of isolated people and departments; the execution of activity could not take place because no one would know what, when, how, or why to do anything; and the controlling process would not exist because there would be no feedback mechanism for measuring performance with expectations.

Communication depends upon the formal establishment of channels and networks for transmitting information in all directions within the organization and upon the recognition and utilization of these channels. This is a very large and very important task for the manager. In highly complex organizations such as those dealing with health care delivery, communication is multidirectional and requires movement downward, upward, and horizontally. People communicate facts, ideas, feelings, and attitudes while working and solving problems. If this communication is adequate, the work gets done more effectively and the problems are solved more efficiently. In any organized effort, communication is essential for people to work together because it permits them to influence and react to one another.

COMMUNICATION DEFINED

We will define communication as *the creation or exchange of understanding between a sender and a receiver.* Clearly, this definition does not restrict the concept to words alone; it includes all methods (verbal and nonverbal) through which meaning is conveyed to others. Even silence can convey meaning and must be considered part of communicating.

---

[1]George R. Terry, *Principles of Management*, 6th ed. Homewood, Illinois: Richard D. Irwin, Inc., 1972, p. 168.

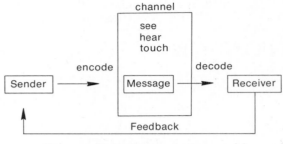

Figure   13–1 Communication model.

An important part of this definition is the word "understanding." A sender wants the receiver of the message to understand what was sent. This means that he or she wants the receiver to interpret the message exactly as it is intended. Unfortunately, communication seldom results in complete understanding because there are so many barriers that can prevent it. Many of these barriers will be discussed later. It is important for the manager to realize that information can be transmitted to others but they cannot be *made* to understand it.

Communication activity can be diagrammed easily, as seen in the model presented in Figure 13–1. The reader should note the feedback loop in this activity. When a sender encodes and transmits a message via a channel (oral, written, or tactile) to a receiver who decodes the message and indicates understanding by giving feedback, effective two-way communication occurs. This is important for the manager because good two-way communication is an absolute necessity for effective management. Furthermore, it greatly increases the likelihood that directives from the manager will be completely understood. A number of studies have shown that the accuracy of work and, almost as importantly, the employees' confidence in the accuracy of their work are improved when effective two-way communication is practiced between participants in the health care organization.[2] There are occasions, of course, when two-way communication is not possible because time is too critical.

For a function so vital to success, communication receives all too little attention from managers. For example, the relationship between effective communication and morale, performance, and even patient recovery rates has been well established.[3] It has also been stipulated that communication is a major intervening variable in the physician–patient relationship.[4] However, a study conducted by one of the authors indicated that communication was not totally effective. The communication between superiors and subordinates in 17 large general hospitals was measured based on the degree of agreement on five basic aspects of the subordinate's function.[5] The assumption was that if there was suc-

[2]Harish C. Jain, "Supervisory communication and performance in urban hospitals." *Journal of Communication, 23*:109, March, 1973.

[3]*Ibid.* p. 105.

[4]Harold C. Walker, "Communication and the American health care problem." *Journal of Communication, 23*:349, December, 1973.

[5]Beaufort B. Longest, Jr., "A look at upward communication in general hospitals." *Atlanta Economic Review, 24*:14, September–October, 1974.

Table 13-1   Percentage distributions of ratings assigned to superior–subordinate pairs on five basic areas of the subordinate's job.

	0 ALMOST NO AGREEMENT ON TOPICS	1 AGREEMENT ON LESS THAN HALF THE TOPICS	2 AGREEMENT ON ABOUT HALF THE TOPICS	3 AGREEMENT ON MORE THAN HALF THE TOPICS	4 AGREEMENT ON ALL OR ALMOST ALL THE TOPICS
Methods of upward communication	12.5	0.0	6.3	12.5	68.7
Job duties	0.0	0.0	0.0	31.3	68.7
Job requirements (subordinate's qualifications)	6.3	0.0	6.3	31.3	56.1
Future changes in subordinate's job	75.0	0.0	18.7	0.0	6.3
Obstacles in way of subordinate's performance	43.7	18.7	12.5	12.5	12.5

(Source: Beaufort B. Longest, Jr., "A look at upward communication in general hospitals." *Atlanta Economic Review, 24*:17, September–October, 1974. Used by permission of the publisher.)

cessful communication about these factors, then there would be a high level of agreement about them. Table 13–1 contains the results of this study. As can be seen, there is little agreement on such things as future changes in the subordinate's job and the obstacles in the way of the subordinate's performance. This is empirical evidence of the extent of the communication problems existing in hospitals. Other types of health care organizations experience the same types of problems. It is imperative, therefore, that managers, regardless of their level in the hierarchy, understand the principles and concepts of communication within health care organizations.

ORGANIZATIONAL COMMUNICATION

Traditional organization theorists felt that communications should be structured and go through "authorized channels." This was necessary, in their view, to ensure unity of command and support their principle of a structure based on hierarchy (see Chapter 7 for a full presentation of these concepts).

The largest area of research in communications has concerned the communication networks, defined as "a system of decision centers interconnected by communication channels."[6] Figure 13–2 illustrates the most common communication networks. The classic network studies were made by Alex Bavelas and Harold Leavitt.[7] The value of these studies is that they show the influence of at least one variable (organized communication patterns) on performance

---

[6] William G. Scott, *Organization Theory.* Homewood, Illinois: Richard D. Irwin, Inc., 1967, p. 165.

[7] Alex Bavelas, "Communication patterns in task-oriented groups." *Journal of Acoustical Society of America, 22*:725, 1950. Reprinted in D. Cartwright and A. F. Zander, eds., *Group Dynamics: Research and Theory,* 2nd ed. New York: Row, Peterson and Company, 1960, pp. 660–683; and Harold J. Leavitt, "Some effects of certain communication patterns on group performance." *Journal of Abnormal and Social Psychology, 46*:38, January, 1951.

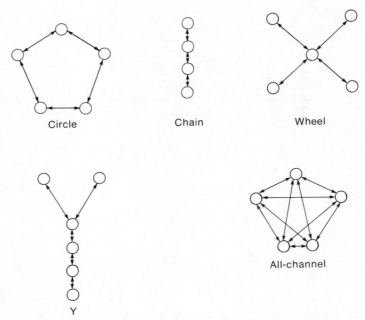

Figure 13–2 Common communication networks.

and satisfaction. For example, one study suggested the results that appear in Table 13–2 for three types of networks.[8]

The reader can see from these findings that one type of network might be desirable in a given situation (for example, wheel when speed and accuracy are needed) and another might be best in a different situation (circle, for example, when morale and flexibility are needed). When the communication involves a surgical team performing a complicated operation, it is easy to visualize the necessity of the wheel arrangement with the surgeon at the center. On the other hand, an administrator meeting with department heads to discuss the impact of a new service might find that the flexibility and morale boost inherent

---

[8]Alex Bavelas and Dermot Barrett, "An experimental approach to organizational communication." *Personnel*, 27:370, March, 1951. Copyright © 1951. Adapted by permission of the publisher.

Table 13–2 Sample of results from classic network studies.

	TYPES OF NETWORKS		
	Circle	*Chain*	*Wheel*
Speed of performance	Slow	Fast	Fast
Accuracy	Poor	Good	Good
Emergence of leader	None	Marked	Very pronounced
Morale	Very good	Poor	Very poor
Flexibility to job change	Very fast	Slow	Slow

in a circle pattern is best. The point of importance is that one is likely to find a multitude of communication networks existing simultaneously in health care organizations.

COMMUNICATION FLOWS

As we stated earlier, communication in health care organizations is multidirectional and flows downward, upward, and horizontally. Typically, the downward flow is the communication between manager and subordinates; upward communication operates through the same channels but in the opposite direction. Horizontal flow is usually between manager and manager or worker and worker. We will examine the specific nature of each of these flows.

DOWNWARD COMMUNICATION FLOW

Communication flows downward in the health care organization from a higher to a lower authority. The downward flow of communication is emphasized in most health care organizations, as it is in many other organizations. In the executing process, for example, it is necessary for superiors to convey a great deal of information to subordinates. Others have summarized the objectives of the downward communication flow in the following way:[9]

1. To give specific task directives about job instructions.
2. To give information about organizational procedures and practices.
3. To provide information about the rationale of the job.
4. To tell subordinates about their performance.
5. To provide ideological information to facilitate the indoctrination of goals.

Downward communication flows through many channels.[10] Most often it consists of verbal orders or instructions from a superior to a subordinate on a one-to-one basis, but other channels include speeches to groups of employees, meetings, and public address systems. The myriad of written methods such as handbooks, procedure manuals, newsletters, bulletin boards, and the ubiquitous memorandum are also downward channels of communication. Computerized information systems contribute substantially to the downward flow of communication in many health care organizations.

One result of the use of these multiple channels has been the saturation of employees with certain types of communication to such an extent that much of it is ignored, misinterpreted, or lost. There are other potential pitfalls in the downward flow of communication. All too often, the manager understands what is being communicated but the employees, with their extreme diversity in education, background, and sociocultural status, may or may not understand. Also, any downward communication that does not provide for feedback will not be very conducive to a feeling of participation on the part of organization

---

[9] Daniel Katz and Robert L. Kahn, *The Social Psychology of Organizations.* New York: John Wiley & Sons, Inc., 1966, p. 239.

[10] For a good discussion see Edwin B. Flippo, *Management: A Behavioral Approach.* Boston: Allyn and Bacon, Inc., 1970, pp. 394–395.

members. As has been suggested, just because there is a very active downward flow of communication does not mean that the information is accurate or that it is received, understood, or accepted.[11]

UPWARD COMMUNICATION FLOWS

In the health care organization, upward communication flows from a lower to a higher authority and it is becoming more important as organizational complexity forces managers to delegate more. Upward communication provides the manager with decision-making information, reveals problem areas, provides data for performance evaluation, indicates the status of worker morale, and generally underscores the thinking of subordinates in the organization.

Furthermore, the upward flow helps "to meet the needs of the human ego."[12] It permits those in positions of lower authority to make their opinions and perceptions known to those of higher authority; as a result, they feel a stronger sense of participation in the health care organization. Of course, for upward communication to be effective, the fear of reprisal must be eliminated.[13]

A number of methods can be used for upward communication. The hierarchical structure is, of course, the main formal method used by organizations to communicate upward. However, this method can be supplemented by such methods as the following, suggested by Luthans:[14]

1. *The grievance procedure.* Provided for in most collective bargaining agreements, the grievance procedure allows an employee to make an appeal upward beyond his immediate superior. It protects the individual from arbitrary action from his direct superior and encourages upward communication.

2. *The open-door policy.* Taken literally, this means that the superior's door is always open to subordinates. It is a continuous invitation for a subordinate to come in and talk about anything that is troubling him. Unfortunately, in practice the open-door policy is more fiction than fact. The boss may slap his subordinate on the back and say, "My door is always open to you," but in many cases both the man and his boss know the door is really closed. It is a case where the adage that actions speak louder than words applies.

3. *Counseling, attitude questionnaires, and exit interviews.* The personnel department can greatly facilitate upward communication by conducting nondirective, confidential counseling sessions, periodically administering attitude questionnaires, and holding meaningful exit interviews for those who leave the organization. Much valuable information can be gained from these forms of upward communication.

4. *Participative techniques.* Participative-decision techniques can generate a great deal of upward communication. This may be accomplished by either informal involvement from subordinates or by formal participation programs.

5. *The ombudsman.* A largely untried but potentially significant technique to

---

[11]Fred Luthans, *Organizational Behavior: A Modern Behavioral Approach to Management.* New York: McGraw-Hill Book Company, 1973, p. 250.

[12]Flippo, op cit. p. 396.

[13]Robert M. Wendlinger, "Improving upward communication." *Journal of Business Communication, 10*:17, Summer, 1974.

[14]Luthans, op. cit. p. 253. Used by permission of the publisher.

enable management to obtain upward communication is the use of an ombudsman. The concept has been used primarily in Scandinavia to provide an outlet for persons who have been treated unfairly or in a depersonalized manner by large, bureaucratic government. It has more recently gained popularity in American state governments, military posts, and universities. (More recently, health care organizations have applied this approach to improve communication between *patients* and the organization. If properly applied, it may very well work in the larger, more complex, and more depersonalized health care organizations as they seek ways to improve upward communication flows from their employees.)

HORIZONTAL COMMUNICATION FLOWS

Management authorities have recently recognized that effective downward and upward communication flows are not sufficient for effective organizational performance. In complex organizations, especially those subject to abrupt demands for action and reaction (such as modern health care organizations), there must also be an effective horizontal flow of communication. Perhaps this is more true when care is being rendered to a specific patient by a variety of personnel from a number of different organizational units. Their actions must be coordinated in an atmosphere that limits upward and downward communication flows in order to meet the requirements of moving all participants toward a common objective. The concept of the hospital as a matrix organization was presented in Chapter 8 and illustrates this phenomenon.

The prevalence of committees in health care organizations can be attributed to the need for horizontal communication flows. Committees provide a mechanism for representatives of organizational units from all levels to sit down together and discuss common problems and potentials face to face. Strict adherence to hierarchical communication flow would never permit this opportunity. As everyone who has been involved with committees realizes, there are some disadvantages to this form of horizontal communication. Committees tend to be time consuming and expensive, and their decisions are often compromises that may represent an ineffectual solution to a given problem. Nevertheless, it is important to note that committees are the main formal mechanism for horizontal communication flows in health care organizations.

BARRIERS TO COMMUNICATION

We have defined communication as the creation and exchange of understanding between a sender and a receiver. On the surface, this may appear to be as easy a task as the model presented in Figure 13–1 would indicate. However, by viewing the expanded model in Figure 13–3, it can be noted that for effective communication to occur, a number of obstacles or barriers must be overcome. These environmental and personal barriers, typically present in any setting, can block, filter, or distort the message as it is encoded and sent, as well as when it is decoded and received. Environmental barriers are characteristic of the organization and work setting; personal barriers arise from the nature of individuals and their interaction with others.

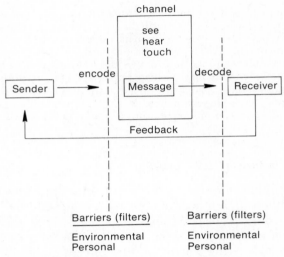

Figure 13-3 Expanded communication model.

ENVIRONMENTAL BARRIERS

Noise, Attention, Time.   Three obvious environmental barriers are (1) noise, (2) competition for attention, and (3) time. The reception and understanding of a message can be greatly affected by the amount of surrounding noise, other demands for the receiver's attention, and the amount of time he has to assimilate the information transmitted. As would be expected, misunderstandings can occur when noise makes it difficult to hear. In addition, multiple and simultaneous demands on the sender may cause him or her to package the message content inappropriately; these demands may also result in the message being filtered or distorted by the receiver. In such a situation, the receiver may hear the message without comprehending it because it is not getting his or her full attention—the receiver is not really "listening." Consider this situation for a moment: the supervisor is very busy, preoccupied with multiple events, and perhaps talking on the phone. Chances are that these competing demands for attention will result in this individual's hearing less than what is sent and not really listening to the content. As a result, understanding may not occur. Finally, time may function as a barrier to effective communication by permitting the sender little opportunity to completely think through and structure the message he or she wishes to convey, and by allowing the receiver an inappropriate amount of time to fully ascertain the meaning of the message.

Philosophy, Levels, Power–status.   Another set of environmental barriers which can filter, distort or block a message consists of (1) the administrative philosophy of the organization, (2) the multiplicity of hierarchical levels, and (3) power–status relationships. Administrative philosophy can often inhibit, as well as promote, effective communication.[15] Viewing it in the negative sense, an administration (or manager) that is not interested in promoting com-

---

[15]Harold Stieglitz, "Barriers to communication." *Management Record, 20*:3, January, 1958.

munication upward or disseminating information downward will, as a rule, establish procedural and organizational blockages. The requirement that all communication "flow through channels," the inaccessibility of superiors, the lack of interest in employees' frustrations, complaints, or feelings, and the insufficient time allocated to receive information are symptoms of an administrative philosophy that tends to retard communication flows. Furthermore, the lack of action[16] with regard to complaints, ideas, problems, and the like will serve as a signal to those who may wish to communicate upward and, as a result, will tend to discourage the free flow of information.

Multiple levels in an organization hierarchy tend to cause message distortion.[17] As the message is transmitted up or down through many people at many levels, there is a likelihood that each person will interpret the message according to his or her frame of reference and vantage point in the organization. When multiple links exist in the communication chain, information will be filtered, dropped, and added, and emphasis will be rearranged as it is transmitted to other receivers. As a result, a message sent through many levels has a good chance of being distorted or perhaps even totally blocked by one of the links. For example, very often a message sent from the administrator to employees through several layers of the organization is received in quite a different form than that which was originally sent. Or, a report prepared for the administrator that is passed through the hierarchy possibly may not reach its destination because it sits on someone's desk and is, in essence, blocked.

Power–status relationships can also distort or inhibit the transmission of a message.[18] A discordant superior–subordinate relationship can dampen the flow and content of information. Furthermore, depending on past experiences, an employee may be inhibited about communicating for fear of reprisal, negative sanctions, or ridicule. Have you ever witnessed a situation where, as a result of poor superior–subordinate rapport, the subordinate does not inform the superior that he or she is doing something wrong or that a plan will not work? "I'm not going to stick my neck out—let him find out for himself."

Power–status communication barriers are particularly prevalent in health care organizations, where a number of professionals must interact with each other. In the doctor–patient relationship the doctor is typically held in awe and little upward communication may occur because of his or her status. People hesitate to question their doctor. Furthermore, status relationships among professionals create a complex situation. How often does the head nurse with 20 years of experience tell the resident that a procedure or treatment might not be efficacious. How is the nurse's message encoded—bluntly or obliquely? The point is, status and role conflicts, particularly among professionals, can serve as a major barrier to effective communication.

Terminology and Complexity of the Message. When messages require the use of specific (1) terminology unfamiliar to the receiver and are (2) complex, there may be a breakdown in communication. Most professionals

---

[16]Alfred Vogel, "Why don't employees speak up?" *Personnel Administration, 30*:22, May–June, 1967.

[17]Stieglitz, op. cit. p. 5.

[18]Charles Blagdon and Lucian Spataro, "Organizational communication." *The American Business Communication Bulletin,* Part 2, *36*:12, September, 1973.

have their own set of terminology. Those on the administrative side of the health care organization may use a completely different set of terminology than those responsible for direct patient care. Terminology is important, since words mean *specific* things to those familiar with them and tend to minimize misunderstanding. However, interaction between those in the health care organization who have different sets of terminology can result in ineffective communication.[19]

When the complexity of the message is such that understanding must be precise, and when it is linked with terminology that may be unfamiliar to the receiver, there is a good chance that understanding will not occur. When messages are complex, care must be taken to use terminology which the receiver will understand, using, perhaps, multiple channels such as oral and visual and relying on feedback to ensure that the message was decoded as intended.

PERSONAL BARRIERS

In addition to environmental barriers to communication, another set, personal barriers, exists when people communicate with each other, whether it is upward, downward, or horizontally.

Frame of Reference, Beliefs, Selective Perception. When people encode and send messages or decode and receive them, they tend to do so according to their (1) frame of reference and (2) beliefs, and they consciously or unconsciously engage in (3) selective perception.[20] The sum of one's socio-economic background and previous experiences can shape the manner in which one receives and interprets communication. For example, someone with a cultural background of "don't speak unless spoken to" and "never question elders" may be inhibited in communicating. Other people, who may be more naive, accept all communication at face value and do not filter out erroneous information or puffing. In contrast to this, aggressiveness and the dissemination of self-edifying information could result in the transmission of a message distorted for personal gain. Furthermore, unless one has had the same experiences as others, it is difficult to completely understand the meaning of their message. The wealthy may have a difficult time understanding hunger. Those who have never experienced pain or childbirth or witnessed death may not be able to truly comprehend them.

Closely related to one's frame of reference are beliefs, values, and prejudices. They can cause messages to be distorted or blocked either in transmission or reception. This occurs because people differ, their personalities differ, and their backgrounds differ; they have preconceived opinions, prejudices, and listen with a reflective ear.[21]

Without being oblique in our message, it can be said that people have preconceived opinions pertaining to a multitude of areas such as politics, ethics,

---

[19]Bradford B. Boyd, "An analysis of communication between departments—roadblock and by-pass." *Personnel Administration, 28*:35, November–December, 1965.

[20]William E. Pride and O. Jeff Harris, "Psychological barriers to the upward flow of communication." *Atlanta Economic Review, 24*:30, March, 1971.

[21]Stieglitz, op. cit. p. 2.

religion, union–management, sex, race, and life style. These biases, beliefs, and values filter and distort communication. For example, these beliefs will cloud and filter messages: female physicians are not as proficient as male physicians; administrators who are not M.D.'s cannot manage a health care organization; ward assistants are less worthy as people than R.N.'s. Furthermore, the tone of a message serves as a cue to the receiver and shapes the way he or she will receive the sender's message. A sender's arrogant attitude can convey the fact that the receiver is thought to be inferior, lazy, or stupid, and will cause the receiver to react, perhaps by ignoring the message.

Selective perception is one of the most difficult personal barriers to overcome, both for the sender and receiver. We all tend to screen derogatory information and amplify words, actions, and meanings that flatter us. In other words, we tend to screen out the "bad" of a message and retain the "good." Selective perception can be conscious or unconscious. When it is conscious, intentional distortion results. For example, the supervisor with high turnover may receive that as a message and (a) amplify the idea that the turnover is due to low wages over which he or she has no control and, therefore, no responsibility, and (b) delete, diminish, or not admit that the real cause is the supervisory style. Unfortunately, selective perception is a part of human nature.

Jealousy, Fear. Two additional personal barriers to communication are (1) jealousy and (2) fear.[22] We previously touched on fear as an environmental inhibitor to full and free communication flow. Jealousy, when coupled with selective perception, may result in conscious efforts to filter and distort incoming information or transmit misinformation, or both. For example, the supervisor with an extremely able assistant who makes him or her look good, may tend to block or distort information that would reveal the situation to other sources. Furthermore, petty personality differences, the feeling of professional incompetence or inferiority, and sheer greed can lead to jealousy and communication distortion.

Evaluate Source, Maintain Status Quo. When people receive messages from others, there is a tendency for the receiver to (1) evaluate the source (sender).[23] Furthermore, conditions often exist where there are incentives to (2) maintain the status quo. Evaluation of the source is frequently necessary in order to decide whether some of the message should be filtered out or discounted. Obviously, a health care equipment salesman will have an incentive for praising the product. However, an impediment to communication can occur if, after the source is evaluated, a decision that is not warranted is made in order to discount the information. For example, a hostile union–management atmosphere may result in the employees ignoring messages from the administration. Another situation could have the supervisor never listening to the employee who continuously gripes or complains. As we mentioned, source evaluation is important for coping with the barrage of communication directed at us daily; however, one must be cognizant of the fact that source evaluation carries with it the hazard that legitimate messages will not be received or understood. This dilemma is not easy to solve.

---

[22]Boyd, op. cit. p. 36.
[23]Blagdon and Spataro, op. cit. p. 13.

The status quo barrier denotes a conscious effort by the sender or receiver to filter out information either in sending, receiving, or retransmitting that would upset the present situation.[24] In other words, the status quo. Basically, this implies the transmission of information that the sender thinks the receiver wants to hear. Environmental conditions which promote "fear of sending bad news"—superior displeasure, lack of candor in the organization, and insufficient confidence in the superior–subordinate relationship—will tend to foster the erection of this barrier.

Semantics, Symbols, Empathy.   The three remaining personal barriers to communication to be presented are (1) semantics, (2) symbols, and (3) empathy. We previously discussed terminology as an environmental barrier. Closely related to terminology is semantics. Since words mean different things to different people, and different people have different backgrounds, care must be taken to communicate in a vernacular that is easily understood. The use of overly complex vocabulary and idioms can impede the understanding of a message.

In health care organizations, symbols are very important and play a major role in the communication activity. They can be characterized by physical things, pictures, and actions. For example, the use of different uniforms by personnel not only denotes status but also enables others to immediately evaluate the source. The nurse wears a white uniform, the LPN may wear a yellow uniform, and the doctor wears a long white coat. In this sense, physical symbols serve a functional purpose.

Pictures or visual representations are another type of symbol. They can be quite helpful in communicating, and greatly increase understanding. Think of how many words would be needed to explain the organization structure in lieu of a pictorial chart of the organization. Or imagine the difficulty of completely describing the message contained in a single X-ray film so that it will be understood.

Finally, action is a symbol that can be used to communicate. A friendly smile or a pat on the back can have meaning. A promotion or a pay increase conveys a great deal to the recipient and to others. Furthermore, lack of action can have symbolic meaning in messages. One writer notes that the

> failure to act is an important way of communication. The manager has communicated when he fails to compliment someone for a job well done or fails to take a promised action. Since we communicate both by action and lack of action, we communicate almost all the time at work, whether we intend to or not. Being at one's desk has meaning, but being away also has meaning.[25]

Action can reinforce and can also be a barrier to communication. When the action is inconsistent with the words, two contradictory messages are transmitted. For example, the supervisor who tells a subordinate, "I have confidence in your ability, your performance is excellent, and I want to expand your duties by delegating more to you" would not be consistent if he or she went into a

---

[24]*Ibid.* p. 14.
[25]Keith Davis, *Human Behavior at Work: Human Relations and Organizational Behavior*. New York: McGraw-Hill, 1972, p. 391.

rage because of a small technical error. Or the receiver who says, "I am listening" to the sender and then proceeds to look at his or her watch impatiently or
starts to walk away would construct a symbolic action barrier to effective communication.

A lack of empathy can impair communication. Empathy basically means
being sensitive to the world of the other people in the communication chain.
Being sensitive to the other person's frame of reference or state of emotions
can promote better understanding. Empathy can help the sender to decide how
to encode the message and help the receiver to interpret its meaning. For example, a subordinate who empathizes with his or her supervisor may discount
an angry message because the subordinate is aware that extreme pressure and
frustration have caused the supervisor's state of·mind. Have you ever had a bad
day and displaced your frustrations on someone or something by word or action? If the receiver of the message empathizes with the sender, it will be interpreted in a much different way than if he or she does not. By the same
token, if the sender is sensitive to the receiver, he or she can decide whether or
not to communicate and how to encode the message. If, for example, the
receiver has had a "bad day," a mild reprimand may be interpreted as being
stronger than it actually is. Or if a receiver has just emerged from a traumatic
experience, such as a family illness or financial setback, the sender may decide
to wait to communicate bad news until a later date.

RESPONSIVE STEPS

We have presented some of the environmental barriers to communication
that are characteristic of the organization and the work setting, as well as
various personal barriers. The awareness that these barriers exist will certainly
contribute to minimizing their impact, as will positive efforts to eliminate them.
The net effect will be more effective communication between the sender and
receiver.

Although the necessary steps to improve communication flows, decrease
distortion and filtering, and eliminate blockages will depend upon particular
circumstances, some general steps can be suggested.

With regard to environmental barriers, efforts on the part of the receiver
and sender to ensure that noise is minimized, that adequate attention is being
given to the message, and that time is devoted to really "listening" to what is
being communicated will be helpful. In addition, an administrative philosophy
that encourages communication flow would be constructive. Efforts taken to
reduce the number of links (levels in the organization hierarchy) through which
messages pass are important. The power–status barrier is much more difficult
to deal with and is greatly affected by interpersonal and interprofessional relationships. Conscious efforts to tailor terminology so that it is understandable
are important. Finally, the use of multiple channels to reinforce complex messages will certainly decrease the likelihood that misunderstanding will occur.

In considering personal barriers, a conscious effort by sender and receiver
to understand the other's frame of reference and beliefs will help to promote
effective communication. Recognition of the fact that most people engage in
selective perception and are prone to jealousy and fear is a first step toward the
elimination, or at least the diminishing, of the impact these barriers can have.

The cautious use of symbols, the reinforcement of words with consistent action, and empathy toward others are obviously necessary steps.

INFORMAL COMMUNICATION

Coexisting with formal organization communication flows is an informal communication flow commonly known as the *grapevine*. This term, by the way, arose during the Civil War, when telegraph lines were strung between trees much like a grapevine. The messages transmitted over these flimsy lines were often garbled and, as a result, any rumor was said to come from the "grapevine."[26]

By definition, the grapevine, or informal flow of communication, in health care organizations consists of those channels which rise out of the interpersonal relationships of organization participants.[27] The informal communication flows in an organization are as natural as the patterns of social interaction that develop. Like the informal organization (see Chapter 7), the informal communication flows coexist with the formal patterns established by management.

The manager must realize that good or bad the grapevine is a fact of organization life. "It cannot be abolished, rubbed out, hidden under a basket, chopped down, tied up, or stopped. If we suppress it in one place, it will pop up in another."[28]

Informal communication channels can be misused. For example, a male R.N., realizing that he is going to be passed over for promotion to supervisor in favor of a more qualified female, might start a rumor that the Director of the Nursing Service does not like male nurses and that she had said she "would not have one as a supervisor." This rumor would not be true but it could cause others to think that the Nursing Director was discriminating against male nurses.

Some authorities believe that the grapevine serves no useful purpose to the organization. John Miner, for example, has said,

> There is very little that can be done to utilize the grapevine purposefully as a means of goal attainment. As a result, rumors probably do at least as much to subvert organizational goals as to foster them. They may well stir up dissension.[29]

However, other authorities suggest that the informal communication flows are useful, if properly managed. When concerned with downward flow, the informal system tends to be much faster than the formal; for upward and horizontal flows, it is essential. In a health care organization, much of the coordination occurring between the units does so through the informal give-and-take information exchange. In the case of upward flow, informal communication can act as a rich source of information about the performance, ideas, feelings, and attitudes of people in the organization. Because of its potential usefulness,

---

[26]*Ibid.* p. 261.

[27]Jay T. Knippen, "Grapevine communication: Management and employees." *Journal of Business Research.* 2:49, January, 1974.

[28]Davis, op. cit. p. 263.

[29]John B. Miner, *Personnel Psychology.* New York: The Macmillan Company, 1969, p. 259.

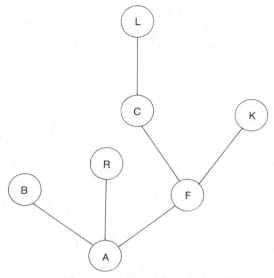

Figure 13–4 Cluster chain, the normal grapevine pattern. (Source: Keith Davis, *Human Behavior at Work,* 4th edition. New York: McGraw-Hill Book Company, 1972, p. 265. Used by permission of the publisher.)

and because of its pervasive existence, managers should try to understand informal communication flows and use them to advantage.

Keith Davis, one of the foremost authorities on informal communication, has suggested that

Managers occasionally get the impression that the grapevine operates like a long chain in which A tells B, who tells C, who then tells D, and so on, until twenty persons later, Y gets the information – very late and very incorrect. Sometimes the grapevine may operate this way, but research shows that it generally follows a different pattern, which works something like this: A tells three or four others (such as B, R, and F), as shown in Figure 13–4. Only one or two of these receivers will then pass on the information, and they will usually tell more than one person. Then as the information becomes older and the proportion of those knowing it gets larger, it gradually dies out because those who receive it do not repeat it. This network is a "cluster chain," because each link in the chain tends to inform a cluster of other people instead of only one person.[30]

In essence, informal communication flow is present in every organization and has the potential for being either good or bad for effectiveness. Part of the manager's job is to utilize this flow advantageously to achieve organization objectives.

Another important aspect of the informal communication flow in the health care organization is its relationship to patient care. As we have seen in previous chapters, a team of people is increasingly responsible for the care rendered to individual patients. These teams are not always highly structured,

---

[30]Davis, op. cit. p. 264.

which would mean that formal channels would be sufficient; instead, they tend to be loosely knit and have a high level need for informal communication flows. Harold L. Walker has suggested that

> As the administration of medicine moves more fully into the arena of team effort, problems will increase since the matrix will continue to expand and networks never before conceived will develop. Societal health will be treated by a melange of professionals from nurse to doctor to social worker to sociologist to nutritionist to computer scientist to administrator. We will have to cope with this explosion of communication patterns.[31]

SUMMARY

We have defined communication as the creation or exchange of *understanding* between a sender and a receiver. The communicating activity itself is simple, but the environmental and personal barriers to good communication often make it a demanding management activity.

Organizational communication flows downward, upward, and horizontally in the health care organization. It also flows through the informal channel called the grapevine.

A major point for the manager to consider concerning the communicating activity is that messages are conveyed through many modes or means—such as sound, sight, touch, smell, and action. Finally, without communication, organization activity cannot be executed. Ineffective communication will detract from organization effectiveness; effective and appropriate communication is the responsibility of all employees.

The manager must remember that unless *what* is to be done, *how* it is to be done, by *whom* it is to be done, and *why* it is to be done can all be effectively communicated, the chance of adequately carrying out the management processes is greatly reduced.

DISCUSSION QUESTIONS

1. What does it mean to say that "communication is a means, not an end"?

2. Discuss the importance of feedback in communicating.

3. Discuss the various types of communication networks and describe the advantages and disadvantages of each.

4. Discuss the purpose of the downward communication flow in a health care organization. How can it be improved?

5. Discuss the purpose of the upward communication flow in a health care organization. How can it be improved?

6. Discuss the role of committees in relation to communication in a health care organization.

---

[31]Walker, op. cit. pp. 356–357.

7. What are barriers to communication? How can they be overcome?

8. Discuss the role of symbols in communication. What problems do they present?

9. Discuss the advantages and disadvantages of the informal communication flow (grapevine) in a health care organization.

INCIDENTS

1. THE LETTER

As administrator of the ABC Nursing Home, you have been confronted by some behavior and leadership problems with your new Director of Nursing Service. She has been on the job approximately three months and you have had several meetings with her. You have now decided to put some of your thoughts in writing. Following is a letter that you have written to her.

Dear Mrs. Jones:

You have mentioned to me that you have been having a difficult time getting your employees to work together as a team. You also mentioned that you have felt frustrated because administration hasn't acted on your suggestions and backed you up. The purpose of this letter is to strongly suggest that you look to yourself as a source of these problems, rather than the administration. It is important that you avoid complaining about things that aren't being done for you, and start doing things on your own. Don't always look to others as the source of your problems. Working with people is a difficult challenge, and the upper management must indicate its strength so that a system of sound leadership will permeate the entire organization. You have to stand or fall on your own. You cannot expect to have your administrator settle all the problems that arise. You have to develop faith and confidence in yourself and learn to work with your peers and the personnel within your department. If your problems persist, it will be necessary to replace you.

A. What might Mrs. Jones do after having received this letter?

B. How will she feel about this letter and how will she interpret it? What was communicated?

C. Do you think the administrator will be surprised at the result that this letter has on Mrs. Jones?

D. What other way could the administrator have communicated with Mrs. Jones?

2. DIRECT COMMUNICATION*

At 4:45 P.M. on Friday, Mary Hite, an employee in the Business Office, walked into the office of Henry Staffs, Business Office Manager, and asked to see him privately. Ms. Hite told Mr. Staffs that she had been elected by the other employees of the Business Office to speak on their behalf about practices that they wished modified or eliminated. One practice concerned the employee evaluation system, which the employees thought was unfair, poorly executed, and used as an excuse for not paying higher salaries. A

---

*Source: Beaufort B. Longest, Jr. in *Business Management of Health Care Providers.* Chicago: Hospital Financial Management Association, 1975. Used by permission of the publisher.

second practice not accepted well was the arbitrary way in which management determined employee vacation time. Ms. Hite said that one employee was given two days' notice before he received his first week of vacation and five days' notice before his second week. Mr. Staffs listened attentively and told Ms. Hite that since it was so late in the day, he would consider these requests the first part of the next week. During the following week, Ms. Hite noticed that Mr. Staffs was out of town and that no action had been taken concerning her remarks. However, her fellow employees tended to treat her like a heroine for representing them before Mr. Staffs.

When she picked up her check the next Friday afternoon, Ms. Hite was shocked to find a discharge notice and two weeks severance pay in the envelope.

A. What should Mr. Staffs have done when Ms. Hite came to see him?

B. What message did Mr. Staffs communicate to Ms. Hite and the other employees? How did he communicate it?

C. What will be the outcome of the action he took?

D. Is there any way that Mr. Staffs can improve communication in the Business Office?

3. GOOD WORK IS EXPECTED*

A 600 bed general hospital, located in a large urban city in the Eastern U.S., brought in an outside management consulting firm to analyze its operations. After five weeks, the consultants made their report to management. One of the areas they had investigated was communication between superiors and subordinates. To their dismay, management learned that there were numerous discrepancies between what superiors said they did and what their subordinates said the superiors did. For example, when the consultants conducted a confidential questionnaire survey with 20 per cent of the managers and workers, they received the following responses to the question "Do you tell your subordinates when they do a good job?"

	TOP MANAGEMENT SAYS OF ITSELF	MIDDLE MANAGEMENT SAYS OF TOP MANAGEMENT	MIDDLE MANAGEMENT SAYS OF ITSELF	LOWER-LEVEL MANAGEMENT SAYS OF MIDDLE MANAGEMENT	LOWER-LEVEL MANAGEMENT SAYS OF ITSELF	WORKERS SAYS OF LOWER-LEVEL MANAGEMENT
Always	93	82	95	63	98	39
Often	7	14	5	15	2	23
Sometimes		4		12		18
Seldom				6		11
Never				4		9

Management was quite upset by the findings. As a result, at the next meeting of the Board of Trustees, the chairman proposed that the hospital bring back the consultants to advise them how to deal with this problem. The resolution was passed unanimously.

When the middle and lower level managers learned of this action, they expressed surprise. One of them noted, "Just because the data indicate poor communication is no need to get excited. After all, workers say lots of things that aren't accurate." A fellow colleague explained, "Look, I expect subordinates to do a good job. I only tell them when they are doing a poor one. If I praised them every time they did something right, they'd all have swelled heads. My approach is to say nothing."

A. What do the responses to the question, "Do you tell your subordinates when they do a good job," indicate?

---

*Source: Adapted from: Richard M. Hodgetts, *Management: Theory, Process and Practice.* Philadelphia: W. B. Saunders Company, 1975, pp. 303–305. Used by permission of the publisher.

B. What do you think of the comments from the two managers? Are they valid?

C. What types of recommendations would you expect from the consultants? Explain.

4. ESTABLISHING CURRENT REPORT CONTENTS*

Lares Hospital, a 250 bed, general acute hospital is located in a midwestern city of 300,000 population. A nonprofit institution, the hospital is governed by a board of trustees composed of fifteen members. The majority of board members are young and alert executives. To maintain a predominance of young men on the board has always been a policy, as the hospital received its start and support from the city's younger set. Five members are elected each year for three years and may succeed themselves for one term. John Dodge, president of the board, is thirty-five years old. Other members vary in ages from thirty-seven to fifty-five. There are only three members over fifty. Five of the board members have had no previous contact with hospitals.

The board members remarked to the president that they could not evaluate the internal processes of the hospital on the basis of the reports and information given them by the director.

Clyde Munter, director of Lares Hospital for four years, had deliberately refrained from presenting complete information or statistical data to the board. He felt that the members of the board were too busy in their respective businesses and too occupied with community social events and country club activities to be burdened with information other than financial statements. The hospital's continued operation without a deficit, apparently with the good will of the public, seemed to justify his approach. The hospital's condition may perhaps be illustrated by its 93 per cent average occupancy over the past year, of which Mr. Munter is quite proud. Mr. Munter, a man in his sixties, was of the opinion that the board members were too immature to appreciate the complicated hospital problems. The board sensed this attitude, and there was growing agitation to replace the director with a younger qualified director. The board was hesitant to act as Mr. Munter had been a board member himself, is an influential citizen in the community, and has only three years left before he retires. The board finally decided to make another attempt to work with the director. The members very pointedly informed him that they would insist upon the submission of adequate written reports at board meetings so they could be as fully informed as a board should be on the activities of the hospital.

Mr. Munter now calls for numerous reports from his department heads and passes most of the information directly to the board. He submits a detailed annual report in addition to a monthly report given the board members at their regular meetings. He also sends them weekly reports of food and laundry costs. Food costs at Lares Hospital are average for the area, but laundry costs have been increasing, and a change may have to be effected.

The board is notified of each change in personnel on the staff. Reports of intradepartmental meetings are sent to the board, which also receives a copy of the monthly medical statistical summary. Since the board set up a special fund for landscaping, it is given a weekly progress report on grounds improvement.

Mr. Munter has always had daily conferences with each of his department heads. Once a week, on Friday afternoons, all department heads participate in a joint conference.

The following reports are submitted to the director by the department heads:

Daily

1. Raw food cost
2. Surgery list

---

*Source: James A. Hamilton, *Decision Making In Hospital Administration and Medical Care.* Minneapolis: University of Minnesota Press, 1967, pp. 266–268. Used by permission of the publisher.

3. Trial balance
4. Admissions and discharges
5. Weight of laundry processed
6. Fuel consumption

Weekly

1. Balance sheet
2. Percentage of uncollectibles
3. New employees, discharges, and resignations
4. Number of meals served, by type of patient
5. List of critically ill

Monthly

1. Outpatient visits
2. Narcotic balance sheet
3. Nursing hours per patient day
4. Census reports
5. Total occupancy
6. Physicians index
7. Cost per served meal

Mr. Dodge is pleased to have more information but agrees with the rest of the board that the individual members are too busy to give all the reports sufficient attention. The department heads' reports are of interest to the board but are far too detailed. Having received the reports for several months, Mr. Dodge decides that the board should specify what reports it wishes to receive from Mr. Munter and at what intervals. Mr. Dodge therefore asks you, as chairman of the board's finance committee, to be chairman of a special board committee of five members with the assignment of preparing appropriate instructions on the subject for Mr. Munter. Mr. Dodge also asks Mr. Munter to explain to the board what reports a director should receive from the department heads. Both reports are to be presented to the board at its next regular meeting.

A. At the present time, are there too many reports? If so, what is the effect?

B. What reports do you think the Board of Trustees of Lares Hospital should receive from Mr. Munter, and how frequently should they be received?

C. What reports do you believe Mr. Munter should receive from his department heads?

Part V

ORGANIZATION CONTROL AND CHANGE

In the preceding parts of this text, we described the health care setting, presented the management of health care organizations from an input-conversion-output point of view, presented a management model and its characteristic processes, examined the organizational design and structure of health care organizations, and discussed organizational dynamics.

This last part *ORGANIZATION CONTROL AND CHANGE,* contains two chapters. In Chapter 14, Control and Control Techniques, we will focus on the controlling process. Subsequent to the formulation of objectives, the structuring of the organization, and the execution of activities, methods must be employed to ensure that desired output is being attained. This is the purpose of the controlling process.

In Chapter 15, Facilitating Change, we will supplement our discussion of internal organizational change (see Chapter 8) by looking at the environment as a force that imposes change on health care organizations. Viewing the management model presented in Figure 2–3 (reproduced in Chapter 14), it can be noted that the implementation of the management processes of planning, decision-making, organizing, and executing will result in output. Whether the output is acceptable (desired) is determined through control. Furthermore, the output generated and the resulting effectiveness and efficiency of the health care organization will have an impact on the whole delivery system. Consequently, this last chapter will conclude our efforts with a presentation of "perspectives" on the future of health care organizations and the possible changes that will be imposed on them by external forces.

This Chapter Contains:

- Introduction

- Need For And Nature Of Control

- The Controlling Process
    Closed and Open Loop Systems
    Control and The Linkage to Planning
    Control Points, Standards, and Measurement
        Output Control
        Activity Control
        Input Control
    Comparison
    Cause

- Control Considerations

- Control Techniques

- Summary

- Discussion Questions

- Incidents

Chapter 14

CONTROL AND CONTROL TECHNIQUES

"Although clearly a professional need of health care personnel and institutions, quality assurance is even more a public need to ensure the credibility of the health care delivery system."

(John D. Porterfield, III)[1]

INTRODUCTION

In the preceding statement the Director of the Joint Commission on Accreditation of Hospitals focuses on one particular area that requires control: quality assurance, or the monitoring of the quality of patient care provided by health care organizations. Although he does not mention other control areas which require attention, such as inputs, resource utilization (manpower and otherwise), organization activity, or resulting efficiency and effectiveness, he does raise several very interesting observations which are germane to our purpose. It can be construed that control is the responsibility of health care managers as well as of professional health care personnel. Moreover, it can be construed that the purpose of control is not only to ensure the delivery of quality patient care but also to demonstrate to the public that health care managers are endeavoring to fulfill their responsibility to society. Porterfield stipulates that the health care organization's constituents should be aware that the controlling process is activated. This control should be visible in order for the health care delivery system to retain its "credibility" in the eyes of its constituents.

At this point, we may raise a number of questions that need to be answered. First, why are controls necessary and what is the importance of controlling? Second, what should be controlled? Last, are health care organizations unique to the degree that they require a different controlling process than other types of organizations? As we address these questions in this chapter, we will include the following: (1) a discussion of the need for and nature of control, (2) a description of the controlling process, (3) several control considerations, and (4) an overview of various control techniques.

---

[1]John D. Porterfield, III, "To defense of the system." *Hospitals*, *48*:47, March 1, 1974.

THE NEED FOR AND NATURE OF CONTROL

NEED FOR CONTROL

In Chapter 1, we discussed some of the phenomena that have contributed to the managerial revolution in health care organizations. Among them were changes in the health care delivery system; the increased role of federal assistance programs; broader third-party health insurance coverage among the nation's population, and the resulting increase in demand; changes in consumer expectations with regard to the quality, availability, and cost of health care; increased resource costs and technological advances; and finally, the rising cost of health care. The net effect of these phenomena on health care organizations and their managers has been a societal demand for greater accountability and increased organization efficiency and effectiveness.

Just as these factors have precipitated a managerial revolution, they also have become the basic reasons for control. First, society demands it. Second, without control there is no guarantee that the health care organization will accomplish its objectives, channel organization resources into the most constructive and contributing endeavors, or ensure that its basic responsibilities are being discharged. We might also add, parenthetically, that if health care managers do not exercise appropriate control over the quality of care and costs, other parties, such as the government, may intervene and impose control standards and methods. Finally, the absence of control will almost assuredly result in inefficiency and ineffectiveness.

It was also mentioned in Chapter 1 that one purpose of this text was to serve as a vehicle to help present and future managers make health care organizations more effective and efficient. It was further indicated that efficiency and effectiveness were two different terms, that efficiency denotes doing something "at the lowest cost for a given quality level," and that effectiveness implies doing what should be done "and doing it well." One of the expectations of the public and the government is greater efficiency and effectiveness on the part of health care organizations. It goes without saying that quality patient care is another of society's expectations. How can health care organizations and their managers fulfill these expectations? One way is to improve controls. Another way is to communicate to society the fact that these organizations are making the improvements.

NATURE OF CONTROL

Before we can fully demonstrate the importance of the controlling process with regard to the management of health care organizations, it is first necessary to describe what this process is. Basically, "control" is a generic term used to denote the monitoring of activities in order to ensure that what is supposed to occur is occurring, and if it is not, why. For our purpose, we will define the controlling process *as the comparison of actual results (performance) to expected results (desired output) and the taking of corrective action if warranted and feasible.*

It was indicated in Chapter 2 that management serves as a conversion mechanism for the transformation of inputs to outputs (see Fig. 2–1, The

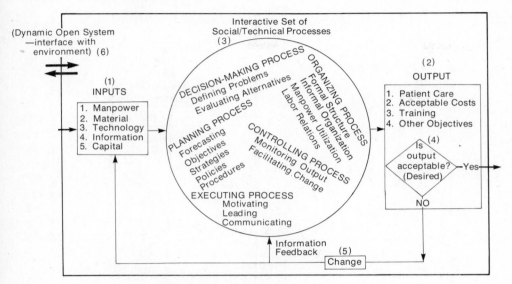

Figure 14-1 Management model.

input-conversion-output model and Fig. 2–3, The management model). The processes characteristic of the management model, reproduced in Figure 14–1, are (1) planning, (2) decision-making, (3) organizing, (4) executing, and (5) controlling. Once input resource requirements have been identified and acquired (subsequent to the determination of the organization's objectives), it is necessary to provide the means (plans and setting) for executing or intitiating activity in order to generate output. To be certain that the output attained is what is desired, it is necessary to continuously monitor the activities of the organization. Furthermore, by viewing the management model presented in Figure 14–1, it can be noted that if output (results) does not correspond with objectives, corrective action and change may be necessary. To make the point in a negative sense, if control is not practiced, there is no guarantee that objectives will be accomplished or that efficiency and effectiveness will occur.

In Chapter 2, controlling was defined as a process that is technical in nature and concerned with monitoring the organization activities. The predetermination of objectives, the gathering of resources, and the utilization of resources resulting from initiated action should all lead to the accomplishment of those objectives. This can only be ensured if control is exercised.

THE CONTROLLING PROCESS

How does one determine if the organization's primary, secondary, and individual departmental objectives are being accomplished? How is it possible to know if the quality of patient care is at the level it should be, or that the care provided is at reasonable cost? How is it possible to determine whether there are too few or too many employees? How can one know if policies and procedures are serving their intended purpose, if plans are being carried out, or if

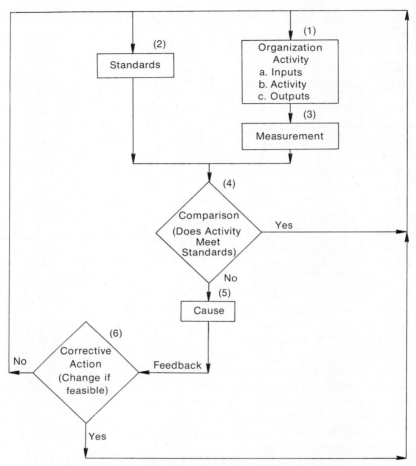

Figure 14–2 Control model.

payroll expenditures are too high? These are examples of situations with which health care managers should be concerned. In order to answer these questions, there are several basic controlling activities which must be activated. Each of the preceding questions implies an awareness of expectations, desired results, levels of performance, and so on. We may classify these as *standards* representing expectations for *organization activity*. Further, in order to determine if expectations, desired results, objectives, or levels of performance are being attained, *methods for measuring actual results* will have to be developed. Third, the *comparison* of actual results with standards should indicate whether there is *deviation*. This leads to an examination of the *cause* and feedback information[2] which should lead to *corrective* action if it is necessary and feasible to ensure that future results will meet expectations or standards. We have just described the

[2]For an interesting discussion of feedback control applied to the health care delivery system see John P. Van Gigch, *Applied General Systems Theory.* New York: Harper and Row, 1974, pp. 364–369.

basic activities characteristic of the controlling process as presented in Figure 14–2. In our dicussion of the controlling process we will refer to this model and its numbered cells.

CLOSED AND OPEN LOOP CONTROL SYSTEMS

Within the design of the means for monitoring an organization's activity, there are two basic control systems: closed loop control and open loop control.[3] The difference between the two is that the latter requires human intervention before corrective action can take place.

Closed loop control systems contain the basic control activities of a predetermined standard representing the results that are expected: a measuring device to determine what results are occurring, a means of comparing actual results to the standard that is expected, and a mechanism by which alteration or change can occur, if necessary. The simplest example of this is a heating system. In this case, the thermostat incorporates both the standard and the measuring functions. If the room is too hot, *comparison* to the standard (desired temperature) results in the automatic shut-off of the furnace. If the room is too cold, the furnace is automatically turned on. Additional examples of closed loop control systems would be incubators for infants or a facility's auxiliary power system, which comes on line automatically if normal power is interrupted. In all instances, *no human intervention* is required since the control system is self-correcting.

An open loop control system, on the other hand, requires human intervention to correct results that are deficient in comparison with the pre-established standard. An example would be heart monitoring equipment that signals the absence or irregularity of a heart beat (a deviation from the standard). The mechansim then notifies those who are responsible for monitoring performance and they can take the appropriate action.

Closed loop control systems seldom exist in dynamic organizational settings. For the most part, control systems are open loop; the remainder of our discussion will focus on them.

CONTROL AND THE LINKAGE TO PLANNING

The primary purpose of the controlling process is to ensure that the results of organized activity correspond to what is expected. By nature, control is directly linked to planning. Planning process activities involve the formulation of the objectives of the health care organization, the determination of the requisite input resources, the means or strategies that will enable objectives (desired output) to be accomplished, and the formulation of policies and procedures that will guide the behavior of those employed by the health care organization. In a sense, planning facilitates the establishment of standards that can be expressed in terms of objectives, costs, efficiency of activities, and input resource utilization.

---

[3]Richard M. Hodgetts, *Management Theory Process and Practice*. Philadelphia: W. B. Saunders Co., 1975, p. 196.

CONTROL POINTS (1), STANDARDS (2), AND MEASUREMENT (3)

There are three primary points upon which control is focused. They are (a) input control, (b) activity control, and (c) output control.[4] The model in Figure 14–2 applies for each control point.

Output Control.   Output control is the type with which we are most familiar. Generally, it is concerned with primary, secondary, and departmental objective accomplishment such as providing the range of services that should be provided, and having the level of quality care what it should be. In other words, is the ouptut what we desire or expect? Output standards are easily established, since they tend to mirror objectives. In order to make standards operational in terms of measurement, it is possible to convert to numerical measures, such as number of admissions, days of patient stay, occupancy rate, and out-patient visits. Deviation from standards, such as decline in average census, an increase in length of stay, or increase in death rate, can be readily recognized from regular reports, retrospective audits, and utilization reviews. In an open loop control system, the feedback information would indicate a deviation from the standard and signal the decision-maker that intervention is required.

Activity Control.   The transformation of output requires organization activity. Characteristics of this activity are (1) strategies–plans; (2) organization structuring reflected by departmentation, coordination, delegation, manpower acquisition and maintenance, and labor relations; and (3) execution facilitated by motivation, leadership and supervision, and communication flows.

Activity control is much more difficult to implement than output control. How does one, for example, determine whether a change in organization structure or a realignment of the medical staff and administrative relationships would be more efficient and effective in terms of accomplishing objectives, or whether existing leadership and supervisory styles could be improved. Obviously, standards of activity in terms of the number of personnel and expenditures needed to provide a given level and quality of care can be established from historical data. If costs and the number of employees exceed expectations, then the controlling process should register that deviation. Additional standards for activity control can be formulated in terms of overtime budgets, turnover rates, supply consumption, maintenance costs, and the like. However, because of the difficulty of establishing standards for many activities, control will tend to focus on input and output, with the assumption that if the two are in agreement with standards, the activities that transform the one into the other will be appropriate.

Input Control.   A question was initially raised as to whether health care organizations are so different from other types of organizations that they require a different controlling process. The answer is both yes and no. The basic open and closed loop control systems apply to all types of organizations, as does the basic control model; however, the distinction for health care organizations lies in the relative importance of the control points. Because of the service they provide, health care organizations should focus on output and input

---

[4]Don Hellregel and John W. Slocum, Jr., *Management: A Contingency Approach.* Reading, Massachusetts: Addison-Wesley, 1974, p. 245.

control to a greater degree than other types of organizations. Because patient care is final, with little opportunity to rectify product deficiency (through recall, for instance), and carries high implied economic considerations (the value of life), output control is a major responsibility and should command the appropriate attention. Furthermore, the uniqueness of the health care delivery system forces attention on input control. As a result of the importance of quality care, the quality (skills) of manpower input resources is controlled through the mechanism of licensing and certification legislation.[5] Other input resources require control, such as the distribution of drugs and the accreditation of physical facilities.

COMPARISON (4)

Whether control is being focused on inputs, activities, or outputs, or all three, a comparison of expectations (standards) to actual results should indicate if deviation has occurred or is occurring. Should results correspond to expectations, one can assume that what is being controlled (monitored) is under control. However, if results exceed or fall short of expectations (standards), an investigation as to the cause is warranted. At this point in the open loop control system, the person responsible for intervening should ask what the cause of the deviation is.

CAUSE (5)

It can be assumed that a negative deviation from standard is a signal that something is wrong. By the same token, a positive deviation from standard may also be symptomatic of something being wrong. For example, activity control in the monitoring of the Nursing Service payroll expenditures may reveal that those expenditures (results) are below budgeted levels (standards). On first glance, this may appear to be beneficial; yet, one should examine the cause. Is it because staffing levels are below authorized strength, perhaps causing a deterioration in quality of care that could appear later at the output control point; or is it due to a high turnover of experienced personnel who are being replaced by less experienced, lower paid nurses? Another example could be less than expected maintenance and equipment expenditures, perhaps at the cost of shifting expenditure burdens to future years by not practicing preventive maintenance or replacing obsolete equipment.

The cause of negative deviations from standard should be examined. By construction, a negative deviation means that expected results are not being met; however, the question of "why" should again be asked. Feedback information should indicate that corrective action is warranted. Yet, there may be instances when the cause of the deviation is beyond the control of the manager. For example, supply expenditures might exceed budgeted levels (standard) because of inflation, increased supplier prices, or the unavailability of less costly replacements. Increased payroll expenditure may be due to a recently negotiated labor contract over which the departmental manager has no control; an

---

[5]Porterfield, op. cit. p. 48.

increase in the accounts receivable collection period may be due to slow payment by third-party payers.

If the expected results of whatever is being monitored (quality of care, census, cash flow, dietary expenditures, volume of ancillary services, number of personnel, turnover rates, overtime payments, or drug distribution) are not being reached, it does not necessarily mean that change can rectify the situation. Whenever possible, steps should be taken so that expectations are compiled within the constraints present. If change cannot be implemented owing to factors beyond the organization's control, standards and the activities being measured may have to be re-evaluated. For example, if the average length of stay is increasing because of a high use of ambulatory surgery, this increased length of stay would be regarded as beneficial to the hospital.

CONTROL CONSIDERATIONS

When deciding what to control, when, and how, several considerations should be taken into account: (1) the significance of the input, activity, or output to be controlled, (2) the net economic benefit that results from control, and (3) the timeliness of the feedback denoting deviation from standard.

SIGNIFICANCE

When referring to the significance of the acti ity to be controlled, we mean its importance or priority relative to all things to be controlled.[6] For example, high on the control priority list of health care organizations would be output control as well as input control. Making certain, through the licensing mechanism, that professional people have the appropriate qualifications is a control activity that not only fosters quality care but also minimizes negligence liability. By the same token, there are times when the item (input, activity) to be controlled may not warrant immediate attention because there are other, more important activities. For example, it would make little sense to control the consumption of paper towels in the wash room at the expense of the attention due the dispensing of narcotic drugs.

ECONOMIC BENEFIT

At times, the cost of controlling may exceed the savings to be derived. In such a situation, there may be larger net benefit for the organization if attention, time, and resources are focused on more significant control items. For example, if Purchasing has a petty cash box with an average balance of $50 for small purchases, the man hours needed for control, to the penny, may not be appropriate. Another example might be the controlling of the number of visitors allowed in patients' rooms. On the rare occasion when more than the specified number of people visit a patient, it may not be economically justifiable

---

[6]William H. Sihler, "Toward better management control systems." *California Management Review, 14*:38, Winter, 1971.

to employ floor monitors just to control the number of visitors. In an exceptional case when a patient cannot be allowed to have many visitors at any one time, the nursing station personnel can exercise control.

TIMELINESS

Another consideration that should be built into the development of control is the timeliness of information feedback.[7] If feedback registering deviation is not timely, the control may not be effective. It would make little sense for quality care deviations to be communicated long after the fact.

CONTROL TECHNIQUES

There are a number of control techniques available to the manager. We will present several of them.

BUDGETS

Probably the most familar control technique is the budget. In health care organizations, there are various kinds of budgets: payroll budgets, supply budgets, equipment budgets, revenue budgets, capital expenditure budgets, maintenance budgets, food budgets, and so on. An obvious question to ask would be, why are there so many budgets? The reason is that a budget is simply a plan expressed in numerical terms[8] which can be used as a standard. For example, the overtime budget for the Nursing Service would indicate the planned number of overtime hours required during a given period of time to accomplish specific results. There are ways to decrease the amount of budgeted overtime. One way would be to hire additional personnel; however, it may be found from cost benefit analysis that it is more efficient to utilize overtime temporarily instead of hiring additional personnel.

Budgets are used as mechanisms for controlling expenditures. In a sense, they become the planning expression, in numerical terms, of what the organization is attempting to do. In other words, they become the standards in the controlling process. With budgets, it is easy to compare results to the standard. and if there is deviation, to determine why.

PPBS, NETWORK PROGRAMMING

Other control techniques available to health care organization managers are PPBS and Network Programming, which were presented in Chapter 5. The specific purpose of the Planning, Programming, Budgeting System developed for federal agencies in the mid-1960's is to systematically require the decision-maker to formulate objectives, evaluate alternatives, and allocate resources on a cost benefit basis. PPBS is also a control system. Although it does not control ac-

---

[7]*Ibid.* p. 38.

[8]David J. Cherrington and J. Owen Cherrington, "Participation, performance, and appraisal." *Business Horizons, 17:39, December, 1974.

tivities over a long period of time, it does serve a control purpose by ensuring the development of standards, the estimation of costs required to accomplish specific objectives, and the determination of the benefits to be derived from various alternatives. In this manner, it serves as a control mechanism in the allocation of resources.

Network programming includes the Performance Evaluation Review Technique (PERT) and the Critical Path Method (CPM). Both are planning and control techniques. In our discussion of PERT and CPM in Chapter 5, it was indicated that these techniques were useful in the planning, scheduling, and control of large complex projects.

RATIO ANALYSIS

Another very useful control technique for any health care organization manager is ratio analysis. Basically, ratio analysis is nothing more than comparing the results of activities as expressed in numerical measures to other types of numerical measures. Examples of pertinent ratios previously cited are average length of stay, turnover rates, and cost per bed. Typically, ratio analysis is fairly straightforward. For example, the ratio "occupany" is determined by dividing the census by the number of beds. This ratio is an excellent control indicator because it identifies the capacity at which the hospital or long-term-care facility is functioning. Knowing that the costs of an empty bed are almost as much as one that is filled, an important control item should be occupancy level. Any sharp change, say from 92 per cent occupancy to 68 per cent occupancy, should indicate that something is wrong.

Although ratio analysis is easy to perform, the reader should be cautioned to compare only appropriate measures. For example, the ratio of total employee accidents to the number of births makes little sense. Furthermore, unless one understands the causes of deviation from standards, ratio analysis can be misleading. A fairly common indicator (ratio) for hospitals which, in a broad sense, measures efficiency is the ratio of the number of employees per 100 beds. When compared to previous time periods, this ratio could signal whether there is control or a lack of it over the number of employees (which can be translated into payroll cost) in relation to a given level of output. However, first glance analysis could be misleading. Consider: last year's "employees/100 beds" ratio was 200; this year's is 230. Does that mean that there are too many employees? Perhaps, but not necessarily. An examination of the cause may reveal that the Out-patient Department had a volume increase from 10,000 visits to 30,000 visits. Although more employees would be required to service more out-patients, the bed size of the facility remained the same, and therefore an examination of "employees/100 beds" ratio alone would be misleading.

SUMMARY

In this chapter, the controlling process was presented. It was described as being technical in nature, concerned with monitoring the inputs, activities, and outputs of the health care organization. A control model was presented which included the basic activities characteristic of the controlling process: the development of standards which represent expectations, the measuring of actual results, the comparison of results to the standard, the identification of the cause of any noted deviation, and the taking of corrective action and implementation of change, if feasible, to ensure that results meet expectations.

The closed loop and open loop control systems were described along with various control considerations. Lastly, several control techniques were presented.

DISCUSSION QUESTIONS

1. Why is it important to have controls? Do health care organizations have too many?

2. Discuss how the controlling process is related to the other processes as presented in the management model (Fig. 14–1).

3. Would you agree that health care organizations should focus more on input and output control than on activity control? Support your position.

4. Several control considerations were discussed in this chapter. Think of others that you feel are important and be prepared to support your points.

INCIDENTS

1. UNEXPECTED SURPLUS

Your hospital's annual budget is approximately $30 million and after ten months, the year-to-date figures show that there is an excess of $1.5 million in revenue. The major reason for this is that virtually all the services, including in-patient days, are quite a bit above what was predicated at the beginning of the year when the revenue and expense budgets were estimated. As a result, department heads are requesting significant increases in personnel to handle the increased workload for the following year; overtime costs come to $500,000. It is difficult to say whether or not this increased level of activity will continue in all departments, and there is some hesitation on the part of administration to approve the increase in personnel budget for the following year for all the requesting departments.

A. What factors would you consider when making a decision whether or not to authorize an increase in the number of personnel?

B. If the personnel additions were approved, and next year's revenues were less than this year's, what would happen?

2. SAFETY MARGIN*

David Yost was assigned the special task of making up a budget for the next fiscal year. After reviewing past budgetary requests, he submitted the proposal to his superior. While waiting for the superior's response, David prepared his defense of each item on the budget. The meeting, however, did not quite go according to his expectations.

"Dave, I've examined your budget request and would like to talk to you about a few items. For example, under administrative expenses you estimate $47,612."

"Yes sir. I can show you the worksheet I used if you'd like."

"Oh, that's not necessary. The only reason the figure caught my eye was that it was such an odd amount. Look, let's round it off to $50,000."

"Okay."

"There are a few other budget estimates I see here that also need to be rounded off, so I'll just change them also."

"How much of an estimate does that make it?"

"It's exactly $210,000."

"Well, that's a bit higher ($22,476) than what I budgeted. Are you sure it's okay?"

"Sure, don't worry about it. You can never tell when something is going to cost just a little bit more than you initially thought."

"It's all right with me if it's all right with you."

"Fine. And oh, by the way, how did you arrive at these other estimates?"

"Well, I worked back from what I thought my department would be doing this fiscal year to how much it would cost to get this work done. There's a manual that was sent to me, and I took my basic format from it."

"That certainly is one way to get a handle on it, Dave. But let me suggest that you be sure to add some safety margins to each of your requests."

"Safety margins?"

"Sure. You know, a little something extra just in case things go wrong. Besides, you never know when management is going to cut around here, and it always pays to have asked for a little more than you need. Do you know what I mean?"

"I think so."

"Fine, well here's your budget back. Add in 10 per cent across the board and send it back in to me. I'll forward it from here."

A. Is David's superior right or wrong in suggesting that he change his budget requests? Explain.

B. What are the dangers in overestimating budget requests? Be specific. What does it do to the controlling process?

C. Why do you think this conversation occurred? Explain.

3. THE DEFICIT THAT SNUCK UP

Donald Smith, a self trained controller in a 100 bed hospital requested an emergency meeting with his administrator, Mr. Miller. At the beginning of their conversation, the first words out of Mr. Smith's mouth were, "Don't get excited boss, but a deficit just snuck up on us. I learned by chance (I was just playing with some numbers from the files with my new calculator) that our occupancy rate last month was 79 per cent, so I checked the figures for the last six months and found that the occupancy rate has been declining two percentage points each month from our level of 91 per cent. Boss, even if we stabilize it, we will have a substantial deficit this year."

---

*Adapted by permission from the publisher from Richard M. Hodgetts, *Management: Theory Process and Practice.* Philadelphia: W. B. Saunders Co., 1975, p. 217–218.

Mr. Miller's question to Donald was, "How could this happen without your knowing about it?"

A. Discuss the control implications of this situation.

B. Who was at fault?

This Chapter Contains:

- Introduction
- Consumerism
- Institutionalization
- Cost Effectiveness
- Quality Control
- The Change Process
- Our Greatest Challenge
- Summary

Chapter 15

FACILITATING CHANGE

"We may not recognize it or otherwise be cognizant of it; we may oppose it or we may even try to accelerate it. No matter what our position may be, change makes its course in the evolution of human effort. Change may take place so slowly that it is not perceptible in one generation or even two, or it may occur with such rapidity that we are left somewhat breathless in the waves."

(Blair Kolasa)[1]

INTRODUCTION

The concepts, principles, and practices that have been presented in this book will be useful to the health care manager only to the extent they are applied. A complication is that these concepts, principles, and practices must be applied in a dynamic setting where the only actual constant is change. The reader must realize that the health care delivery system exists in an environment that is constantly changing as well. Changes in this environment will affect the health delivery system of the future. During the past decade, a substantial amount of attention has been devoted to change in health care literature.[2] Gordon L. Lippitt, in his award-winning article, cites some of these environmental changes:

...the greatly increased standard of living in the U.S. and throughout the world; an increasing gap between the powerful rich, and the powerless and poor; a rapid

[1]Blair J. Kolasa, *Introduction to Behavioral Sciences for Business.* New York: John Wiley and Sons, Inc., 1969, p. 348.

[2]For examples see
S. D. Promrinse, "The crisis in the health care system." *Hospital Administration, 19*:10, Winter, 1974;
H. A. Singer, "The changing role of administrators in the 1970's." *Hospital Administration, 11*:40, Summer, 1966;
Richard L. Johnson, "Changing role of the hospital's chief executive." *Hospital Administration, 15*:21, Summer, 1970;
Leonard A. Duce, "The administrator: Today and tomorrow." *Hospital Administration, 13*:7, Fall, 1968;
Everett A. Johnson, "Giving the consumer a voice in the hospital business." *Hospital Administration, 15*:15, Spring, 1970;
Paul J. Gordon, "Administering the 'field' of administration." *Hospital Administration, 16*:27, Spring, 1971;
Charles E. Odegaarid, "Crisis in American health care." *Hospital Administration, 9*:67, Summer, 1969.

increase in the world population; continued changes in value systems; the greater
expectation of people for services in general, but for health care in particular; the
increased influence of local, state, and federal governments; an increasing desire
for power by minority groups; a continued increase in the influence of mass media;
the extensive development of education as it applies to continued growth and
development at all ages; a shift from a production to a service economy; a continued increase in technology; an increased confrontation by consumer; the development of new avocations and vocations in society; an increased international
interdependence; a continuation of ecological concerns; an increased mobility of
people with a lessening of commitment to an organization or community; an increased size of the social systems of mankind so that there will be a greater feeling
of powerlessness on the part of members of such institutions; a continued explosion of knowledge; and a desire for quality, not just quantity, as a goal in life.[3]

John D. Porterfield, III, Director of the Joint Commission on Accreditation
of Hospitals, has suggested that the health care system is "at a crossroads in
time and place. Where we go from here...will make the difference in finding
reasonable solutions to health care problems."[4] In an effort to illuminate the
road ahead, this chapter will examine several issues[5] that will face the health
care field in the next decade. Hopefully, you the reader will reflect on some of
the factors which contribute to the dynamic state of the health care industry
and how they affect you, your organization, and your management of them. Finally, the chapter concludes with a section on change and the role of the manager as a change agent.

CONSUMERISM

Nothing will have a greater impact on the delivery of health services in the
decade ahead than the expectations of consumers and the dictates of the federal government. The people served by the health care industry have changed;
this fact will in turn change health care delivery.

Ray Brown has pointed out that the United States has become a "health
conscious nation whose health aspirations have kept ahead of medical advances
and whose health sense is becoming as sophisticated as the activities behind the
'no visitors' sign in the inner sanctums of the hospital."[6] The people of the
United States, through their vote, have produced Medicare, Medicaid, PSRO,
PL 93–641, and other health related programs and legislation. The people have
demonstrated their willingness to pay on a group basis for what they perceive
as quality medical care. They are aware of the qualitative differences in health
care and the inequalities of a health delivery system that offers several levels of
care. Much of the current consumer movement is aimed at giving meaning to
the cry that "health care is a right," rather than a privilege.

---

[3]Gordon L. Lippitt, "Hospital organization in the post-industrial society." *Hospital Progress,*
50:55, June, 1973. Reprinted with permission. Copyright © by the Catholic Hospital Association.
[4]John D. Porterfield, III, "To the defense of the system." *Hospitals, 48*:49, March 1, 1974.
[5]These issues have been suggested by William L. Kissick and Samuel P. Martin, "Issues of the
future in health." *The Annals of the American Academy of Political and Social Science, 399*:159, January
1972.
[6]Ray E. Brown, "The hospital redefined." *Hospital Progress,* November, 1966, p. 71.

Melvin Glasser has stated that

> There is mounting evidence that the consumer of health services is no longer content to leave the planning for and organization of his health services solely in the hands of the professional, doctors, hospital administrators, health insurance executives—yes, even health planners. The consumer wants in—he pays for the programs, he is the beneficiary of good contributions and the sufferer from their inadequacy, and increasingly he is insisting that his voice be heard and that he be included in the councils of those who plan for and offer health services.[7]

Consumers must be brought into the mainstream of decision-making concerning their health care services and the institutions that provide them. Health care providers must develop a depth of social responsibility that will be measured in part by involving consumers in the major decision-making roles in our health care system. There are dangers here, of course, but these dangers are vastly overrated by an overly conservative health care delivery system that may fear that its decisions will be attacked by "outsiders." This challenge can be turned into a major assest; the modern health care manager must develop sound strategies, and give consumerism a high priority in future decision-making.

INSTITUTIONALIZATION

As Anne Somers has said, "The need for reorganization and rationalization of the delivery system is now widely recognized."[8] Implicit in her words is the thought that the problems of reorganizing and rationalizing the delivery of health services are somehow new. They are not. The following quotation was taken from the *Journal of the American Medical Association*, the May 8, 1897 issue:

> The Future Physician—The doctor as a private physician working for himself will more and more find his position disappearing. There will be general practitioners in out-of-way places; there will be men of rare talent and ability who will remain individualistic in their work. But the great mass of town physicians may be obliged to adapt themselves to other conditions, and either become salaried employees of State and private institutions or form mutual and cooperative hospitals and dispensaries, thereby employing themselves; which plan or plans will soonest find adoption the future alone will tell; but the general physician will probably not remain as he is, and sooner or later he will be obliged to choose between the old and new paths.

This quotation, written in the previous century, seems perfectly appropriate in today's context of prescriptions for reorganizing and rationalizing health care organizations. It also illustrates just how slowly these institutions change.

---

[7]Melvin A. Glasser, "What the consumer expects in coordinated planning for health." Paper presented before the Fourth Annual Institute for Staffs on Areawide Health Facility Planning Agencies, Center for Health Administration, Graduate School of Business, University of Chicago, Chicago, Illinois, December 12–16, 1966, p. 13.

[8]Anne R. Somers, "The nation's health: Issues for the future." *The Annals of the American Academy of Political and Social Science*, *399*:163, January, 1972.

Partly related to the demands of consumerism described previously, and intertwined with the issues of efficiency, effectiveness, and quality control, which will be discussed later in this chapter, the institutionalization of health services is currently and will in the years ahead be an issue of major importance.

Concern over the problems of providing health care to all U.S. citizens has produced several alternatives in recent years. Not one of them is universally accepted at this point, but all bear the mark of one similarity: greater and greater institutionalization of health care delivery. Among the recent proposals for reorganizing the health delivery system are the health maintenance concept, the American Hospital Association's concept of the Health Care Corporations,[9] White's idea of "personal health service systems,"[10] and Somers' proposed system based on a state franchised hospital as the primary[11] coordinating unit in the health care system.

It is still open to debate whether the way to rationally institutionalize the delivery of health services will be one of those already mentioned or another; perhaps no approach will emerge at all. In any case, the issue of institutionalization of health care delivery is a live one and it will affect health care managers in the decade ahead. Hepner and Hepner have described the objectives of any suitable reorganization of the health delivery system as follows:[12]

1. Easy access to care
2. Better financing and cost containment
3. Availability of comprehensive care
4. Quality care
5. Better utilization of health manpower

A goal which all health care managers must share is the development of an institutional framework in which their objectives can be met. Furthermore, there is a growing recognition of the fact that not all health services must be made available through the traditional institutional mechanisms (including the traditional doctor–patient relationships). There is a growing recognition of the importance of self-help and mutual aid groups like Synanon, Mended Hearts Inc., Committee to Combat Huntington's Disease, Emphysema Anonymous, and Alcoholics Anonymous. These groups exist to further the development of ways beyond the traditional institutional modalities to improve health, both mental and physical. If the efforts of these groups are somehow tied into an expanded role of the traditional institutional provider, both approaches will be improved.[13]

---

[9]*Ameriplan* Report of a Special Committee on the Provision of Health Services, American Hospital Association, Chicago, 1970.

[10]Kerr L. White, "Personal health services system: Desiderata." *Journal of the American Medical Association, 218*:1683, December 13, 1971.

[11]Anne R. Somers, *Health Care in Transition: Directions for the Future.* Chicago, Ill.: Hospital Research and Educational Trust, 1971, Chapter 7.

[12]James O. Hepner and Donna M. Hepner, *The Health Strategy Game: A Challenge for Reorganization and Management.* St. Louis: The C. V. Mosby Company, 1973, p. 294.

[13]For the readers who may be interested in exploring self-help groups further, see Leonard D. Borman, *Explorations in Self-Help and Mutual Aid.* Evanston, Ill.: Center for Urban Affairs, Northwestern University, 1975.

COST EFFECTIVENESS

Perhaps no issue has stirred more criticism of the health delivery system than that of soaring costs. After several years of skyrocketing medical costs, the providers and consumers of health services are alarmed. These increasing costs cannot be fully rationalized—in many cases they cannot even be explained. In the decade ahead, one of the issues affecting all health care managers will be the efficiency—cost effectiveness—of not only the present system but also any future delivery system that may evolve.

This problem is related to the larger question of total resource allocation in a society. In western countries, the private market system essentially determines resource allocation, *except* in the case of health care where the system does not function very well. When the private market system does not work, a systematic cost benefit or cost effectiveness approach is needed to allocate scarce resources; however, this approach has not been taken. Considering the fact that health services literature contains considerable treatment of the importance of cost benefit analysis for improving the allocation of resources to and within the health field, it may, as Klarman has suggested, "prove to be a source of astonishment that relatively few complete cost-benefit studies of health programs have been carried out."[14]

In view of the limited resources available for the delivery of health services, the cost benefit approach will be taken more and more, at both the level of the individual institution and the total health care delivery system. For example, a careful analysis of the cost of averting death (by programs of examination, detection, and treatment of cases found) for several types of cancer was made over the period from 1968 to 1972. Table 15–1 contains the results of this analysis. Under limited resource conditions, decision-makers could use resources for programs that would avert the most deaths per dollar of expenditure. As can be seen in Table 15–1, this would be uterine-cervical cancer. The costs of head and neck cancer and colon-rectum cancer are so high that limited

---

[14]Herbert E. Klarman, "Application of cost-benefit analysis to the health services and the special case of technologic innovation." *International Journal of Health Services*, 4:329, 1974.

Table 15–1 Cancer Control Program, 1968–1972

	UTERINE-CERVIX	BREAST	HEAD AND NECK	COLON-RECTUM
Grant costs (in thousands)	$97,750	$17,750	$13,250	$13,300
Number of examinations (in thousands)	9,363	2,280	609	662
Cost per examination	$ 10.44	$ 7.79	$ 21.76	$ 20.10
Examinations per case found	87.5	167.3	620.2	496.0
Cancer cases found	107,045	13,628	982	1,334
Cost per case found	$ 913	$ 1,302	$13,493	$ 9,970
Cancer deaths averted	44,084	2,936	303	288
Cost per death averted	$ 2,217	$ 6,046	$43,729	$46,181

Source: *Analysis and Evaluation of Public Expenditures: The PPB System.* Joint Economic Committee, 91st U.S. Congress, 1969, Vol. 3, p. 1212.

funds might be better spent on further research instead of detection–treatment programs.

Of course, cost effectiveness analysis has a serious limitation. Although this type of analysis is useful in deciding between various approaches to the same or similar benefits, it does not answer the broader question of what benefits should be achieved. This is answered in terms of solution criteria and constraints imposed internally, by the organization, and externally, by society.

QUALITY CONTROL

The health care field is in the middle of a major shift in quality control that will surely last into the 1980's. Kissick and Martin, in describing this shift, have stated,

> The old concept of individual responsibility for the quality of health care was an ideal of the era of the single practitioner and his patient. With the rapid growth in the size and diversity of participants in care, together with institutionalization of the system, quality control will undoubtedly enter a new phase where it will involve all the health care team and be shared with the patient and the body politic.[15]

The benefits of quality control are clear. Appropriate control of the quality of care will reduce needless suffering and deaths.[16] The characteristics of a good control system have been delineated (see Chapter 14, also). Avedis Donabedian has suggested the following characteristics of control:

a) It is continuing.
b) It is systematized by virtue of having several components that are interrelated and mutually reinforcing rather than being an assemblage of random, ad hoc activities.
c) It includes monitoring of the outcomes as well as the process of care.
d) It is linked to action, so that deviations from expected performance result in investigation and appropriate action, which is preventive and rehabilitative rather than mainly punitive.
e) It preferably has external, in addition to internal, components.
f) It is formalized, but it is supported by many informal features of the organization and by shared values and objectives.[17]

What is not clear, and what is going to be an issue in the years ahead, is *how* to ensure quality. The present approaches to licensure, the voluntary accreditation of facilities, peer review (which is increasingly being formalized by such programs as PSRO), and the ever present possibility of malpractice litigation have been effective to a degree. However, the solution to the problem of controlling quality has not been found. While we cannot predict the exact nature of the activities that will pertain to this issue in the years ahead, the reader

[15] William L. Kissick and Samuel P. Martin, op. cit. p. 158.
[16] Abraham Gerber, *The Gerber Report.* New York: David McKay Co., 1971, p. 235.
[17] Avedis Donabedian, "Models for organizing the delivery of personal health services and criteria for evaluating them." *Milbank Memorial Fund Quarterly, 50*:120, October, 1972, Part 2.

can rest assured that there will be changes imposed by society that will affect the manager in the health care organization.

THE CHANGE PROCESS

The issues previously mentioned (along with many others) will make it necessary for all health care organizations to change. There are many types of changes that take place within health care organizations. A very important distinction between these changes is whether the change is imposed on the organization (a government regulation, for example) or made without direct, perhaps coercive, external pressure. Both situations are organizational changes, but the latter, as suggested in Chapter 8, is an innovative organizational change. The open system view of organizations suggests that they interact with, react to, and influence their environment. The health care organization that only reacts to its environment, that only changes when literally forced to by external pressures, cannot be thought of as an innovative organization. In Chapter 8, we suggested that the best definition of innovation was given by Lloyd Rowe and William Boise: "Organizational innovation refers to the successful utilization of processes, programs, or products which are new to an organization and which are introduced as a result of decisions made within the organization."[18]

The role of the manager in this activity has been described as "change agent." This role is not an easy one to fulfill. People resist change for many reasons. Among the most common are the following:

1. Insecurity. This is the most obvious reason why humans resist change. People are generally comfortable with the status quo. Change often is viewed as a threat to their security.
2. Economics. A very practical reason why persons, especially in the lower levels of an organization, oppose change is that they are afraid of possible economic loss. Being replaced by a machine is a real threat to most workers. Today, with the increasing use of the computer, many middle managers are also beginning to experience the same fear.
3. Sociopsychological. Although insecurity and economics are partly sociopsychological in nature, there are also perceptual, emotional, and cultural barriers to change. Perceptually, wrong interpretations of the change may lead to resistance. Persons may react emotionally to a change by bringing fears and prejudices to the surface. Persons facing change in an organization are influenced by their cultural values which they bring to the situation with them.[19]

The problem of maintaining a viable organization—one that can function effectively, efficiently, *and* change over time—is a complex one. A balance between the appropriate maintenance of the status quo and "progressive" change should be the goal of the change agent manager. The state of the art does not permit us to suggest a universal or easy approach to change. A great deal of work remains to be done before the change process can be fully understood.

---

[18]Lloyd A. Rowe and William B. Boise, *Organizational and Managerial Innovation: A Reader.* Pacific Palisades, California: The Goodyear Publishing Company, 1973, p. 6.

[19]Edgar G. Williams, "Changing systems and behavior." *Business Horizons, 12*:55–56, August, 1969. Used by permission of the publisher.

Larry Greiner has suggested that the following actions are a logical beginning point:

1. We must revise our egocentric notions that organization change is heavily dependent on a master blueprint designed and executed in one fell swoop by an omniscient consultant or top manager.
2. We too often assume that organization change is for "those people downstairs," who are somehow perceived as less productive than "those upstairs."
3. We need to reduce our fond attachment for both unilateral and delegated approaches to change.
4. There is a need for managers, consultants, skeptics, and researchers to become less parochial in their viewpoints.[20]

In light of the inevitability of change, the reader might reflect for a moment on Kast and Rosenzweig's summary of organizations and the factors they feel will affect organizations in the future:

1. Organizations will be operating in a turbulent environment which requires continual change and adjustment.
2. They will have to adapt to an increasing diversity of cultural values in the social environment.
3. Greater emphasis will be placed on technological and social forecasting.
4. Organizations will continue to expand their boundaries and domains. They will increase in size and complexity.
5. Organizations will continue to differentiate their activities, causing increased problems of integration and coordination.
6. Organizations will continue to have major problems in the accumulation and utilization of knowledge. Intellectual activities will be stressed.
7. Greater emphasis will be focused on suggestion and persuasion rather than coercion based on authoritarian power as the means for coordinating the activities of the participants and functions within the organization.
8. Participants at all levels in organizations will have more influence. Organizations of the future will adopt a power-equalization rather than power-differentiation model.
9. There will be greater diversity in values and life styles among people and groups in organizations. A mosaic psychosocial system will be normal.
10. Problems of interface between organizations will increase. New means for effective interorganizational coordination will be developed.
11. Computerized information-decision systems will have an increasing impact upon organizations.
12. The number of professionals and scientists and their influence within organizations will increase. There will also be a decline in the proportion of independent professionals with many more salaried professionals.
13. Goals of complex organizations will diversify. Emphasis will be upon satisfying a number of goals rather than maximizing any one.
14. Evaluation of organizational performance will be difficult. Many new administrative techniques will be developed for evaluation of performance in all spheres of activity.[21]

---

[20] Larry E. Greiner, "Patterns of organization change." In Gene Dalton and Paul Lawrence eds., *Organizational Change and Development*. Homewood, Ill.: Richard D. Irwin, Inc. and the Dorsey Press, 1970, pp. 227–228.

[21] Fremont E. Kast and James E. Rosenzweig, *Organization and Management: A Systems Approach*. New York: The McGraw-Hill Book Company, 1974, pp. 617–618. Reprinted by permission of the publisher.

If the health care organization manager is to function, even survive, in the years ahead, his or her approach to management must include flexibility, a devotion to innovation and creativity, and the development of power bases for warding off inappropriate change thrusts. We may take a case in point to demonstrate this. By drawing on Kast and Rosenzweig's points (1) "Turbulent Environment" and (8) "Power Equalization Model", we have constructed "Our Greatest Challenge."

OUR GREATEST CHALLENGE

The greatest challenge facing health care leaders is "government by unyielding dogmaticism", a phrase coined recently by John Alexander McMahon, the President of the American Hospital Association.

Cost controls are rapidly replacing quality controls. Through consumerism, health care has become, justifiably, the right of every American, instead of a service priced in the open marketplace. This has increased demand...and cost. With the arrival of Medicare in 1966, the federal government steadily began to increase its purchases of health care; as a result, cost pressures have accentuated. In this turbulent environmental setting, programmatic health care expenditures are closely linked to politics and must compete with other projects for the allocation of governmental dollars. As a result, the slant seems to be toward cost instead of quality.

Management in health care organizations is now being put to perhaps its greatest test. Will health care managers and their spokesmen unite to meet these challenges? Will cost controls weigh more heavily than quality assurances in the future? As we head toward national health programs, will the managers of our nation's health care organizations have a voice in the shaping of external forces, trends, solution criteria, and solution constraints which emanate from the environment to the organization? Will the role of the manager in the formulation of organizational objectives and strategies to accomplish them be constricted in the future? Will *inputs* be molded in such a way that they will define *desired output*, and therefore render the *conversion mechanism* a set of mechanical nondynamic processes?

Hopefully, these raise additional questions in the minds of the readers. Realistically, there is little the health care organization manager can do, independently, to alter the external environment or hold back the inevitable changes, be they good or bad. However, the manager can try to be responsive to society's needs and fulfill his or her responsibilities by managing effectively and efficiently. Then, in aggregate, constructive progress will hopefully occur.

SUMMARY

This chapter serves as a conclusion to the book by suggesting that the concepts, principles, and practices that have been presented will be useful to the manager in the health care setting only to the extent they can be applied. It was pointed out that the setting is dynamic and faces many changes in the decade ahead. Aside from environmental changes that will affect the health care organization, there are a number of specific areas of change that the health care manager faces: consumerism, institutionalization, cost effectiveness, quality control, and strong governmental intervention.

The role of the health care manager as a change agent was described and one of the great challenges of the future was presented. With this final note, we leave it to the reader to consider our presentation of the management processes, the activities characteristic of each, and their inter-relationship as portrayed by the management model (Fig. 2–3, page 22). Hopefully, considered reflection and implemenation of these processes in the managing of health care organizations will enable both the new and the experienced manager to contribute constructively to organization effectiveness and efficiency and to cope with the environment of the future.

INDEX